Next Saturday April 14
Committing to ① Having Complete Oncology
② Rough draft of Resume

ONCOLOGY NURSING
CARE

③ Work daily of Forgiveness

Wednesday Eve –
Oncology

Edited by

Gloria York, RN, MAed

** Private Home*
Decorating

Telomerase – } find CA early
Protein
CA cells – make telomerase
It makes tumors thrive i.e
cell divide over over 5 succumbing
to normal aging + death

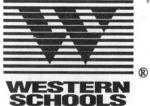

**WESTERN
SCHOOLS
PRESS**

CA Board of Regist
Sacramento
CA Nursing Assn.
916-488-4059
CA License Vocation
916-444-6901

1 Renew License
916-322-3350 –
Need # 412664
Form to Renew – $117⁰⁰ ($80⁰⁰)

12-31-98

7840 El Cajon Blvd. Ste. 500
San Diego, CA 91940-3617
1-619-469-2121

Books from Western Schools Press are designed to provide current information which will assist you in providing comprehensive nursing care to clients in a variety of clinical settings. All our books are designed for quality and excellence and are reviewed by experts to meet your professional development needs.

WESTERN SCHOOLS' courses are designed to provide nursing professionals with general information to assist in their practices and professional development. The information provided in these courses and course books is based on research and consultation with medical and nursing authoritites and is, to the best of WESTERN SCHOOLS' knowledge, current and accurate. However, the courses and course books are offered with the understanding that WESTERN SCHOOLS is not engaged in rendering legal, nursing, or other professional advice. WESTERN SCHOOLS' courses and course books are not a substitute for seeking professional advice or conducting individual research. In applying the information provided in the courses and course books to individual circumstances, all recommendations must be considered in light of the unique circumstances of each situation. The course books are intended solely for your use, and not for the benefit of providing advice or recommendations to third parties. WESTERN SCHOOLS disclaims any responsibility for any adverse consequences resulting from the failure to seek medical, nursing, or other professional advice or to conduct independent research. WESTERN SCHOOLS further disclaims any responsibility for updating or revising any programs or publications presented, published, distributed, or sponsored by WESTERN SCHOOLS unless otherwise agreed to as part of an individual purchase contract.

Copy Editor: Barbara Halliburton, PhD
Typesetter: Gwen Nichols
Graphic Designer: Kathy Johnson
Cover Designer: Dunn and Associates
Proofreader: John Wolf, MA

About the Editor:

Gloria York, RN, MA Ed, is an educational technologist and continuing education consultant. Ms. York has been a nurse for over 20 years and has worked in the field of continuing education for the past 12 years. She has developed numerous instructional products and contributed the chapter, "Continuing Education for Relicensure" to *Issues and Trends in Nursing,* a Mosby Year Book. Ms. York recently developed *Supervisory Skills for Nurses* a continuing education course published by Western Schools Press.

About the Authors:

Theresa W. Gillespie RN, MA, OCN, wrote chapters 1-3, 5, 7, and 9 of this book. She is the Assistant Director of the Winsip Cancer Center at Emory University School of Medicine, Atlanta. In her 15-year nursing career she has held clinical, research and administrative positions. She currently holds a concurrent appointment as an Instructor in the Department of Community & Preventive Medicine at Emory University School of Medicine, and has also taught at two schools of nursing. She is the author of numerous publications and is listed in *Who's Who in American Nursing.*

Myra Woolery-Antill RN, MN wrote chapters 8 and 13 of this book. She is a pediatric clinical nurse specialist in the Cancer and Human Genome Nursing service at the National Institutes of Health in Bethesda, Maryland. She is a certified pediatric oncology nurse. She has been a clinical nurse specialist for 8 years working with children and young adults with cancer and/or HIV infection. She has numerous presentations and publications related to cancer care.

Theresa Moran RN, MS wrote chapters 10-12. She is a clinical nurse specialist in AIDS/Oncology in the outpatient department of San Francisco General Hospital. Ms. Moran has cared for Oncology patients for the past 18 years and during that time has authored numerous articles and chapters. In addition, she has co-edited a book on the nursing care of AIDS patients entitled *AIDS: Concepts in Nursing Practice.* Ms Moran is also an Assistant clinical professor in the Department of Physiological Nursing of the University of California, San Francisco.

Donna Wright RN, BSN, MS wrote chapters 4, 6, and 14 of this book. She is a nurse educator at the University of Minnesota Hospital and Clinic at Minneapolis, MN. She has her Masters Degree in Nursing Education from the University of Minnesota and has worked in oncology for 13 years. Donna holds an adjunct faculty position at the University of Minnesota School of Nursing. She also works as a speaker/consultant for Professional Education Systems, Inc. in Eau Claire, WI. Donna has authored and presented nationally on many topics including competency, oncology, and creative training techniques.

About the Subject Matter Expert:

Cindy Jones, MS, RN, ONC has been the oncology clinical nurse specialist at the Veterans Affairs Medical Center in San Diego, CA for the past 15 years. She has published on oncologic complications and is a noted speaker on oncology related topics at the state, national and international level. She is a member of the Oncology Nursing Society, served as the founding president of the San Diego chapter, and is active at the national level. In 1995, she was the recipient of the Oncology Certified Nurse of the Year award by the Oncology Nursing Certification corporation.

TABLE OF CONTENTS

208 page 14 chapt

PRETEST

Begin by taking the pretest. Compare your answers on the pretest to the answer key (located in the back of the book). Circle those test items that you missed. The pretest answer key indicates the chapters where the content of that question is discussed.

Next, read each chapter. Focus special attention on the chapters that cover the questions for which you made incorrect answer choices. Study questions are provided at the end of each chapter so you can assess your progress and understanding of the material.

1. Cancer incidence is defined as:

   Specified pop
   specified time

   a.) The number of new cases of cancer diagnosed in a specified population during a specified time period
   b. A measure of the existence of disease at a certain point in time
   c. The number of patients with cancer who survive 5 years or more
   d. The number of patients with cancer who have died during a specified time period

2. Neoplasm is defined as:

   a. A malignant tumor
   b. Hyperplasia
   c.) New growth
   d. Benign atypia

   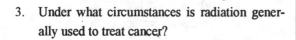
   radiation localized early stage

3. Under what circumstances is radiation generally used to treat cancer?

   a. When the tumor has metastasized to multiple organ sites.
   b. When the tumor is a hematologic cancer at an advanced stage.
   c.) When the tumor is localized or at an early stage.
   d. When the tumor is poorly differentiated at the time of diagnosis.

4. Pathologic examination of a patient's biopsy specimens shows a small tumor with clear margins and no lymph node involvement. Radiologic examination shows a possible tumor in the right lobe of the liver and several nodules in the lower lobe of the left lung. On physical examination, an enlarged supraclavicular lymph node was palpated. If all the suspected sites are areas of malignant tumor, the patient's cancer would be classified as:

   a. Localized
   b. Regional
   c. Distant involvement
   d. Minimal

5. Which of the following is done in an excisional biopsy?

   a. Cells are removed for cytologic examination.
   b. A CT scan may be used for visualization.
   c. A piece of the tumor is surgically removed.
   d.) The entire tumor mass is removed.

6. In what percentage of cancer patients is surgery alone considered curative?

    a. 10
    b. 30
    c. 50
    d. 60

7. Because of the area it affects, radiation therapy is characterized as what kind of treatment?

    a. Localized
    b. Systemic
    c. Generalized
    d. Superficial

8. At what time do side effects related to radiation therapy usually occur?

    a. Minutes after treatment
    b. 1–2 days after treatment
    c. 10 days to 6 months after treatment
    d. Rarely, if at all

9. Cytotoxic chemotherapy refers to which of the following?

    a. Cell killing
    b. Cell kinetics
    c. Cellular proliferation
    d. Cell growth

10. Higher doses of chemotherapeutic drugs may be more effective than lower doses because higher doses do which of the following?

    a. Overcome drug resistance
    b. Increase the sensitivity of tumor cells to the drug
    c. Kill a greater proportion of tumor cells
    d. Prevent tumor growth between cycles

11. Biotherapy enhances the bodys own immune system through which of the following?

    a. Bone marrow transplant
    b. Radiation and chemotherapy
    c. Biological response modifiers
    d. Pain management

12. Bone marrow transplantation is characterized as which of the following?

    a. Investigational treatment only
    b. Standard treatment only
    c. Neither investigational nor standard treatment
    d. Both investigational and standard treatment

13. One category of commonly used unproven methods of cancer therapy is:

    a. Surgery
    b. Physical therapy
    c. Drugs or natural products
    d. Travel

14. Psychoneuroimmunology refers to which of the following?

    a. A type of high-fiber diet
    b. A field of cancer quackery
    c. A mind-body link
    d. Cancer chemotherapy

15. Inadequate management of which of the following side effects is more likely to cause a cancer patient to discontinue treatment of the cancer?

    a. Nausea and vomiting
    b. Anemia
    c. Sepsis
    d. Stomatitis

16. Which of the following statements about pain due to cancer is true?

    a. Achieving adequate pain control is usually difficult.
    b. Most patients receiving opioids become addicted.
    c. Pain is a cancer-related problem feared by patients and their families.
    d. Pain is always manifested by overt signs.

17. Which of the following is a true oncologic emergency?

    a. Hypercalcemia of cancer
    b. Referral to hospice care
    c. Metastases to the hip
    d. Diagnosis of breast cancer

18 One reason for giving heparin to patients with disseminated intravascular coagulation is to do which of the following?

    a. Promote bleeding
    b. Deplete circulating coagulation factors
    c. Restore balance to the coagulation system
    d. Enhance thrombocytopenia

19. Which of the following is a risk factor for melanoma?

    a. Having blond or red hair and a fair complexion
    b. Residing in Canada
    c. Eating large amounts of red meat
    d. Smoking tobacco

20. Palliative care includes all of the following except:

    a. Treatments that prolong life
    b. Treatment that alleviates suffering
    c. Aggressive management of signs and symptoms
    d. Treatment aimed at promoting a painless death

21. Which of the following statements about advance directives is correct?

    a. Advance directives are federally mandated for hospice programs, clinics, and health care agencies.
    b. If advance directives are not filled out before a patient enters a hospice program, care will be denied.
    c. Advance directives limit patients' rights.
    d. Once signed, an advance directive cannot be revoked.

22. Approximately how may new cases of cancer in children less than 15 years old are diagnosed each year?

    a. 6,000
    b. 6,800
    c. 7,000
    d. 7,800

23. What is the most common cancer in children?

    a. Acute myelocytic leukemia
    b. Rhabdomyosarcoma
    c. Acute lymphocytic leukemia
    d. Brain tumors

24. Ethical principles associated with clinical trials include all of the following *except:*

    a. Justice
    b. Autonomy
    c. Unlimited resources
    d. Nonmaleficence

25. What is described as an extreme outcome of unrelieved stress related to excess demands on energy, strength, and resources?

    a. Stress
    b. Moral conduct
    c. Grieving
    d. Burnout

CHAPTER 1

BIOLOGY OF CANCER

CHAPTER OBJECTIVE

After completing this chapter, the reader will be able to relate what is generally known about the etiology of cancer, carcinogenesis, tumor nomenclature, and current trends in the epidemiology of cancer.

LEARNING OBJECTIVES

After studying this chapter, the reader will be able to

1. Recognize cancer statistics and epidemiologic trends.

2. Specify the major components of carcinogenesis.

3. Recognize current theories about the etiology of cancer.

4. Specify characteristics of malignant cells versus benign cells.

5. Name various kinds of tumors.

INTRODUCTION

Although more people in the United States actually die from cardiovascular disease, a diagnosis of cancer carries with it an enormous fear and is generally equated with a death sentence by most Americans. Cancer is the second highest cause of death in adults in the United States, and it affects three of every four families. The mortality rate of lung cancer has been increasing for the past 50 years, and this type of cancer now reigns as the number one cause of death due to cancer for both men and women. Other cancers, however, have higher incidence rates: Breast cancer in women and prostatic cancer in men have the highest rates.

The incidence of cancer varies according to a person's sex, age, risk factors (including diet, environmental exposures, and geographic location), and genetic makeup. Although much progress has been made in understanding how some cancers originate, grow, and spread, little is known overall about the exact etiology of cancer as a broad-based disease. Consequently, public education on how to prevent cancer is limited, although certain risk factors (e.g., tobacco, radiation) have been well documented.

EPIDEMIOLOGY

Understanding cancer as a disease requires comprehending the nature of the problem. Cancer epidemiology focuses on populations and patterns of distribution within those populations rather than on cancer occurring in individuals. Cancer epidemiology tracks the incidence of cancer (number of new cases diagnosed in a specified population during a specified time period), mortality rates (deaths over time), survival rates (usually based on survival 5 years after diagnosis), and new trends observed. Trends over the past decade include the marked increase in melanoma rates among Caucasians, a sharp increase in certain cancers in African-Americans, and the overtaking of breast cancer by lung cancer as the number one cause in women of deaths due to cancer. Cancer epidemiology also notes differences in patterns of occurrence between geographic locations, ethnic and cultural backgrounds, and the two sexes.

Incidence and Mortality

According to estimates, cancer is diagnosed in 1 million persons in the United States each year; more than half of the cases occur in the elderly. Cancer tends to be a disease of older persons, perhaps because of hormonal changes for certain cancers and the decreased functioning of the immune system with age. Cancer is second to cardiovascular disease as the leading cause of death in America, although for certain age groups (e.g., young women 35–54 years old), it is the number one cause of death. As the incidence of infectious disease has declined over the past century because of immunizations and improvements in sanitary and social conditions, the incidence of chronic diseases, such as cancer, has increased. This pattern is true in the United States and in other industrialized countries but not necessarily for developing nations, where infectious diseases, malnutrition, and other public health issues are prevalent.

The estimated number of deaths due to cancer is 500,000 per year in the United States, and current 5-year survival rates are approximately 50%. However, mortality and survival rates vary according to age, sex, race, tumor site, and stage of disease at diagnosis. In general, cancers diagnosed during the early stages of disease have the best prognosis, and the reverse is true for cancers detected at advanced stages. Types of cancer with generally poor prognosis include tumors of the lung, esophagus, and pancreas; tumors with a generally favorable prognosis include testicular and uterine cancers and childhood leukemia. Although cancer remains a serious health problem for children and is the number two cause of death (after accidents) for young persons (birth to 34 years), cancer mortality rates in children have been declining for the past 40 years.

Patterns of Occurrence

Patterns of occurrence for certain cancers that vary from one country to another may be linked more to behavioral, cultural, and dietary factors than to racial or ethnic differences. Studies have shown that the incidence of cancer increases in immigrants to the United States as these persons are assimilated into the population and adapt to their new environment. Over time, sometimes two to three generations, the incidence rates approach or equal those of the United States rather than reflect those of the immigrants' native countries. One exception to this principle is skin cancer, which is associated with race and skin type. Examples of geographic differences in the incidence of cancer include Australia, where skin cancer rates among fair-skinned residents of European descent are the highest in the world; primary liver cancer, which is prevalent in China, Africa, and Southeast Asia but rare in the United States and Europe; breast cancer, which tends to be more prevalent in the United States and Europe and less prevalent in Japan; and colorectal cancer, which has high rates in the United States and Great Britain and much lower rates in Africa, China, and Japan.

Incidence rates can also differ according to ethnicity, culture, and sex: The rate of cervical cancer in black women is nearly twice the rate in white women; Hispanics have a lower overall incidence of cancer than Caucasians do but an increased incidence of certain cancers (e.g., stomach, cervical, and gallbladder); Seventh-Day Adventists and Mormons have significantly lower rates of gastrointestinal and lung cancers; rural Southern women who use snuff have higher rates of oral and pharyngeal cancers.

Help me to forgive, Dear God!

Risk Factors

Although an unequivocal etiology of all cancers has not yet been determined, certain risk factors have been studied, and their role in certain cancers has been clearly recognized (Table 1-1).

CARCINOGENESIS AND PATHOPHYSIOLOGY OF CANCER

Carcinogenesis

Studies of the relationship between certain risk factors and specific cancers have helped determine possible causes of cancers. Knowledge that tobacco use is correlated with lung cancer led to the study of how tobacco can act as an agent to initiate carcinogenesis or promote transformation, the changes that a normal cell undergoes as it becomes malignant. Other risk factors such as ionizing radiation (x-rays), ultraviolet radiation (exposure to the sun), or industrial chemicals also can act as initiators.

Carcinogenesis involves a continuum of events and may speed up, slow down, or even go in reverse, depending on what factors are at work. Initiators may mutate DNA or otherwise regulate the proliferation of cells. Initiating factors besides those just mentioned include viruses and oncogenes, which may enhance or suppress certain carcinogenic changes. Over time, transformation may occur, a multistep process affected by initiators, promoters, and reversers. Promoters act after initiators

mutate DNA

path of cancer affected by viruses & oncogenes

Table 1-1
Risk Factors for Various Cancers

Risk Factors	Potential Cancers
Viruses: Herpes simplex virus type 2, human papilloma virus, Epstein-Barr virus, cytomegalovirus, hepatitis B virus	Burkitt's lymphoma, Kaposi's sarcoma, hepatoma
Environmental factors: Benzene, asbestos, cadmium, ethylene oxide, iodizing radiation	Leukemia; lung, prostatic, stomach, skin, liver, brain, breast cancers
Medical factors: Chemotherapy, hormones, immunosuppressive therapy	Leukemia, uterine cancer, lymphoma
Tobacco and alcohol	Lung, bladder, kidney, oral, head and neck, cervical cancers
Diet: Obesity, dietary fat, preservatives, cured or smoked foods, low fiber	Colon, breast, prostatic, ovarian, uterine, esophagus, stomach cancers
Heredity and genetic predisposition	Neuroblastoma, Wilms' tumor, familial polyposis and colon cancer, breast and ovarian cancers
Hormones and factors related to sexual development: Early menarche, late menopause, undescended testes, childbearing, use of exogenous hormones, multiple sexual partners	Breast, testicular, cervical, ovarian cancers

to enhance cellular changes toward neoplasia, and extensive long-term exposure may be required. Certain factors may act as either initiators or promoters, depending where the exposure occurs in the carcinogenesis continuum. Finally, certain reversing factors may actually inhibit or destroy the action of promoters. Potential reversers include certain chemopreventive agents (e.g., actinomycin D, β-carotene, tamoxifen), enzymes (glutathione), and dietary factors (vitamins A and C).

Neoplasia

Neoplasia, the abnormal growth of new tissue caused by abnormal increases in the size of cells (hypertrophy) or the number of cells (hyperplasia), may be benign rather than malignant. A neoplasm, or tumor, is not malignant unless it has the characteristics of malignant lesions. Neoplastic growth may be metaplastic, in which one mature cell type is replaced by another mature type, or dysplastic, in which a mature type of cell is replaced by a less mature type. Understanding the significance of certain tumors and their malignant potential requires understanding how tumors are classified. Classification is based on both the tissue or origin of the tumor and the malignant or benign nature of the growth. For example, the suffix -oma is used for both benign (e.g., papilloma, cystoma) and malignant (sarcoma, carcinoma) tumors. Sarcomas originate from connective tissue (bone, muscle), whereas carcinomas originate from the epithelium. Hematologic malignant tumors can be traced to hematopoietic stem cells in the bone marrow. Terms such as lympho- or myelo- may be used to describe the origin of hematologic cancers (e.g., myeloblastic leukemia).

Alterations in Cell Biology

Changes in the biology of the cell associated with carcinogenesis can take various forms. Anatomic changes include abnormal size and shape of cells; increased rates of mitosis (cell division) in malignant cells; and modification of the cell structure itself, including the cell membrane, organelles (mitochondria), and, particularly, the nucleus. Often malignant cells have enlarged nuclei, chromosomal changes, or multiple mitoses that pick up the standard stains used in histopathologic examinations; consequently, cancer cells often appear blue on microscopic examination. Biochemical changes can produce increases in the concentrations of enzymes on the cell surface and of prostaglandins or decreases in the concentrations of certain growth factors or oxygen needed for cell division.

Kinetic changes refer to changes in the growth and division of the cells. Proliferation rates may vary from tumor to tumor and from one patient to another. The cancer doubling time indicates the length of time for division of all tumor cells present; it may range from hours to months, or even years. On average, approximately 30 doubling times are required for a tumor to be clinically detectable (about 10^9 cells). Tumor doubling time, and therefore cancer growth rate, may be controlled by the following:

- Vascularization of the tumor, so that the cells have adequate nutrition for growth.

- Presence of tumor necrosis, or dead cells, that may interfere with uptake of nutrients and with growth.

- Expression of tumor antigens, which influences escape from immune surveillance.

- Genetic factors, which can enhance or suppress tumor growth.

Changes in cellular differentiation affect the process by which a cell's specific structure, function, and rate of division are established. Low-grade tumors have well-differentiated cells that deviate least from normal cells; high-grade tumors, which are more malignant, have poorly differentiated cells and less resemblance to normal cells. Anaplastic cells have an atypical tissue structure and growth pattern and bear the least resemblance to normal cells of the specific tissue involved.

Characteristics of Malignant Tumors

As mentioned, cell growth alone is not sufficient to classify a tumor as malignant, because benign lesions also are neoplastic. However, several characteristics differentiate malignant changes from nonmalignant ones:

[handwritten top margin: oncogenes – regulate the proliferation process.]

- **Invasiveness:** Malignant neoplasms have the capacity to expand and to invade and destroy normal adjacent tissue.

- **Rapid growth:** Although benign, or even normal, cells can grow and divide rapidly, highly malignant cells have an enhanced competence for proliferation.

- **Decreased contact inhibition:** Even when normal cells do grow and divide quickly, they are able to stop growing when they reach adjacent tissue. Malignant cells lack this innate ability to know when to stop growing.

[handwritten: to grow in adjacent tissue]

- **Dissemination:** Malignant cells usually have the capacity to spread or metastasize throughout the body, often through known patterns of dissemination. Tumor dissemination can occur through contiguous spread, via the lymphatic system, through the bloodstream, by transabdominal seeding, and by transplantation (e.g., through mechanical means such as surgery). Although metastasis is rare with some malignant tumors (e.g., brain tumors), most have this capacity. Factors that may contribute to increased metastatic spread include high rate of tumor growth, trauma, necrotic tissue, heat, radiation, and use of chemotherapy. Factors that may decrease metastases include use of anticoagulants (e.g., aspirin, heparin), radiation, presence of ascites, and chemotherapy. Cancers often have a set pattern of metastasis based on the organ of origin (e.g., lung cancer tends to spread to liver, bones, and brain), but the most common sites of metastases from solid tumors are lung, liver, central nervous system, and bone.

[handwritten left margin: lymphatic / bloodstream / transabdom / seeding / transplant]

[handwritten left margin: 1. 2. liver / bones / 3. brain]

[handwritten left margin: common / sites of metastases / lung, liver, CNS, bone]

A more recent area of investigation is angiogenesis, the process by which cells and tissues develop vascularity and the ability to take in nutrients, as well as possibly spread malignant cells, through blood vessels. The development of increased vascularity may lead to enhanced tumor growth and may indicate a higher metastatic potential for a particular tumor. The role of oncogenes in angiogenesis and how genetic factors affect the development of cancer and the spread of cancer remain to be elucidated.

Role of the Immune System

The role of the host's immune system in carcinogenesis, metastasis, and response to therapy is not yet clear. The theory of immune surveillance argues that although transformation of cells occurs often, an intact, fully operational immune system has no problem detecting the abnormal cells and destroying them. However, in both the very young and the very old, the immune system operates at less than optimal levels, and it is in these age groups that increased rates of cancer are observed. It has been proposed that factors that suppress recognition of tumors, such as the development of fibrin coats around tumors or the production of antibodies to the tumors, allow tumor cells to escape routine immune surveillance and continue to proliferate. This concept supports the idea that the use of anticoagulants may enhance immune surveillance and inhibit metastatic spread of malignant tumors.

[handwritten: anticoagulants may enhance surveillance]

Genetics and Cancer

Certain neoplastic disorders have a genetic aspect to their development, for example, retinoblastoma, for which the contributing gene has been identified, and familial polyposis coli, in which the prevalence of colon cancer is thought to be 100% if the disease is not treated. The genetic basis for carcinogenesis proposes that the changes associated with initiation, promotion, and transformation are caused by genetic alterations. These alterations affect oncogenes, which promote uncontrolled cellular proliferation, and anti-oncogenes, or suppressor genes, which generally regulate oncogenes and would cause cancer only if present in the recessive state. More than 50 oncogenes have been identified, and the expression of these genes through mutation, chromosomal deletions, or other genetic changes is thought to result in an increased susceptibility to specific cancers or groups of cancers or to the malignant changes that produce such cancers.

Individuals may not always inherit a "cancer gene"; instead, they may inherit a susceptibility, as well as possibly a resistance to certain cancers. Most cancers are not

[handwritten bottom margin: angiogenesis – cells + tissues develop vascularity]

directly inherited, although certain genes have been associated with the prevalence of colon, prostatic, breast, and ovarian cancers; leukemia; and other cancers. Family history may be important and may require careful assessment along with assessment of other risk factors for cancer. However, genetic screening and the significance of biomarkers are still being investigated, and the clinical implications of these findings are debatable. Still, a strong family history of certain cancer(s) may be the basis for encouraging a person to pursue recommended screening activities on a regular basis or to avoid known risk factors for cancer.

Viruses Associated with Human Cancer

Like the role of immune, genetic, and environmental factors, the role of viruses in the development of cancer is not clear. Specific viruses, for example, herpes simplex virus (types 1, 2, and 6), human cytomegalovirus, Epstein-Barr virus, and human T-cell leukemia virus, have been studied. The family of papovaviruses, which includes human papilloma virus, has been strongly linked to cervical cancer, and human immunodeficiency virus is known to be associated with the development of malignant tumors. The prevalence of hepatitis B virus (HBV) in certain countries (e.g., China) has been correlated with the high incidence of primary hepatoma in these areas.

Although the exact mechanism of the viral etiology of cancer, or which cancers can be specifically tied to viral factors, has not been totally resolved, the relationship between viruses and human cancers appears to be strong. One way to determine a direct causal link between agent and host is to attempt to prevent the disease through vaccination. Use of the hepatitis B vaccine will contribute important information over the next several decades about the connection between HBV infection and the development of hepatomas. If HBV is a cause of cancer, prevention of hepatitis B through use of a vaccine may also prevent the development of cancer. The study of viral etiology also raises the question of disease transmission, and whether cancer can be spread from one person to another as other viral conditions can. Considerable inquiry will be necessary before any conclusions can be reached or any changes in the standard practice of cancer care should be recommended.

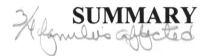

SUMMARY

Cancer is an important public health problem: It affects three of four families in the United States, with 1 million new cases and 500,000 deaths each year. Overall, it is second to cardiovascular disease as a cause of death. The incidence of cancer varies widely according to age, sex, ethnic background, and multiple risk factors. Carcinogenesis and the exact etiology of all cancers are not known, but generally accepted theory describes a continuum over which cancer develops over time and requires factors that cause changes in normal cells. These factors may include environmental, genetic, viral, immune, or other changes, which lead to initiation, promotion, and eventual transformation of normal cells to malignant cells. Malignant cells are invasive, have increased rates of proliferation, and can metastasize to involve distant sites. Determining and assessing potential risk factors associated with the cause and progression of cancer are important, although the clinical significance of such findings is questionable.

STUDY QUESTIONS

Chapter 1

Questions 1–8

1. The primary cause in women of death due to cancer is:

    a. Breast cancer
    b. Lung cancer
    c. Ovarian cancer
    d. Cervical cancer

2. Cervical cancer has been associated with which of the following viruses?

    a. Hepatitis B virus
    b. Epstein-Barr virus
    c. Human papilloma virus
    d. Human immunodeficiency virus

3. Which of the following cancers is less prevalent in Japan than in the United States?

    a. Gastric cancer
    b. Esophageal cancer
    c. Melanoma
    d. Breast cancer

4. A malignant tumor arising from glandular epithelium would be called:

    a. Adenocarcinoma
    b. Adenoma
    c. Lipoma
    d. Chondroma

5. Hyperplasia is defined as an abnormal:

    a. Increase in cell size
    b. Increase in the number of cells
    c. Number of less mature cells
    d. Decrease in the number of cells

6. An example of a possible reversing factor in carcinogenesis is:

    a. Angiogenesis
    b. Tobacco
    c. Ultraviolet radiation
    d. Glutathione

7. A benign tumor arising from the smooth muscle would be called:

    a. Rhabdomyosarcoma
    b. Chondrosarcoma
    c. Choriocarcinoma
    d. Leiomyoma

8. Genes that can contribute to the process of malignant transformation when in the recessive state are termed:

    a. Oncogenes
    b. Suppressor genes
    c. Tumor susceptibility genes
    d. Promoter genes

CHAPTER 2

OVERVIEW OF CANCER THERAPY

CHAPTER OBJECTIVE

After completing this chapter, the reader will be able to specify the four major methods of treatment used in cancer therapy and the general indications for use of each therapeutic approach.

LEARNING OBJECTIVES

After studying this chapter, the reader will be able to

1. Specify the mechanisms of action of the four major methods of treatment used in cancer therapy.

2. Indicate the bases of choice for the various methods of treating cancer.

3. Recognize grades of tumors.

4. Specify the side effects of various types of cancer therapy.

INTRODUCTION

Cancer and cancer treatment were first described by the ancient Egyptians as early as 5,000 years ago. As long ago as 2,500 B.C., Egyptian medical practice included the use of surgery, drugs, physical manipulation, and magic to treat cancer. The beginning of Western medicine, which can be traced to early Greek and Roman civilizations, also addressed ways to treat cancer. The philosophy of the four "humors" of the body held that all illnesses, including cancer, resulted from an imbalance among the humors and that cancer could best be treated by being left alone. However, the Roman physician and surgeon Galen, although agreeing in principle with the concept of leaving tumors alone, also advocated the surgical removal of various cancers.

TYPES OF TREATMENT

Treatment of cancer consists of four major methods: surgery, radiation therapy, chemotherapy, and biotherapy.

Surgery

Modern cancer therapy has evolved from critical developments in the late 19th and early 20th centuries. The use of anesthesia contributed to the advance of surgery and its dominant role as the primary approach to treatment of cancer. William Halsted and the Halsted radical mastectomy influenced the care of cancer for a century. Halsted's work led to a fundamental axiom of cancer therapy, that for the best chance of cure, the primary objective should be to remove the tumor and all related tissue. For localized solid tumors, surgery generally is the initial method used, if only to obtain a biopsy specimen of the cancer for diagnostic purposes.

Radiation Therapy

The discovery of radium, also in the late 19th century, and the use of radium and x-rays to treat some tumors, led to the development of radiotherapy or radiation oncology. Now, with the use of high-speed and computer-directed sources of radiation, radiation therapy may be the primary method of treatment for some solid and hematologic tumors (e.g., some lung cancers, early-stage Hodgkin's disease). Because radiation can only be directed to specific areas of the body at one time, radiation therapy, like surgery, is considered a local treatment. It is most useful in early-stage disease in which the cancer has not spread (i.e., the tumor is "localized"); as adjunctive therapy to surgery or chemotherapy or both; and for relief of symptoms, such as body pain from metastases.

Chemotherapy

Early in the 20th century, using scientific principles and new technology, researchers began the search for chemicals to treat cancer. However, it was the use of nitrogen mustard gas in World War I and the observation of its effect on soldiers' bone marrow that led investigators to limited success with chemotherapy. In the 1940s, nitrogen mustard was first used to obtain a brief remission in a patient with lymphoma. Since then, a variety of drugs, both natural and synthetic, have been tested on all types of tumors, and clinical trials, which are often used to evaluate combinations of chemotherapeutic agents, continue in attempts to detect the most effective treatments. Many cancers now considered highly curable (e.g., childhood leukemia, Hodgkin's disease, testicular carcinoma) are successfully treated by using a combination of chemotherapeutic drugs that kill the cancer cells ("cytotoxic" drugs).

Unfortunately, many cytotoxic chemotherapeutic agents also kill normal cells, particularly rapidly dividing cells, such as those in the hematopoietic system (bone marrow), the lining of the digestive tract, the skin, and hair. Consequently, such drugs generally cause toxic side effects. Bone marrow suppression with anemia (low red blood cell count), neutropenia (low white blood cell count), and thrombocytopenia (low platelet count); gastrointestinal effects, such as mucositis, diarrhea, nausea, and vomiting; and loss of body hair may occur. Although chemotherapeutic drugs may be given as single agents, usually several drugs are given together during the same cycle, perhaps at different times. This practice maximizes the number of cells killed, minimizes overlap of toxic effects, and prevents or diminishes resistance of the cancer cells to specific drugs.

Chemotherapy is generally used for tumors that have metastasized, are at more advanced stages, or have spread beyond the point at which local control is effective. Chemotherapy is also used for hematologic tumors (e.g., leukemias, lymphomas, multiple myeloma); tumors for which systemic treatment is required because of the nature of the cancer, such as bone marrow involvement; and cancers that have recurred after use of other therapies (e.g., surgery or radiation therapy).

Although its mode of action is different from that of cytotoxic chemotherapy, hormonal therapy is usually classified with chemotherapy because both methods are a systemic approach to treatment of tumors. Hormonal therapy is used for breast, gynecologic, urologic, and other tumors that respond to various hormones or whose growth may be controlled by the use of drugs that bind certain hormonal factors.

Biotherapy

The fourth method of treatment is biotherapy, or use of biological response modifiers. This therapy involves using the body's own immune system to treat tumors. Patients are given additional amounts of substances normally produced by the immune system or agents that stimulate the immune system to fight the cancer on its own. Biotherapy is still considered investigational on some levels, because a complete explanation of the workings of the immune system and the system's role in the etiology and development of and response to cancers remains to be elucidated.

Both biotherapy and chemotherapy are most often used for systemic treatment of advanced cancers or hematologic tumors. However, unlike chemotherapeutic agents, biological response modifiers are not cell cycle–specific in their function, and the cytotoxic effects are a result of the immune system's actions. Thus, the common side effects experienced with immunotherapy often resemble immune responses to other conditions (e.g., a flulike response accompanied by fever, chills, malaise, and fatigue). Although biological response modifiers can cause some of the same adverse effects that chemotherapeutic drugs do, myelosuppression is usually not the dose-limiting toxic effect.

A type of biotherapy currently under investigation is gene therapy. Similar to the situation for use of biological response modifiers two decades ago, the development of this approach depends on the accumulation of new information. Knowledge of the genetics of cancer may lead to interventions that cure, or even prevent, certain cancers.

THERAPEUTIC DECISION MAKING

Regardless of the type of cancer therapy available or being considered, the basis for the therapeutic approach is the same and includes determination of the following:

1. Type of cancer, including specific cell type and grade.

2. Stage of the disease.

3. Goal of therapy: cure versus control versus palliation (relief of signs and symptoms).

Type and Grade of Cancer

Until the invention of the microscope in the 16th century, medical scientists could only guess about the nature of cancer. When it became possible to actually look at specific cancer cells, it became apparent that cancer is not one disease, but many different diseases, each with certain characteristics related to its tissue of origin and organ site. Thus, for example, researchers eventually determined that lung cancer includes multiple types of tumors, including some categorized as small-cell or oat cell carcinoma and others categorized as non–small-cell carcinoma, such as squamous cell carcinoma, adenocarcinoma, large cell carcinoma, and even sarcomas. Each of these terms refers not only to the tissue of origin but also to the associated patterns of metastasis and potential prognosis for that type of tumor. Even when a cancer spreads to another organ (e.g., lung cancer that metastasizes to the bone or liver), the tumor at the new site is still lung cancer, rather than bone cancer or liver cancer, and the characteristics of the new tumor are the same as those of the primary tumor, in this case, a lung tumor.

The importance of having an accurate diagnosis based on histopathologic or cytopathologic criteria cannot be overemphasized. Otherwise, decisions about staging tests, choices of therapy, goals of therapy, and the long-term prognosis will be incorrect and inappropriate. Tumor tissue obtained through a variety of diagnostic procedures (e.g., excisional biopsy, needle aspiration, bone marrow biopsy) requires careful histopathologic or cytopathologic examination, including use of appropriate stains, genetic markers, or other techniques, and the findings must be correlated with the clinical picture to make a differential diagnosis.

Besides showing the actual cell type of the tumor, pathologic examination is also used to determine the grade of a tumor, the degree to which the tumor cells resemble normal cells from the same tissue. Well-differentiated tumors are considered low grade (grade 1), and the malignant cells in the tumors still resemble normal cells in some important ways. Poorly differentiated, or high-grade (grade 3), tumors often have lost all normal characteristics and are said to be anaplastic. The grade of a tumor can also be related to the estimated growth rate of the malignant cells, on the basis of the mitotic rate or other criteria for "malignant potential." Higher grade tumors are thought to be more aggressive or to proliferate faster, perhaps with higher rates of metastasis; however, these tumors may also be more responsive to cancer therapy because of those same malignant properties.

Staging of Cancer

Information gained from the diagnosis will assist clinicians in planning a staging examination. Staging is a standardized means of determining the extent to which a cancer has spread (local, regional, or distant). Two types of staging are used in oncology: clinical staging, which is based on diagnostic, radiologic, and physical parameters determined before definitive treatment is started, and pathologic staging, which is done at the time of surgical resection and is based on the examination of surgical specimens, such as margins of the tumor, lymph nodes, or biopsy specimens of other organs. The cell type of the tumor and the primary organ site (e.g., lung, breast, colon) determine the standard staging workup that may be done. The workup may include radiologic studies (computed tomography, magnetic resonance imaging, chest radiography, bone scanning), laboratory and organ function tests (complete blood cell count, chemistry studies, pulmonary function studies), and physical evaluation, with assessment of any conditions such as enlarged lymph nodes or masses.

Results of the staging tests coupled with the pathologic data are used to determine the extent of the cancer, indicate the options that could be pursued with therapy, and allow standardized comparisons between patients or groups of patients. Because cancers that have spread beyond the local or regional stage are not usually curable by localized therapies, such as surgery or radiation alone, the results of staging may show that systemic therapy (i.e., chemotherapy or immunotherapy) is needed.

A variety of staging methods in oncology exist, but the method most widely used and most highly recommended is the TNM method, proposed by the International Union Against Cancer and the American Joint Commission on Cancer. The *T* refers to the tumor itself, including the tumor's size, invasiveness, and other characteristics. The *N* refers to the status of the lymph nodes, that is, whether the regional nodes are involved with cancer. The *M* refers to the presence or absence of distant metastases. The information obtained with the TNM method is most often used to classify a tumor as stage I, II, III, or IV; each successive stage represents increasing extent of disease involvement. Other staging systems are used for specific organ sites (e.g., for gynecologic and urologic cancers). Regardless of the system, all methods of staging attempt to define the extent of the disease by using a representative, uniform approach.

Therapeutic Goal

One consideration in choosing possible treatment options is the goal of the therapy. Cancers that are localized at the time of diagnosis likely may be cured by localized therapy, such as surgical excision. Disease that has recurred or is widespread at the time of detection may not respond to any known form of therapy, and a goal of palliation may be appropriate. Some cancers, although not amenable to cure, may be controlled for extended periods (e.g., breast cancer treated with hormonal therapy).

SUMMARY

Cancer is defined by its specific cell type and organ of origin. These pathologic characteristics, combined with the clinical and pathologic staging of disease, delineate the extent of the clinical problem, the possible prognosis, and the potential options for therapeutic intervention. Therapeutic methods in oncology include localized treatments, such as surgery and radiation therapy, and systemic approaches, such as chemotherapy and immunotherapy. Therapeutic goals may include cure, control of the disease, or palliation of symptoms, and these goals may change over the course of the disease. Cancer in most cases is a long-term, chronic disease. Therapeutic and clinical decision making is important at multiple points along the cancer continuum and must be repeated as needed because of new findings about the disease, the success of the therapy, and the patient's response to the disease and the treatment

STUDY QUESTIONS

Chapter 2

Cytotoxic chemotherapeutics

9. The main mechanism of action of cytotoxic chemotherapeutic agents is:

    a. Killing of rapidly dividing cells
    b. Binding with hormone receptors
    c. Causing an increase in cell numbers
    d. Causing nausea and vomiting

10. In cancer treatment, chemotherapeutic drugs are usually given in combination in order to do which of the following?

    a. Improve palliation
    b. Avoid drug resistance
    c. Cause greater bone marrow suppression
    d. Bind with hormones that support tumor cell growth

high-grade tumor

11. A high-grade tumor could also be described as:

    a. Histopathologically stable
    b. Benign
    c. Poorly differentiated
    d. Well differentiated

12. Which of the following side effects is most commonly associated with use of biological response modifiers?

    biological response modifiers → SE

    a. Myelosuppression
    b. Gastrointestinal distress
    c. Hormonal imbalance
    d. Flulike syndrome

CHAPTER 3

SURGERY FOR CANCER THERAPY

cornerstone of CA care

CHAPTER OBJECTIVE

After completing this chapter, the reader will be able to relate general principles of surgical oncology, the rationale for surgical intervention in cancer as correlated with the stage of the disease, common surgical procedures used in cancer therapy, and nursing implications associated with cancer surgery.

LEARNING OBJECTIVES

After studying this chapter, the reader will be able to

1. Specify general principles underlying surgical intervention in treatment of cancer.

2. Specify how surgery can be related to the stage of disease in cancer patients.

3. Recognize common types of surgery used in cancer therapy.

4. Indicate the implications of cancer surgery on the nursing care of patients with cancer.

5. Specify complications associated with surgery for treatment of various cancers.

INTRODUCTION

Surgery is the oldest form of cancer therapy and is still the foundation for other techniques used in modern medical approaches in oncology. From the initial procedure used for diagnosis of the tumor to intervention for palliation or pain control in the late stages of disease, surgery is the cornerstone of cancer care.

surgery of palliation + pain control

SURGERY FOR DIAGNOSIS AND STAGING

The initial step in any clinical decision about cancer therapy is to obtain an accurate diagnosis and determine the exact type of tumor. Surgical biopsy can be classified in several ways.

Fine-needle aspiration

Fine-needle aspiration involves using a small-gauge needle and syringe device to remove cells from a palpable mass, placing the cells directly on a slide, and examining the cells to make a cytologic diagnosis (cells are examined individually). The accuracy of this procedure depends on the skill of the operator, who may be a surgeon, cytopathologist, or other specialist, and on the

palpable

type and amount of material obtained. If adequate material is acquired, the slide can be interpreted quickly, and a diagnosis of malignant or benign tissue can be made in a brief time. Additional diagnostic or pathologic procedures may be necessary to establish the specific tumor type.

Needle biopsy c̄ radiologic vis.

A needle biopsy is a variation of fine-needle aspiration. Specialized needles of various sizes are used to obtain a core of tissue for pathologic examination. If the tumor is not directly accessible but can be seen on radiologic examination, a needle biopsy can be accomplished by using radiologic visualization for obtaining the tissue specimen (e.g., a CT-directed biopsy).

Incisional biopsy (>3cm diam)

Incisional biopsies are used for masses that are palpable on physical examination, are accessible via surgery, and do not involve potentially lethal sites (e.g., a major blood vessel). A piece of tumor is surgically removed from the main mass and examined. The findings are used to make a pathologic diagnosis. Incisional biopsy is particularly useful for large tumors (3 cm or more in diameter). Care must be taken not to contaminate other parts of the tissue with tumor cells when the biopsy specimen is removed.

Excisional biopsies

Excisional biopsies are used for palpable masses that are accessible via surgery and small enough to be totally removed at time of initial surgery. The tumor is completely excised during the surgery. Excisional biopsies are often used for small skin lesions for which pathologic diagnosis is not needed to plan the surgical intervention. Sometimes, a fine-needle aspiration is done initially for diagnosis, and the excisional biopsy is the definitive surgery (e.g., for a lumpectomy in breast cancer). A disadvantage of this technique is that it can be used for only relatively small tumors. Also, a plan must be established for subsequent care so that wider excisions and more extensive surgery can be done at a later time if needed.

Staging refers to classification of a tumor according to the extent of involvement of local, regional, and distant tissues. Generally, the classification includes information on whether just the primary cancer or adjacent tissues, lymph nodes, and metastatic sites contain malignant tissue. Standardized staging systems are used for reporting cases of cancer, comparing cancers between persons or groups, and determining optimal cancer therapy.

Surgical intervention allows the clinician to judge the stage of the cancer on the basis of the clinical diagnostic stage and the surgical evaluative stage and to obtain tissue for pathologic examination and determination of the postsurgical pathologic stage. Surgical exploration for staging may involve multiple biopsies of various organs, removal of lymph nodes at distinct sites, detection of occult tumors by palpation and physical examination, and resection of entire organs. All tissues removed are examined pathologically for evidence of tumor involvement. The clinical, surgical, and pathologic data are then combined to define the tumor stage.

SURGERY AS THERAPY

Surgery has definite advantages over other therapeutic methods:

- The cancer is immediately removed from the body; the effect is immediate rather than delayed as with chemotherapy or radiation.

- The cancer can be completely removed in a localized area, with clear surgical margins.

- Unlike radiation and chemotherapy, surgery does not suppress the patient's immune system.

- In some cases, even large tumors can be excised all at once, or extensive tumors can be "debulked" so that subsequent chemotherapy or radiation therapy will be more effective.

- Staging of the tumor and therapeutic surgery can often be done at the same time.

tumors cured c̄ surgery early stage, thin melanoma, early cervical

Despite widely held cultural views that having surgery can speed a person's demise due to cancer ("exposure to the air through surgery"), no solid data support this perception.

Surgery also has distinct disadvantages:

- Some tumors (e.g., hematologic malignant neoplasms) cannot be treated with surgery.

- The location and extent of some tumors make surgical intervention impossible or highly risky.

- Some patients are poor candidates for surgical resection because of other medical conditions for which surgery or anesthesia is contraindicated.

- Tumor resection may require extensive surgery, resulting in disfigurement, loss of function, or other associated illness.

- Surgery itself can result in death.

- Resection is not appropriate for cancers that have spread, including micrometastatic disease, at the time of diagnosis or surgery. Often, patients in this category require the addition of chemotherapy, radiation therapy, or other combined therapies to treat the systemic aspects of the cancer.

Surgery as a Definitive Cancer Therapy

If the first axiom of oncologic care is, "When in doubt, cut it out," the caveat to that is, "If you cut it out, get it all out." Resections in which the margins of the removed tumor contain malignant cells are not curative. The residual tumor in the body can be a site of further cancer growth; the tumor may recur at the site of resection. If a tumor cannot be completely removed, a plan must be in place to use additional radiation therapy or chemotherapy.

Certain tumors may be considered "cured" as a result of complete surgical removal. These include early-stage, thin melanomas; basal cell carcinomas; and early-stage cervical cancers. Other tumors may be partially removed and subsequent chemotherapy or radiation therapy used for a curative approach, which contributes to improved function as well as cosmesis. Examples are early-stage breast cancer and early-stage sarcoma.

Because surgery can be associated with "seeding" of tumor cells (e.g., into the abdominal cavity), or spread of cancer via physical manipulation of the tumor, care must be taken to ensure that the tumor is handled minimally and not allowed to shed cells as it as being removed. One technique used to avoid tumor seeding is *en bloc* resection. The tumor, involved adjacent tissue, and regional lymph nodes are removed at one time, along with any sites of biopsies. To decrease further the risk of contamination with tumor cells, surgical instruments are changed for each biopsy site, and instruments used to remove tumors are replaced before new tissues are manipulated. If the margins of the resected tissue might include tumor cells, pathologic examination of "frozen sections" of the resected tissue are done to determine if the tumor site still has tumor cells. **?**

With advances in understanding the biology of cancer, the age-old assurances given by the surgeon to the patient, "We got it all" and that is the "end of the story," have become less and less the standard of care. The concept that micrometastases are probably present in lymph nodes, blood vessels, or other organs, even when no evidence of tumor spread can be found clinically, has shattered the idea that for the majority of cancers, surgery can be considered definitive therapy. With solid tumors, surgery can be considered curative (i.e., the surgeon did get all the tumor) in only about 30% of patients. *30% solid cured*

Surgery in Combination with Other Therapies

Frequently, surgery is combined with other treatments, such as radiation therapy and chemotherapy. This approach is used when (1) the margins of the resected tumor contain tumor cells, and a more extensive re-excision is not an option; (2) tumor spread to other regional or distant sites has already occurred or is likely; and (3) a large tumor or one with extensive local involvement requires debulking to increase the probability that other nonsurgical methods will be effective. Treatment given in addition to a primary therapy, such as chemotherapy given after removal of a breast cancer, is termed adjuvant therapy. Additional therapy given before the primary intervention is called neoadjuvant therapy. Commonly, surgery is the primary therapeutic intervention, and radiation or chemotherapy or both are given as adjuvant therapy.

Surgery as Palliative Therapy

Surgery is often used in cases even when the chances of cure are considered remote. Surgical biopsy may be used for an initial diagnosis or may be repeated to confirm recurrence or spread of cancer. Surgery is also used to debulk tumors that are causing signs and symptoms, discomfort, or loss of function; to relieve pain from large tumors or tumors in specific locations; to prevent or alleviate an obstruction; to provide cosmesis in the case of tumors that are difficult to control in terms of odor, leaking of fluids, hemorrhage, and so forth; and to provide a tumor-free period, although this time may be brief, and recurrence is considered highly probable.

Sites of a single focus of metastatic spread may also be amenable to surgical resection. These include pulmonary, hepatic, and brain metastases. Excisional biopsy or wedge resection of these single foci, although often not ultimately curative, may result in relatively long disease-free periods. As with other instances of surgical intervention, particularly when the goal is palliation, the risk-benefit ratio should indicate that the anticipated benefits in terms of time gained for the patient or prevention or relief of signs and symptoms outweigh the potential risks of morbidity and mortality associated with the intervention.

Surgery as Rehabilitation and Reconstruction

Although surgery can sometimes leave physical deformity and loss of function, it can also restore abilities and reconstruct tissues to improve both cosmesis and function. Prime examples of tumors for which plastic and reconstructive surgery are often beneficial are breast cancer, head and neck cancers, and some gynecologic tumors. Just as advances in understanding carcinogenesis and improvements in cancer treatment have led to increases in the of length of life of cancer patients, advances in therapies have enhanced the quality of cancer patients' lives. Surgical intervention can heighten pain control, particularly in cases of nerve involvement by the tumor or specific types of cancers (e.g., pancreatic) that may generate considerable pain. Creation of a feeding jejunostomy can improve nutritional status. Free transfer of tissue, use of flaps, building of continent ileostomies, and construction of artificial organs are ways that surgery has contributed to the rehabilitation and greater quality of cancer patients' lives.

pancreatic of pain

SURGERY FOR BREAST CANCER

Complete removal of the breast has been the gold standard of treatment of breast cancer since the 19th century. Halsted pioneered the concept that removal of the breast tissue as well as the greater and smaller pectoral muscles (musculi pectoralis major and pectoralis minor) and regional lymph nodes, called radical (Halsted) mastectomy, could improve survival. Later, data from comparative clinical trials established the effectiveness of the modified radical mastectomy, in which the breast tissue is totally removed, but the greater pectoral muscle, and often the smaller pectoral muscle, is left intact. At the same time, lymph nodes on the same side as the breast removed are usually resected, or specimens of lymph nodes are removed for pathologic examination. The lymph nodes are obtained to determine regional nodal involvement to aid in staging of the cancer and to remove a sanctuary for tumor cells from which the cells could potentially metastasize. Both the number and the location (level) of the lymph nodes involved are important in predicting prognosis.

More recently, results of clinical trials led to acceptance of another surgical procedure, lumpectomy or segmental mastectomy, that conserves breast tissue in an effort to preserve cosmesis. The surgeon attempts to remove the breast mass completely, leaving a surgical margin free of tumor cells (approximately 1 cm), and axillary lymph nodes are resected, or samples of lymph nodes are obtained through a separate incision. After surgery, radiation is used to treat the remaining breast tissue. This postoperative radiation may involve external-beam radiation therapy as well as electron boosts to the tissue or brachytherapy over a period of 4–6 weeks. The addition of radiation therapy to the primary surgical resection of the tumor is necessary to provide local control of tumor equal to that given by total surgical removal of the breast.

Segmental mastectomy is recommended as an option for smaller tumors (<1cm) when the tumor does not include a marked intraductal component, the location of the tumor is conducive to this approach (e.g., resection of subareolar tumors may not give optimal cosmesis), and the size of the breast is sufficient to accommodate lumpectomy without distortion. In cases in which the tumor is large or the breast is small, or the margins of the resected tissue continue to contain tumor cells, modified radical mastectomy with immediate or delayed reconstruction is the preferred procedure. The patient herself might also choose to have a modified radical mastectomy in order to avoid daily radiation therapy postoperatively or if breast reconstruction is favored. A woman may also choose modified radical mastectomy over segmental mastectomy for psychologic reasons: With a modified radical mastectomy, all the breast tissue has been removed, and therefore "all the cancer is gone, too." It is important that the surgical options be clearly presented to patients and the advantages and disadvantages objectively discussed. If both options are feasible, the choice of treatment should be left to the patient. Although the prevalence of breast cancer in males is quite small (<5% of total cases), similar surgical techniques would be used for treatment.

Nursing Implications

Besides the potential for psychologic and emotional disturbances associated with changes in body image and the diagnosis of cancer, certain physical complications can result from mastectomy. Hematoma and seroma can occur as well as nerve trauma resulting in a pins-and-needles sensation or itching. Patients who have had their entire breast removed may complain of a feeling that the breast is still in place and painful; this feeling is called phantom breast sensation. The most important complications are limitations in mobility due to the surgery itself or to lymphedema of the arm related to the dissection of axillary lymph nodes. Estimates of the prevalence of lymphedema vary, but about 12% of women postoperatively have signs and symptoms ranging from pain and fluid retention and swelling of the arm to limited or painful movement of the arm and shoulder. Cellulitis also can occur in the affected arm. Patients are warned to avoid having needles inserted in or blood pressures taken on the arm on the same side as the mastectomy site to reduce risk of lymphedema.

Treatment of lymphedema is generally long-term and unsuccessful and may involve wraps, mechanical compression, or even surgical intervention. Milder cases may be controlled through positioning and refraining from wearing short-sleeved clothes. Women who receive radiation postoperatively for lumpectomy should be aware that edema and skin changes can continue to occur long-term in the remaining breast tissue after radiation is completed. Rehabilitative exercises and psychologic support can be obtained after surgery through groups such as the American Cancer Society, which has the Reach to Recovery program.

SURGERY FOR LUNG CANCER

Surgery is the treatment of choice for early-stage (I and II) non–small-cell lung cancers and may also be used for some stage III cancers. The extent and type of surgery depend on the stage and what anatomic areas are involved with tumor. Some stage III tumors in which the cancer has invaded the chest wall, pericardium, diaphragm, vertebral body, and parts of the pleura may be completely resected by using an *en bloc* technique.

Knew pre-op pulmonary status

Lobectomy, the removal of the involved lobe of the lung, is the standard surgical approach for early-stage lung cancers. Pulmonary function is generally preserved, and associated mortality is less than 3%. A more extensive operation than a simple lobectomy can be done when both a lobe and the main bronchus are involved. In these cases, a sleeve lobectomy may be done instead of a complete pneumonectomy, and more lung tissue is preserved.

Segmentectomy

Less extensive surgery may also be used. The size of the tumor, the amount of involvement of anatomic structures, and diminished pulmonary function may make some type of limited resection feasible. Segmentectomy involves removal of a specific segment of a lung and may include the relevant bronchus, lung tissue, and pulmonary artery and vein. Small, peripheral lesions, including metastatic nodules, may be removed via a wedge resection. Local recurrence of tumor varies with the stage and extent of resection but may be as high as 12%. However, mortality with limited lung resections is generally quite low, averaging less than 2%, and postoperatively, pulmonary function is usually enhanced.

Pneumonectomy won't 6%

When lung tumors are large or centrally located, pneumonectomy, complete removal of the involved lung, may be necessary. Such surgery is technically demanding, and the resulting compromise of pulmonary function can greatly affect the patient. Mortality rates are about 6% with this procedure. For tumors involving the carina or lower part of the trachea and lung, even more extensive tumor removal is possible with sleeve pneumonectomy. In this procedure, an anastomosis is created between the lower part of the trachea and the opposite main bronchus. Mortality rates are 15–20%.

Laser surgery may be used in conjunction with bronchoscopy to remove a tumor obstructing an airway. Such a procedure is palliative. It may alleviate signs and symptoms, but it does not improve long-term survival.

Nursing Implications

Care of patients who have had surgery for treatment of lung cancer includes the routine postoperative care required by any patient who has had thoracic surgery. In addition, nurses should be aware of the extent of the resection, the amount of lung tissue and pulmonary function remaining, and the preoperative pulmonary status of the patient. Many lung cancer patients have long histories of tobacco use and impaired pulmonary status, including chronic obstructive pulmonary disease. Age may also be a factor, although this consideration is not a sole contraindication for thoracic resection.

To enhance expansion of the remaining lung tissue, patients who have had a lobectomy should avoid prolonged lying on the side that was operated on. In contrast, to allow full expansion of the lung remaining, patients who have had pneumonectomy should not lie on the side opposite the side operated on. Postoperative teaching should address ways of dealing with limitations in pulmonary function and realistic assessment of the impact of prognosis. Because most lung cancers are detected at later stages, 5-year survival is low, and patients may be adjusting to a new diagnosis, poor prognosis, and possible assignment of blame if the cancer is associated with environmental exposures (e.g., occupational hazards or cigarette smoking).

SURGERY FOR
PANCREATIC CANCER

Although the incidence of pancreatic cancer is low, the mortality rate is usually high, partly because the disease is generally diagnosed at late stages. Although surgery is the primary therapy for this cancer, most patients with pancreatic carcinoma are not candidates for curative resection. Only about 20% of patients with pancreatic cancer who undergo laparotomy have resectable tumors.

The standard approach to the most common pancreatic tumor, cancer of the head of the pancreas, has been the Whipple procedure, since 1935. Modern modifications of the procedure have slightly improved mortality (2–4%) and morbidity (25–35%) rates. However, the procedure is still complex and technically demanding and has a tremendous impact on the postoperative activities of

Pancreas → Whipple Procedure

daily living for the patient. During the surgery, a search is made for additional sites of tumor spread, including the liver and adjacent structures. If the tumor is considered resectable, the portal vein and the head of the pancreas are removed; a pancreaticojejunostomy is done, with an end-to-end or a mucosa-to-mucosa anastomosis with the remaining part of the pancreas; the common bile duct is anastomosed to the jejunal loop; a gastrojejunostomy is done; and a vagotomy is done, if the gastric resection is limited. Contemporary techniques may leave the pylorus intact, because nutritional deficits are the primary long-term complication in patients who have had a Whipple procedure.

An alternative surgical approach is total pancreatectomy. Long-term survival (16–30 months) after total pancreatectomy is similar to that for the Whipple procedure. However, if no pancreatic tissue remains after resection, endocrine adjustment after surgery can be quite complex, and establishing control can be difficult.

Nursing Implications

The extensive surgery involved in both the Whipple procedure and total pancreatectomy makes postoperative care a challenge. Nutritional complications are expected and correlate with the extent of gastric resection. Additionally, endocrine problems may occur in patients who have had total pancreatectomy. Stomal ulceration can also occur. Further surgical intervention for palliation may be necessary for relief of pain and of signs and symptoms due to obstruction.

AMPUTATIONS AND LIMB-SPARING SURGERY

Osteo-, Ewing's, chondro-, soft-tissue = sarcoma

The most common cancers involving the extremities for which surgical resection would be an option include osteosarcoma, Ewing's sarcoma, chondrosarcoma, and soft-tissue sarcomas. The type of surgery depends on the type of tumor and the stage of disease. Management

of cancer involving the extremities has changed considerably over the past two decades. Although resection of as much tumor as possible is still the guiding principle of therapy, limb-sparing techniques result in equivalent survival rates.

radiation + chemo shrink primary tumor + clear margins

Adequate tissue margins with no tumor cells are still a requirement to eliminate the need for amputation. Consequently, radiation therapy or chemotherapy is often used before or after surgery to shrink the primary tumor or to clear margins. Both external-beam radiation and implantation of radiation sources at the tumor site have been used as adjuvant therapy. In some studies, local recurrence of tumor was slightly higher in patients who had limb-sparing surgery than in patients who had amputation, but overall survival was the same in both groups.

external beam rad. + implant

Nursing Implications

Even when attempts are made to retain maximal function with limb-sparing procedures, some loss of tissue and functional ability usually occurs. In the case of amputation, considerable adaptation by the patient and relearning of certain skills with the assistance of physical and occupational therapy and rehabilitation medicine are necessary. If radiation therapy is used along with limb-sparing surgery, wound healing can be compromised, especially if radiation is started soon after the surgery. As is the case with other tissue-conserving techniques, patients who have these procedures often have heightened anxiety that the cancer "will come back," because radical surgery to remove the tumor was not done.

SURGERY FOR HEAD AND NECK CANCER

radical = radiation

In a variety of head and neck cancers, surgery, which often is radical and may be combined with radiation therapy, forms the foundation for curative therapy. Surgical oncologists must work in concert with plastic and reconstructive surgeons and specialists in rehabilitation medicine to not only eradicate the cancer but also conserve or restore sufficient functional ability and cosmesis lost through surgical resection. Surgery in the head and neck area directly affects basic skills, such as speech, breathing, and swallowing, and the four senses (smell, sight, taste, hearing), and indirectly affects such things as nutrition and exercise. Because the appearance of the head is intimately linked to body image and self-concept, the repulsive results that can sometimes occur with radical surgery can have devastating psychologic and emotional effects.

Partial laryngectomy or epiglottidectomy may be used for early-stage lesions and total laryngectomy for late-stage tumors. Radiation therapy to the region, including nodal beds if metastases to the lymph nodes are known or suspected, may also be used. In a supraglottic laryngectomy, the anatomic structures lying above the false vocal cords, including the epiglottis, are removed. Postoperatively, patients have difficulty in swallowing but still have their true vocal cords and near-normal speech. Hemilaryngectomy involves resection of one true vocal cord, one false vocal cord, and the adjacent cartilage. After surgery, patients generally have intact swallowing function, but their voices may be hoarse. In a total laryngectomy, the larynx is completely excised from the hyoid bone to the level of the second tracheal ring, necessitating a permanent tracheostomy. Postoperatively, patients cannot speak or perform the Valsalva maneuver, and their sense of smell is diminished. Other surgical procedures for head and neck cancers may involve *en bloc* resection of the oral cavity, muscles, nerves, and lymph nodes in a radical neck dissection or resection of facial bones.

Nursing Implications

Specific nursing care of patients who have had surgery for treatment of head and neck cancer depends on the surgical procedure done and the functional or cosmetic defects that result. Commonly, patients experience difficulty with speech and swallowing, with risk of aspiration, and have shoulder, facial, or mouth droops if certain nerves or muscles are affected. Because many head and neck cancers are associated with lifestyle factors, particularly smoking and use of alcohol, potentially patients must also deal with self-recrimination or, conversely, a desire to continue the habits that may have led to their current condition.

SURGERY FOR GYNECOLOGIC TUMORS

Optimal therapy of gynecologic cancers often involves surgery, sometimes in combination with radiation therapy. The extent of surgery is dictated by the stage of the tumor. Hysterectomy is used for advanced cervical cancer, endometrial cancer, and as part of more extensive surgical resections for vaginal and ovarian cancers. An abdominal approach rather than a vaginal one is often used for the surgery because a thorough assessment of the pelvis and abdominal cavity is less likely with a vaginal approach.

Advances in the use of laparoscopic surgery, including visualization and the ability to obtain biopsy specimens of lesions that may be malignant, have influenced the surgical procedures used in gynecologic cancers. For ovarian cancers, total abdominal hysterectomy and bilateral salpingo-oophorectomy are standard procedures. Treatment of more advanced tumors may include partial bowel resection, omentectomy, and para-aortic and pelvic lymphadenectomy, as well as complete exploration of the pelvic and abdominal cavity and biopsies of adjacent tissues and organs. Surgical debulking is used so that residual tumor is optimally less than 2 cm in size; the small size enhances the effectiveness of postoperative chemotherapy and radiation. More radical surgery, including pelvic exenteration, may be indicated in advanced or recurrent gynecologic cancers and is usually done by gynecologic oncologists, often assisted by urologists or general surgeons. In these cases, total abdominal hysterectomy, bilateral salpingo-oophorectomy, and lymphadenectomy may be combined with resection of the bladder, parts of the bowel, including the rectum, and the components of the pelvic cavity.

Nursing Implications

Nursing care of patients who have had surgery for gynecologic cancer depends on the type and extent of the
surgery performed. In general, nursing care of a woman
who has had a hysterectomy because of cancer is similar to that of a woman who has had a hysterectomy because of benign conditions, except that the cancer
patient may also be receiving adjuvant radiation therapy
or chemotherapy. Radiation therapy can cause immediate and delayed side effects, including skin reactions,
radiation cystitis, enteritis, vaginal or cervical fibrosis
resulting in sexual dysfunction, and vaginal stenosis.

Fistulas involving the vagina, bladder, rectum, or small
bowel can require surgery for repair. Wound separation,
necrosis, and infection are also potential complications.
Patients who undergo lymph node resection are at risk
for leg edema and lymphangitis. When surgical resection has been extensive (e.g., pelvic exenteration or
radical vulvectomy), patients must adapt to multiple
changes in function and need rehabilitation to regain
sexual function on some level.

SURGERY FOR COLORECTAL CANCER

The location and stage of a colorectal tumor dictate the
type and extent of surgery that is recommended. The
goal is to resect the tumor yet preserve function and
avoid the need for a permanent colostomy. Cancers of
the rectum that are sufficiently removed (10 cm or
more) from the anal verge may be treated with a low anterior resection, in which the sphincter is preserved as
long as adequate margins of resection are obtained. Tumors lower in the rectum may require an abdominal-
perineal resection, in which the tumor and other tissue
are removed through an abdominal incision. Postoperatively, patients have a perineal wound, which may be
closed with a drain or left open to heal by granulation,
and a colostomy. Anal cancers that require removal of
the anal canal with anterior-posterior resection may also
require pelvic exenteration if the cancer involves the

bladder and other pelvic structures. In these cases, a colostomy and a urinary diversion (e.g., ileal conduit), if
the bladder or urethra is removed, is done. Other colorectal cancers may be treated by a hemicolectomy, in
which the tumor and both proximal and distal sections
of colon are resected to provide adequate free margins;
a temporary colostomy may be established, but a permanent colostomy may be avoided if the tumor is small
enough to allow resection and anastomosis of the remaining sections of the colon. Dissection of regional
lymph nodes is generally done as well.

Nursing Implications

Specialized nursing care of patients who have had surgery for colorectal cancer may include care related to
the permanent or temporary colostomy, wound care,
and nutritional assessment. Possible complications include leaking at the site(s) of anastomosis, urinary and
bowel dysfunction, poor wound healing or infection,
stomal problems, herniation, and prolapse. Sexual functioning may be impaired in both men and women, because of surgical intervention or because of scarring
from surgery or radiation therapy. An enterostomal
therapist, usually a nurse with specialized training in the
care of ostomies and wounds, may be a valuable member of the health care team for patients who have colorectal surgery. The therapist's role includes
preoperative planning for placement of the stoma, and
preoperative and postoperative teaching of patients, patients' families, and staff members about ostomy care.

SURGERY FOR PROSTATIC AND GENITOURINARY CANCER

Surgery for prostatic cancer is becoming more refined
as the high incidence of this cancer has prompted further research into new and better methods for surgical

intervention that is effective but conserves function. One result of this exploration is that radical prostatectomy, the standard for early-stage prostatic cancer, is considered curative. However, newer techniques call for a retropubic approach to remove the prostate, seminal vesicles, and a small amount of the neck of the bladder and resect or obtain samples of pelvic lymph nodes. When nerve-sparing procedures are used, function of the capsular and periprostatic nerves is retained, resulting in maintenance of potency in most patients and a reduction in incontinence to 1–2%. Other techniques used for prostatectomy may include a perineal or suprapubic approach, although occurrence of urethral strictures may be increased with these approaches. Lymph nodes may be dissected at the time of prostatectomy. Examination of the lymph nodes adds to the staging information, but their removal has not been shown to have a therapeutic effect or to increase survival. Larger lesions (1.5–2 cm) and more advanced stages of disease may be treated by transurethral resection of the prostate, in which the tumor and prostate are removed through the urethra. Adjuvant radiation therapy is used after surgery.

Other genitourinary cancers (e.g., cancer of the bladder), although not as common as prostatic cancer, are treated similarly. Early-stage bladder cancer may be removed via radical cystectomy or treated with intravesical administration of chemotherapeutic agents. A transurethral surgical approach may be used for superficial, low-grade bladder tumors, with the addition of intravesical chemotherapy or laser surgery. In more advanced stages of bladder cancer, radical cystectomy is used routinely. In men, this procedure calls for removal of the bladder, perivesical fat, adjacent peritoneum, prostate, and seminal versicles. Radical cystectomy may also result in impotence. For women, radical cystectomy involves resection of the bladder and urethra, possible hysterectomy and bilateral salpingo-oophorectomy, removal of the anterior wall of the vagina, and pelvic lymphadenectomy. Urinary diversion may consist of an ileal conduit in which the distal portion of the ileum is used to form an external stoma, and ureters are placed into the ileum, allowing urine to flow into the conduit and out via the stoma. An alternative diversion may be a continent ileal reservoir so that urine is stored in an internal intraabdominal pouch; no external ostomy device is used for urine collection.

Nursing Implications

Problems with voiding and sexual function are two potential complications of genitourinary surgery that require nursing attention, that is, assessment and teaching of patients, before and after the procedure. Patients with urinary diversions will be at risk for complications related to the ostomy, formation of fistulas, skin ulcers, and infection. Scarring, surgical intervention, and other therapeutic interventions (e.g., hormonal manipulation in prostatic cancer, radiation therapy) can directly affect sexual functioning. Patients should be informed about potential problems and alternative solutions, including, for men, the possibility of penile implants at the time of surgical resection.

CRANIOTOMY

The primary therapy for gliomas, whether benign or highly malignant, is resection. Depending on the location of the tumor and the general state of the patient, securing tissue for diagnosis, debulking to prevent or relieve pressure, and reducing tumor burden are usually the goals. Unless the tumor is located in the upper part of the brainstem or the pons, surgery consisting of stereotaxic biopsy, at a minimum, or, optimally, removal of the tumor, is generally an alternative. A tissue diagnosis is important before initiation of radiation therapy, which can be effective in brain tumors.

Stereotaxic biopsy may be the definitive surgical treatment when the tumor is located in the thalamus or midline corpus callosum. For this procedure, a head ring with a localizing system is attached to the patient's head with screws; computerized simulation and computation are used to determine the exact technical approach for biopsy. An open craniotomy may be done later for tumor debulking or removal of as much tumor as possible. Because of the nature of brain tumors themselves and the risk of neurologic deficits due to surgery, clear surgical margins are usually not a consideration. Radiation therapy, chemotherapy, or immunotherapy may be given after surgery to reduce further the risk of tumor recurrence.

Nursing Implications

Because of the risk of intracranial hemorrhage, increased intracranial pressure due to cerebral edema, and infection, careful nursing assessment is required for patients who have had surgery for brain tumors. Checks of the patient's neurologic status should be done frequently to ascertain changes in functioning. Acute complications may occur during hospitalization, but patients and their families should be instructed to report signs and symptoms of later occurring complications, such as thrombosis, progressive neurologic deficit, recurrence or increase in frequency of seizures, and indications that intracranial pressure is increasing. For patients who have received radiation therapy, long-term side effects may include necrosis, interference with surgical wound healing, and diminished neurologic functioning.

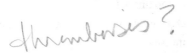

SUMMARY

Surgery provides an essential foundation for other cancer therapies and may be used in conjunction with other therapeutic interventions. The precise surgical approach is usually determined by the size, stage, and location of the tumor. Nurses fill a critical role in detecting potential risks before and after surgery, assessing patients for the presence of these risks or other surgical complications, and instructing patients and patients' families in ways to deal with postoperative changes and detect long-term side effects that require intervention.

STUDY QUESTIONS

Chapter 3

Questions 13 –22

13. What tissues are removed in a segmental mastectomy?

    a. The complete breast
    b. The breast plus the greater pectoral muscle
    c. The breast mass, surrounding tissue, and regional lymph nodes
    d. The complete breast plus regional lymph nodes

14. Nursing interventions after lung surgery for cancer should include:

    a. Positioning a patient who has had a lobectomy so that he or she is lying on the side that was operated on
    b. Positioning a patient who has had a pneumonectomy so that he or she is lying on the side that was operated on
    c. Wound care for the anastomosis
    d. Referral to the Reach to Recovery program

15. The primary long-term complication in patients who have had the Whipple procedure for treatment of pancreatic cancer is:

    a. Nutritional deficits
    b. Chronic anemia
    c. Phantom pain
    d. Delayed wound healing

16. Incisional biopsies are most commonly indicated for which of the following?

    a. Tumors involving major blood vessels
    b. Very small palpable masses
    c. Large tumors
    d. Definitive surgical resection of small tumors

17. One advantage of surgery over other cancer therapies is that:

    a. Tumor staging can take place at the same time.
    b. Surgery can be used to treat every type of cancer.
    c. Associated morbidity is rare.
    d. Surgery is the primary treatment for all tumor types.

18. Cancer therapy given in addition to the primary treatment is termed:

    a. Augmentation therapy
    b. Extension therapy
    c. Tumor suppression therapy
    d. Adjuvant therapy

19. Surgery in which the goal is to relieve cancer-related pain is termed:

    a. Curative
    b. Neoadjuvant   @ primary intervention
    c. Palliative
    d. Reconstructive

20. Patients who undergo which of the following procedures will be unable to speak after surgery?

    a. Epiglottidectomy
    b. Total laryngectomy
    c. Hemilaryngectomy
    d. Supraglottic laryngectomy

21. A permanent colostomy is most often associated with treatment of which of the following cancers?

    a. Ovarian
    b. Colon
    c. Rectal
    d. Anal

22. Nursing interventions after surgery for treatment of prostatic cancer should include assessment of:

    a. Urinary continence
    b. Colostomy care
    c. Pelvic lymph nodes
    d. Abdominal cavity

CHAPTER 4

RADIATION THERAPY

CHAPTER OBJECTIVE

After completing this chapter, the reader will be able to specify the basic principles of radiation therapy, indicate nursing care of patients receiving radiation therapy, and specify ways to ensure the safety of these patients and their families and caregivers.

LEARNING OBJECTIVES

After studying this chapter, the reader will be able to

1. Specify the basic principles of radiobiology.

2. List the common types of radiation therapy used to treat cancer.

3. Describe safety issues associated with teletherapy.

4. Specify safety considerations for patients receiving brachytherapy and for the patients' families and caregivers.

5. List the side effects associated with radiation therapy.

6. Specify nursing care for patients experiencing various side effects of radiation therapy.

INTRODUCTION

About 50% of all cancer patients will receive radiation therapy at some point during their treatment. In this method of treatment, high-energy rays are used to stop cancer cells from growing and multiplying. Radiation is often combined with surgery, chemotherapy, or immunotherapy, but it can also be used alone (Groenwald, Frogge, Goodman, & Yarbro, 1990). The two most common forms of radiation therapy are teletherapy and brachytherapy. Both of these are discussed later in the chapter.

Among the available cancer treatments, radiation therapy is one of the oldest. The history of radiation began in 1895, when Wilhelm Roentgen discovered roentgen rays, now called x-rays (American Cancer Society [ACS], 1990; Ashwanden, Belcher, Mattson, Moskowitz, & Riese, 1990). X-rays penetrate tissue much as a beam of light penetrates glass, and it was quickly realized that they would be useful in diagnosis. Soon after that, scientists discovered that exposure to radiation could shrink tumors.

Two types of radiation are used to treat cancer. X-rays are generated by a man-made source, such as a cathode ray tube. γ-Rays are produced by natural sources, usually cobalt or cesium. Radiation is a localized form of treatment. This means that only the cells exposed to the radiation are affected. Cells outside the field of radiation are not harmed.

PRINCIPLES OF RADIOBIOLOGY

Radiation therapy is based on the ability of radiation to interact with the atoms and molecules of tumor cells and produce harmful biological effects (Groenwald et al., 1990). Radiation kills cancer cells by damaging the cells enough so that they cannot grow or divide. The relationship between radiation dose and cell death is complex (ACS, 1990). Small, individual doses of radiation are relatively inefficient at killing cells because the cells can repair themselves between treatments. In contrast, high doses damage cells to such an extent that small increases in the doses used can kill a relatively high proportion of cells.

This information suggests that the most effective way to kill cancer cells would be to use large, single doses rather than several small doses given at intervals over a long time. However, extensive clinical experience has shown that high doses cause severe injury to normal tissue and are less likely to bring about tumor control (ACS, 1990). Although the goal of treatment is to destroy cancerous tissue, healthy tissue must be preserved (Baird, McCorkle, & Grant, 1991). Therefore, it is more effective to use several small doses of approximately 200 cGy each (ACS, 1990).

Why fractionated, small-dose treatment is more effective than single, high-dose treatment is not entirely understood. Fractionation of a dose is based on the four *R*s of radiobiology (ACS, 1990; Baird et al., 1991; Groenwald et al., 1990):

1. Repair: The goal of fractionation is to deliver a dose that is sufficient to prevent repair of can-

cer cells but allow recovery of normal cells before the next dose is given.

2. Repopulation: Repopulation is the replacement of killed cells by the division and growth of surviving cells. Both normal and malignant tissues are capable of recovery from radiation injury in this way. Repopulation rates vary greatly according to the type of tissue. This may explain why some tissues are more radiosensitive than others.

3. Redistribution: Killing by radiation is more effective during certain phases of the cell cycle. Cells are more sensitive during mitosis and growth than they are during synthesis. After a dose of radiation, cells are redistributed throughout the various phases of the cell cycle. This redistribution is usually more successful for cancer cells than for normal cells. This can be advantageous, because each dose of radiation can capture more cancer cells in vulnerable phases.

4. Reoxygenation: Well-oxygenated cells are more sensitive to radiation than poorly oxygenated cells are. Normal tissue is usually well oxygenated, whereas cancerous tissue is characteristically poorly oxygenated, or hypoxic. When fractionated doses are used, the tumor has time between treatments to reoxygenate and thus become more susceptible to the effects of radiation.

The overall goal of radiation therapy is to eradicate the tumor while sparing normal tissue. Programs that call for daily treatment with radiation are designed to optimize the four *R*s of radiobiology. As these four processes become better understood, more successful treatment regimens may be developed (ACS, 1990).

RADIATION DOSAGE

It is standard practice in radiation therapy to divide the amount of radiation given into small doses and administer these doses over a given period. Until recently, the term used to describe the unit of dosing was *rad,* the acronym for radiation absorbed dose. In 1985, the term *gray* (Gy) was officially adopted to replace the term rad. For conversion purposes, 1 Gy = 100 rads, or 1 rad = 1 cGy (centigray) (ACS, 1988, 1990; Groenwald et al., 1990). The term centigray is most common in treatment regimens. Treatment plans may list *dose rate,* the number of centigrays given in a specified unit of time, and the *dose-time factor,* the total number of centigrays given in a total number of days (Groenwald et al., 1990).

Radiation treatment is usually given on a daily basis. Schedules for some radioresistant tumors may include treating the patient twice daily. In some situations, such as slow growing skin cancer, treatments may be given only two or three times a week (ACS, 1988).

Courses of treatment designed to provide palliation are usually shorter than courses designed to cure, because the goal is to control the cancer rather than eradicate it. The total dose in a palliative course will be relatively low and can be given in a short period. A curative course, however, will use a maximum dose, given over a longer time. Curative treatment usually takes 5–8 weeks or more.

STEPS IN DELIVERY OF RADIATION THERAPY

Radiation therapy can be delivered in several different ways. The initial steps are the same in all cases.

Consultation

A patient's initial visit to the radiation therapy facility involves consultation, assessment, and discussion of the treatment plan. Patients are encouraged to bring along members of their families or significant others to help provide information and to reinforce information given by the caregiver (Baird et al., 1991). During this visit, a complete history is obtained, and a physical examination is done. Diagnostic results and pathology reports are reviewed and discussed with the patient and the patient's family. Patients and their families receive education about the proposed treatment. The education should include the treatment schedule, potential side effects, and the plan of care. This first visit may also include a physical orientation to the facility and resources available to patients and patients' families throughout the treatment.

Simulation

Before radiation treatments are started, several steps are taken to define the treatment target, ensure the accuracy of the setup for daily treatment, and protect healthy tissue from radiation injury as much as possible (Groenwald et al., 1990). These steps involve a process called simulation. In simulation, the tumor target is visualized and defined through x-rays, scans, and physical landmarks. The patient is positioned exactly as he or she will be positioned for the actual radiation treatment. Coordinate points on the body are used to ensure alignment. These points may be physical landmarks or ink markings applied to the body. Such ink markings should not be washed off until the treatment is complete. Small permanent tattoos may also be used later in treatment to ensure longer term accuracy in alignment.

During the simulation, the need for immobilization devices such as casts, head-holders, and restraints is determined. These devices are used to ensure proper alignment during treatment (Baird et al., 1991; Clark & McGee, 1992).

Treatment

When the consultation and simulation have been completed, treatment can begin. The length of an average course of treatment is 2–8 weeks (Baird et al., 1991). Treatment is usually given daily, 5 days a week. The exposure to radiation takes only a few minutes. Most of the time in the treatment room is spent positioning the patient and the machine for appropriate alignment. Some treatments involve multiple angles or changes in the patient's position (Baird et al., 1991). These treatments require more time than other treatments do.

TELETHERAPY

Teletherapy is commonly referred to as external radiation or external-beam radiation therapy (EBRT). This form of radiation therapy is used in most patients. Teletherapy (from *tele*, Greek prefix meaning "at a distance") involves electromagnetic radiation in the form of x-rays and γ-rays. The radiation is supplied by a fixed source located at a distance from the patient (Ashwanden et al., 1990; Baird et al., 1991).

The goal of teletherapy is to deliver a beam of ionizing radiation from an external source to a designated target in the body. This can be achieved with a variety of machines. Early machines used in teletherapy had kilovoltages of 40–150, and they generated x-rays that had minimal penetration because of the rays' low energy. Between 1920 and 1940, orthovoltage equipment with a range of 180–250 kV was developed that could be used to treat deeper tumors. However, the therapeutic value of orthovoltage equipment was limited, because healthy tissue was not spared (Baird et al., 1991).

After World War II, radiation therapy entered the supervoltage era. Atomic reactors made cobalt a more readily available source of radiation for treatment. In the 1950s, cobalt machines became the standard source of radiation for deep therapy. Later, in the 1960s and 1970s, linear accelerators were built (Baird et al., 1991). These machines produce x-rays by accelerating electrons along a radiofrequency electromagnetic wave (Groenwald et al., 1990).

Although they are more complex to operate and maintain than cobalt machines are, linear accelerators are more widely used in health care today. These accelerators have two distinct advantages in treatment: speed and accuracy. Linear accelerators are fast and provide efficient use of time for staff and patients. This means that patients spend less time in awkward or uncomfortable positions. In addition, linear accelerators provide a sharp, defined field of irradiation. This means that less normal tissue is affected by the treatment (Groenwald et al., 1990).

Treatment

Teletherapy requires only a few minutes of actual exposure to radiation and about 10 min in the treatment room altogether (Baird et al., 1991). Most of the treatment time is spent positioning the patient and the machine. The patient is positioned on a treatment couch or table. Teletherapy machines are large and may be noisy. Treatments are given by a registered radiation technologist. It is important to prepare patients for the experience of radiation therapy. They should be assured that there is no pain or sensation during the irradiation. Patients often expect to feel heat, tingling, or some other sensation. This, however, is not the case. Some discomfort may be experienced because of positioning or because of lying on a firm table (Baird et al., 1991).

Accurate setup and alignment of the patient are an essential part of successful teletherapy. Periodic beam radiographs or check radiographs may be taken to evaluate the positioning of the patient and the placement of the machine. Check radiographs are compared with the original simulation radiographs to determine the accuracy. This process takes a few extra minutes during treatment. Patients often mistakenly think that a check radiograph will show changes in tumor size. The process and purpose of the check radiograph should be explained to them.

During a course of treatment, a patient is usually seen by a radiologist or nurse at least once a week. This interaction provides caregivers an opportunity to monitor the progress of treatment, assess reactions, develop interventions, and offer support (Baird et al., 1991).

Safety Related to Teletherapy

Discussions of radiation and precautions associated with its safe use often evoke questions, concerns, and even

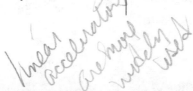

fears. Health care providers should understand the hazards associated with this treatment for both patients and staff.

Exposure to radiation is a part of daily life for everyone and cannot be completely prevented. Persons are constantly exposed to radiation from natural sources such as rocks, uranium and potassium in soil, the sun, and lead and radon in the environment (ACS, 1988). The levels of exposure are usually low. Artificial sources of radiation include diagnostic x-ray examinations and occupational exposure. Workers whose occupations may expose them to radiation include crews of jet aircraft, manufacturers of radiopharmaceuticals, industrial radiographers, uranium miners, and nuclear fuel processors (ACS, 1988). Any occupational environment in which workers may be exposed to radiation should be monitored.

All teletherapy is subject to federal and state regulations and requires both training of personnel in radiation safety and monitoring. In this type of radiation therapy, the source of radiation remains within the machine, and no radioactivity is imparted to the patient (ACS, 1988). Patients never become radioactive when they are receiving external-beam therapy (Ashwanden et al., 1990). Exposure to radiation related to teletherapy depends on the location of the beam and how long the beam is activated. Safety measures often taken by health care personnel during treatment include wearing leaded aprons or standing behind leaded barriers. Patients may also be draped with a leaded shield when vital organs may be exposed. Staff personnel should wear radiation badges to monitor their exposure to radiation. Because the fetus is susceptible to radiation, pregnant patients or staff members should avoid exposure or use shielding.

BRACHYTHERAPY

Brachytherapy is commonly referred to as internal radiation. In this form of therapy, a source of radiation is placed within or on the patient's body (Groenwald et al., 1990). Radioactive isotopes are temporarily or perma-

nently placed in a body cavity, within tissue, or on the surface of the body. Unlike teletherapy (external radiation treatment), which delivers a calculated daily dose of radiation within a short time, brachytherapy delivers a specific dose of radiation continuously over several hours or days (Hassey, 1988).

Brachytherapy is gaining prominence as treatment for a variety of tumors. It is an effective way to deliver a concentrated dose of radiation to a defined area with minimal side effects to the surrounding tissue (Brandt, 1989).

With teletherapy, radiation is distributed evenly to a large area of tissue. With brachytherapy, a highly concentrated dose is provided in or near the tumor site, and the dose diminishes rapidly as it reaches adjacent tissues (Hassey, 1988). Brachytherapy can be used in conjunction with teletherapy for better results. When larger doses are delivered to a tumor site, recurrence of local disease is less likely. The rapid decrease in radiation to the surrounding normal tissues spares them from damage, and the risk of long-term side effects is also reduced (Hassey, 1988). Brachytherapy has been used in combination with surgery and chemotherapy to cure, control, or relieve symptoms of many types of cancer (Brandt, 1989).

Properties of Radioisotopes

A radioisotope is a highly unstable element. As the radioisotope breaks up and decays, energy particles are emitted that penetrate tissue easily (Hassey, 1988). To determine how a radioisotope will be used in treatment, its half-life must be considered. The half-life is the time required for the radioisotope to decay to 50% of its original strength. Half-lives of radioisotopes can vary from several days to more than 1600 years (Hassey, 1988). A particular radioisotope is selected for temporary or permanent use on the basis of its half-life. For example, gold-198 (^{198}Au) has a half-life of 2.7 days. Sources of this radioisotope can be left in the body permanently; they do not need to be removed when treatment is complete. Radium, however, has a half-life of 1600 years. Sources of radium must be removed from the body after the specified treatment period (Hassey, 1988).

Types of Brachytherapy

Brachytherapy can be achieved through implants (en-capsulated radiation) or through radiopharmaceuticals (unencapsulated radiation). Implant therapy is the most common. Sealed sources of radiation in the form of wires, seeds, needles, or ribbons are implanted into the tumor or placed in a body cavity. Because the source is sealed, no body fluids are contaminated by the radiation (Ashwanden et al., 1990).

Implants are the method of choice in a variety of can-cers (Groenwald, et al., 1990). Typical ones are gyne-cologic and eye tumors and cancers of the breast, prostate, lung, esophagus, colon, and head and neck (Ashwanden et al, 1990; Baird et al, 1991; Johnson & Gross, 1985). Many radioisotopes can be used (Groen-wald et al., 1990):

Wires	Tantalum-182 (^{182}Ta)
Ribbons and tubes	Iridium-192 (^{192}Ir)
Needles	Cesium-137 (^{137}Cs)
	Radium-226 (^{226}Ra)
Seeds and grains	Gold-198 (^{198}Au)
	Radon-222 (^{222}Rn)
Capsules	^{137}Cs
	^{226}Ra

The radioisotope selected depends on the site of the cancer to be treated, the size of the tumor, and whether the implant is to be temporary or permanent (Groenwald et al., 1990).

The positions of the implants vary. Intracavitary im-plants are commonly used to treat gynecologic cancers. Cesium implants are placed in the vagina by using a gynecologic applicator. The applicator provides a cham-ber for two vaginal ovoids separated by a spacer. A cen-tral uterine tandem can be added if both the corpus and cervix are treated (Groenwald et al., 1990). Many of these applicators are designed so that the radioisotope can be loaded into the device later. The device may be positioned in the operating room and the capsules added in the patient's room (Groenwald et al., 1990). This method is most desirable, because health care personnel are not exposed to radiation during the time the device is positioned, the recovery period, and transport from the procedure area. Once the capsules are in place, they remain there for 1–3 days.

Interstitial wires or threads are implanted in the tissue to be treated. This method may be used to treat stage I and stage II breast cancer. Two layers of plastic tubes are in-serted into the breast tissue through the affected area and held in place with buttons. After radiographs show the tubes are in the desired position, the tubes are threaded with ^{192}Ir seeds and left in place for several days (Figure 4-1).

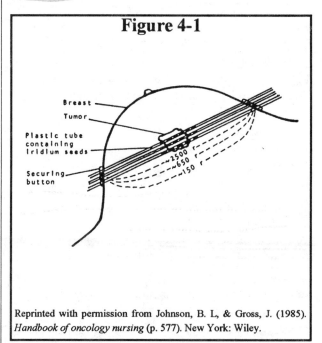

Figure 4-1

Reprinted with permission from Johnson, B. L, & Gross, J. (1985). *Handbook of oncology nursing* (p. 577). New York: Wiley.

In a third method, implants are placed on the surface of the body. An example of this is treatment of eye tumors with strontium (Clark & McGee, 1985).

Use of radiopharmaceuticals in brachytherapy is not as common as use of implants. In this form of internal ra-diation therapy, unsealed sources of radiation are given orally or intravenously or instilled into a body cavity, such as the abdomen or pleural cavity (Johnson & Gross, 1985). The radioactive substance is usually in liquid form. Radiopharmaceuticals are often referred to as metabolized or absorbed forms of radiation (Clark & McGee, 1992). Because the sources are unsealed, body fluids are contaminated with radiation while a source is active (Ashwanden et al., 1990). Sources with short half-lives are therefore used.

Radioisotopes may be selected that are easily absorbed by the organ involved. For example, iodine-131 (^{131}I) is used to treat thyroid cancer. Use of intraperitoneal phosphorus-32 (^{32}P) is being explored as a treatment for ovarian cancer (Ashwanden et al., 1990). Radiopharmaceuticals can also be used to treat bladder cancer, polycythemia, and abdominal ascites (Johnson & Gross, 1985).

Nursing Care

Nursing care of patients receiving brachytherapy differs slightly depending on the type of radioisotope used, whether the source is sealed or unsealed, and whether the implant is temporary or permanent. Knowledge of the specific properties of radioisotopes and the ways they are used helps nurses to provide safe care (Baird et al., 1991). Preparing patients for the experience is an essential part of brachytherapy.

Generally, an implant remains in place 48–72 hr (Ashwanden et al., 1990). The patient should be assigned to a private room. The implant will be inserted there, and the patient will remain in the room for the duration of the treatment. Education can greatly decrease the anxiety or confusion the patient may have about this therapy. Education should include a complete description of the procedure, from the insertion of the implants to their removal. Discussion should also address the plan of care for the treatment period. Nursing care may be slightly different from care the patient may have received before. Special radiation precautions should be discussed with the patient and the patient's family. Areas to include in patients' education before brachytherapy include the following (Groenwald et al., 1990):

- Describe the procedure (from insertion of the implants to their removal).

- Discuss any changes that might occur in the patient's appearance.

- Discuss possible pain or discomfort related to treatment and measures available for relief.

- Review possible side effects.

- Explain restrictions on activities while the radioactive source is in place. For example, patients with cesium implants for gynecologic cancer may be confined to bed for the duration of the treatment.

- Review visiting restrictions.

- Describe the radiation precautions that will be used by health care personnel during the treatment phase.

Many creative approaches have been used to help patients plan suitable activities for the treatment period. Boredom and isolation are sometimes the most difficult part of brachytherapy (Groenwald et al., 1990). Patients can read, do handwork, watch television, talk on the telephone, watch videos, or play video games. Many of these activities can be set up before treatment begins. Preparation for visitors is also important. Because most facilities that offer brachytherapy suggest that patients have no visitors or have minimal visitation in the patients' rooms, activities such as making telephone calls or writing letters should be encouraged as a means of support to the patient. With proper application of the principles of radiation safety and careful attention to the patient's psychosocial needs, the challenges of safe, effective nursing care can be met (Groenwald et al., 1990).

Safety Considerations

Nursing care for patients receiving brachytherapy is a challenge that goes beyond basic medical-surgical theory. It requires an understanding of radiation safety, radiobiology, and the physiologic manifestations of radiation treatment. Rather than fear radiation, health care providers should develop a healthy respect for working with radioisotopes.

Three primary factors should be foremost in the minds of all personnel involved in the care of patients receiving brachytherapy: time, distance, and shielding (ACS, 1988; Baird et al, 1991; Groenwald et al, 1990; Hassey, 1988).

1. Time: The longer a person is exposed to radiation, the greater the dose absorbed. Nursing care must be planned and organized so that as little time as possible is spent in close contact with the patient being treated.

2. Distance: The intensity of radiation decreases by the inverse square of the distance from the source (Figure 4-2). Caregivers should stay as far away from the radiation source as possible. When not providing direct care, they should stop frequently at the doorway to talk with the patient and check on his or her status.

3. Shielding: Placing lead barriers between health care personnel and the source of radiation can greatly decrease the personnel's exposure to radiation. The selection of shielding depends on the type of radiation emitted and the range of penetration.

In addition to applying the principles of time, distance, and shielding, personnel caring for brachytherapy patients should wear some type of monitoring device. Although these devices do not provide protection from radiation, they do provide a record of personal exposure to radiation (ACS, 1988).

Because the total amount of exposure to radiation depends on the duration of exposure and the proximity to the source, personnel should perform their duties expeditiously. Visitors can stay near the door of the patient's room or visit for limited periods only. Once the implant is removed, no residual radioactivity remains. Frequently, patients and their families need to be reassured of this fact (Wittes, 1990).

SIDE EFFECTS OF RADIATION THERAPY

Just as with many other treatments, the response to radiation therapy varies from patient to patient. The onset and severity of radiation side effects are affected by several factors (ACS, 1988).

Radiation factors include the total dose of radiation received and the amount of radiation received each day. Patients who receive higher total doses of radiation have more side effects than patients who receive lower total doses. For example, a patient receiving a total dose of 5,000 cGy will probably have more side effects than a patient receiving a total dose of 3,000 cGy.

The amount of daily radiation also plays a role in the onset and severity of side effects. Patients who receive radiation treatments more often may experience side effects earlier than patients who are treated less often. For example, a patient who is receiving 180 cGy twice a day, five times a week, will probably have an earlier onset of side effects than a patient receiving 180 cGy once a day, five times a week.

Factors related to the patient also affect the onset and severity of side effects. These can include the area of the body treated by radiation, the patient's age, and the patient's health status.

As mentioned before, radiation is a localized treatment, so its effects depend on the area of the body included in treatment. A patient whose abdomen is irradiated may have nausea and vomiting, a decrease in appetite, or diarrhea. This patient, however, will not have loss of hair (alopecia) on the head related to the radiation treatment because the radiation will affect only those cells in the abdominal area. Even more specifically, a patient receiving radiation to the upper part of the abdomen may experience nausea and vomiting, whereas a patient receiving radiation to the lower part of the abdomen may have more problems with diarrhea.

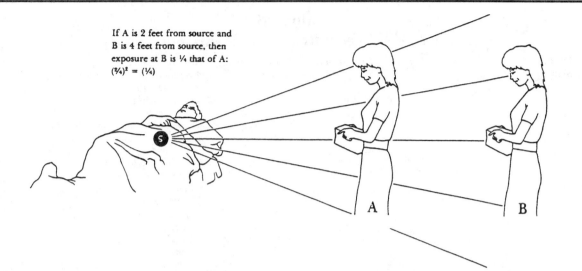

If A is 2 feet from source and B is 4 feet from source, then exposure at B is ¼ that of A:

$$(\tfrac{3}{4})^2 = (\tfrac{1}{4})$$

Figure 4-2. The inverse square law. As distance from a source of radiation increases, exposure decreases by the square of that distance. Reprinted with permission from Groenwald, S. L., Frogge, M. H., Goodman, M., & Yarbro, C. H. (Eds.). (1990). *Cancer nursing: Principles and practice* (2nd ed., p. 225). Boston: Jones and Bartlett.

The patient's age and health status also contribute to the severity of side effects experienced. Generally, patients who are in better overall health, are ambulatory, and are able to participate in their care tolerate radiation therapy better than patients whose health status is diminished.

Other factors related to treatment include combining radiation therapy with other cancer treatments, such as surgery, chemotherapy, biotherapy, and bone marrow transplantation. With a combination of treatments comes a combination of side effects. For example, a patient who receives abdominal radiation may experience nausea, vomiting, and diarrhea. If radiation and chemotherapy are used together, the patient may have other side effects not localized to the radiation site, for instance, loss of hair. The other side effects occur because chemotherapy is systemic and thus affects all areas of the body to some degree.

Certain treatment-related side effects can be expected to develop during radiation therapy (Table 4-1). Most of the effects are site specific and depend on the amount of radiation, dose fractionation, total dose, and individual health factors (Groenwald et al., 1990). Side effects may first occur 10–14 days into treatment and can continue for 6 months after treatment is complete.

NURSING CARE OF PATIENTS WITH SIDE EFFECTS RELATED TO RADIATION THERAPY

Management of radiation-induced side effects is a primary focus of nursing care. Understanding the side effects is essential in planning nursing care and patients' education. Most side effects can be predicted, and patients can therefore be prepared with appropriate self-care behaviors (Baird et al., 1991). Through education, patients will know what to expect and when to expect it. This can reduce their anxiety and help them get through the treatment experience.

Skin Reactions

Regardless of the body site treated, radiation must penetrate the skin to reach its target (Baird et al., 1991). Skin reactions may vary from mild to severe, depending on the radiation treatment and the patient's skin condition. Possible reactions include itching, dryness, erythema,

Table 4-1
Common Side Effects Related to Radiation Therapy

Organ	Response	Dose (rads)	Time to Onset	Nursing Considerations
Skin	Erythema	3000-4000	2-3 wk	Assess skin at regular intervals during treatment.
	Moist desquamation	4500-6000	5-6 wk or within 6 wk from end of therapy	Instruct client to wash skin with only water. Decrease exposure to irritating substances—fabrics, sun, soap, and trauma.
	Telangiectasis	4500-6000	Months to years	
Hair	Loss within treatment area	300-400	Few weeks	Instruct client to avoid excessive shampooing, hair dryers, hot rollers, or curling irons. Encourage planning for hair loss by purchasing wig, scarf, turban, or hat before loss.
Teeth	Caries	4000	Months to years	Encourage pretreatment dental evaluation. Instruct on prophylactic oral care measures.
Mouth/tongue	Mucositis	3000	2-3 wk	Encourage to avoid alcohol, tobacco, and other irritating agents.
	Xerostomia	3000-4000	2-3 wk	
	Taste changes	3000-4000	2-3 wk	
Larynx	Edema	5000-6000	Late in treatment	Monitor for changes in quality of voice.
	Necrosis of cartilage	6500 +	Months or years	Assess difficulty in breathing or talking.
Thyroid	Hypothyroidism	3500-4000	Years	Monitor for signs and symptoms of hypothyroidism.
Lung	Pneumonitis	2500-3000	6-8 wk after	Evaluate pulmonary function before treatment. Monitor respiratory rate, rhythm, and effort.
	Fibrosis	4000	Months to years	Monitor for signs and symptoms of infection.
Gastrointestinal (GI) tract	Nausea Vomiting	125 +	1-2 hr after treatment	Instruct in use of antiemetic agents during treatment.
Small intestines	Cramping	2000-3000	2-3 wk	Begin client on low-residue diet.
	Diarrhea	2000-3000	2-3 wk	Avoid ingestion of food or beverages that increase GI motility.
	Malabsorption	3000-4000	Months to years	Maintain adequate fluid intake.
	Necrosis	6000-7000	Months to years	Monitor stool for signs and symptoms of bleeding.
	Ulceration	6000-7000	Months to years	Evaluate changes in bowel patterns.
	Strictures	6000-7000	Months to years	
Urinary bladder	Cystitis	3000	Few weeks	Monitor for signs and symptoms of bladder irritation or bleeding.
	Fibrosis	6500-7000	Months to years	Evaluate changes in bladder patterns. Assess character of urine.
Ovary	Sterility	500-1000	Days to weeks	Assess ovarian function before initiation of therapy. Evaluate impact of sterility on client/partner.
Uterus	Necrosis	20000 +	Months to years	Monitor for signs of infection or necrosis—discharge, odor, bleeding, or pain.
Brain/spinal cord	Neurological deficits	5000, whole brain	Months to 1 yr	Assess neurological and sensory function.
	Necrosis	6500-7000, smaller areas		Evaluate changes over time.
Bone (child)	Arrested growth	2000-3000	Depends on area	Evaluate growth pattern before initiation of therapy. Instruct parents about potential risks of arrested growth. Monitor growth and development patterns after therapy.

Reprinted with permission from Clark, J. C., & McGee, R. F. (1992). *Oncology Nursing Society core curriculum for oncology nursing* (2nd ed., pp. 324–325). Philadelphia: Saunders.

hair loss, rash, flaking skin, and even wet desquamation (which resembles a second-degree burn) (McGowan, 1989). Patients who are more sensitive to sunburn often have more severe reactions to radiation than other patients do.

Whenever a patient receives radiation therapy, a plan for skin care should be communicated to the patient and the patient's family and to other health care providers. Some general guidelines for patients for skin care include the following (Baird et al., 1991; Groenwald et al., 1990; McGowan, 1989):

- Keep the skin dry.

- Avoid using powders, lotions, creams, or deodorants on the affected area, especially ones that contain alcohol or perfumes.

- Wear loose-fitting garments. Avoid clothing that will bind or rub.

- Do not apply tape to the area when dressings are needed.

- Protect the skin from exposure to sunlight, chlorinated water (e.g., in swimming pools), and extreme temperatures (e.g., extreme temperatures outside, hot water bottles, heating pads).

- Use a mild soap and warm or cool water (not hot water) for washing the affected area. Rinse well and pat dry.

- Shave with an electric razor. Do not use shaving creams or lotions or aftershave.

- To soothe dry skin, use a nonirritating water-soluble moisturizer. Do not apply moisturizer on the treatment day until after treatment is over.

- Do not use cornstarch, which can help prevent itching, to control perspiration or moisture.

Moisture and cornstarch generate glucose, which is an ideal medium for fungal growth.

Alopecia

Alopecia, or loss of hair, is traumatic for most patients. The needless fear of this loss is equally as traumatic. Patients who are receiving radiation therapy that does not include the scalp should be assured that hair loss will not occur as a result of treatment (Groenwald et al., 1990). If radiation does include the scalp, care of the hair and scalp is essential.

Radiation-induced alopecia is not preventable. However, care of the hair and scalp is important to minimize skin reactions (Baird et al., 1991). Guidelines for patients for care include the following (Baird et al., 1991; Groenwald et al., 1990):

- Use a very gentle brush or comb.

- Shampoo as infrequently as possible.

- When shampooing, use a mild shampoo followed by thorough rinsing and gentle towel drying.

- Avoid using hair dryers, curling devices, and any hair chemicals (e.g, hair coloring, styling gels).

- Wear a hat or cap to protect the scalp from sunlight. (The forehead, neck, and ears are also more sensitive to sunlight after radiation treatment.)

Mucositis

Mucous membranes are found in the respiratory, digestive, and genitourinary tracts, and they are highly sensitive to radiation. Mucous membranes undergo continuous proliferation. When cell renewal cannot keep up with cell loss, mucositis occurs (Baird et al, 1990).

Mucositis is characterized by a patchy, white membrane that becomes confluent and may bleed if disturbed. This reaction is easily visible if radiation includes the mouth and oropharynx (Groenwald et al., 1990). Mucositis can be very painful. Soreness in the oral cavity can lead to decreases in nutritional intake and oral hygiene, which will only enhance the severity of the problem.

Patients can use a number of measures to manage mucositis in the oral cavity (Groenwald et al., 1990):

- Avoid alcohol, tobacco, and spicy or acidic foods.

- Avoid very hot or very cold foods and beverages.

- Avoid commercial mouthwashes (even diluted, they are too astringent).

- For mouth rinses, use normal saline or 1 oz (30 ml) of diphenhydramine hydrochloride (Benadryl) elixir diluted in 1 qt (1 L) of water. (Lidocaine and Maalox mixtures are also commonly used.) Dilutions of hydrogen peroxide have been used for years, but they are damaging to tissue if not diluted correctly.

- Do the steps necessary for mouth care every 3–4 hr.

- Take steps to control pain before eating meals and cleaning the mouth.

Xerostomia

Radiation to the head and neck may injure the salivary glands. This can eventually lead to fibrosis and decreased salivary secretions. This condition is referred to as xerostomia (LeVeque, Montgomery, Potter, et al., 1993). Patients with radiation-induced xerostomia produce little or no saliva. The effects of this condition are dose related and permanent (Groenwald et al., 1990; LeVeque et al., 1993). Xerostomia is painful and can lead to oral disease, nutritional deficiencies, and an overall decline in the quality of life.

There is no clearly effective treatment for radiation-induced xerostomia. Saliva substitutes are generally ineffective and are not desired by patients for long-term use. Pilocarpine, a drug that increases salivation and pro-

vides symptomatic relief, has been used with some success (Johnson, Ferretti, Nethery, et al., 1993; LeVeque et al., 1993).

Nausea and Vomiting

Radiation treatment to the abdominal, pelvic, or spinal areas can lead to nausea and vomiting. Nausea and vomiting are more common when large areas are irradiated. However, nausea and vomiting are not inevitable side effects. Even when it is anticipated that radiation will produce them, they can be minimized or even prevented by using antiemetics (Baird et al., 1991).

When nausea or vomiting occurs, antiemetics should be given on a regular schedule. A dose before treatment should be incorporated into this plan. In addition to antiemetics, an eating pattern should be developed so that the radiation treatment is given when the patient's stomach is relatively empty. The patient should delay intake of a full meal until 3 or 4 hr after treatment. Most nausea related to radiation therapy occurs 1–3 hr after treatment (Groenwald et al., 1990).

Diarrhea

Diarrhea, like nausea and vomiting, is not an inevitable side effect of radiation therapy. Radiation-induced diarrhea is most common in patients who are receiving radiation to the abdomen or pelvis. Changes in the epithelial layer of the small bowel result in a flattening or loss of the villi. This in turn decreases the absorption ability of the intestinal surface and leads to diarrhea (Baird et al., 1990).

Diarrhea can usually be controlled with antidiarrheal medications and a low-residue diet. Recovery may take several weeks or even months. The intestinal lining takes some time to recover and return to normal functioning. It is important that the patient maintain a low-residue diet during this period. Foods not part of the low-residue diet should be added back gradually. For some patients, certain foods (e.g., corn, legumes, and milk products) may never be tolerated (Baird et al., 1991).

Fatigue

Fatigue is a common side effect of radiation therapy. Although many patients may be able to maintain their normal daily activities, they will probably require extra rest to do so. It is important to inform patients of the potential for fatigue related to treatment. Encourage them to arrange their daily activities to allow for naps, rest periods, or going to bed early. Patients who are hospitalized or bedridden should also have a time for quiet and rest built into the plan of care for radiation therapy.

Other Side Effects

Other side effects related to radiation therapy include anorexia, radiation-induced caries of the teeth, esophagitis, dysphagia, and bone marrow suppression. Patients should be informed about all side effects, and steps to deal with the effects should be incorporated in the plan of care.

Radiation Recall

Radiation recall is a phenomenon that can occur in a previously irradiated site. A radiation-induced side effect can reappear with the administration of certain chemotherapeutic agents. The side effects that resurface are usually skin reactions and mucositis. Radiation recall can occur in response to chemotherapy from several months to a year after radiation was received.

NURSING CARE ISSUES IN ALL RADIATION THERAPY

It is often the goal in any radiation treatment to maximize killing of cancerous cells and minimize damage to normal cells. To achieve this goal, high-tech equipment is used, and formulas are established to zero in on the cellular potentials of the radiation.This goal is part of the disease experience of a patient. A person's life is the driving force behind all these effects. Part of this process includes attempts by patients and their families to cope with all that is occurring. Nursing care helps patients and their families manage side effects, adjust to the changes in their daily routine, and maintain the quality of their life (ACS, 1988). The essential role of the nurse is to create a plan that focuses on the patient and the impact of radiation treatment on that patient.Figure 4-1. Cross-section of the breast shows placement of iridium-192 seeds and approximate dose of radiation.

BIBLIOGRAPHY

American Cancer Society. (1988). *Nursing management of the patient receiving radiation therapy*. New York: Author.

American Cancer Society, Massachusetts Division. (1990). *Cancer manual* (8th ed., pp. 85–98). Boston: Author.

Ashwanden, P., Belcher, A. E., Mattson, E. A., Moskowitz, R., & Riese, N. (1990). *Oncology nursing: Advances, treatments and trends into the 21st century*. Rockville, MD: Aspen.

Baird, S. B., McCorkle, R., & Grant, M. (1991). *Cancer nursing: A comprehensive textbook* (pp. 246–290). Philadelphia: Saunders.

Brandt, B. (1989). What you should know about radiation implant therapy to the head and neck. *Oncology Nursing Forum, 16*(4):579–582.

Clark, J. C., & McGee, R. F. (1992). *Oncology Nursing Society core curriculum for oncology nursing* (2nd ed., pp. 319–328). Philadelphia: Saunders.

Groenwald, S. L., Frogge, M. H., Goodman, M., & Yarbro, C. H. (Eds.). (1990). *Cancer nursing: Principles and practice* (2nd ed., pp. 200–283). Boston: Jones and Bartlett.

Hassey, K. (1988). *Care of the patient with radioactive implants*. New York: American Cancer Society.

Johnson, B. L., & Gross, J. (1985). *Handbook of oncology nursing* (pp. 567–585). New York: Wiley.

Johnson, J. T., Ferretti, G. A., Nethery, W. J., et al. (1993). Oral pilocarpine for postirradiation xerostomia in patients with head and neck cancer. *New England Journal of Medicine, 329*:390–395.

LeVeque, F. G., Montgomery, M., Potter, D., et al. (1993). A multicenter, randomized, double-blind, placebo-controlled, dose-titration study of oral pilocarpine for treatment of radiation-induced xerostomia in head and neck cancer. *Journal of Clinical Oncology, 11*(6):1124–1131.

McGowan, K. L. (1989). Radiation therapy: Saving your patients skin. *RN, 52*(6):24–27.

Wittes, R. E. (1990). *Manual of oncologic therapeutics* (pp. 60–65). Philadelphia: Lippincott

STUDY QUESTIONS

Chapter 4

Questions 23–32

23. What type of radiation therapy uses an external source of radiation?

    a. Teletherapy
    b. Brachytherapy
    c. Biotherapy
    d. Immunotherapy

24. What type of radiation therapy uses an internal source of radiation?

    a. Teletherapy
    b. Brachytherapy
    c. Biotherapy
    d. Immunotherapy

25. Side effects associated with radiation therapy affect only the tissues and organs in the radiation field because radiation is what kind of treatment?

    a. Localized
    b. Systemic
    c. Generalized
    d. Superficial

26. How long are patients radioactive after they have teletherapy for treatment of cancer?

    a. No time at all
    b. A few minutes
    c. A few days
    d. For the rest of their lives

27. Which form of brachytherapy involves the placement of seeds, wires, or ribbons into a body cavity or directly into the tumor itself?

    a. Radiation implants
    b. Radiopharmaceutical therapy
    c. Teletherapy
    d. Biotherapy

28. Which form of brachytherapy involves oral, intravenous, or intraperitoneal administration of a radioactive liquid?

    a. Radiation implants
    b. Radiopharmaceutical therapy
    c. Teletherapy
    d. Biotherapy

29. Where is loading of radiation implants into a patient done?

    a. In the operating room
    b. In the patient's private room in the hospital
    c. In the radiology department's examination room
    d. In the patient's home

30. Nursing care of a patient undergoing brachytherapy care should include which of the following?

    a. Keeping the door to the patient's room closed.
    b. Spending as much time at the patient's bedside as the schedule will allow.
    c. Completing bedside tasks as quickly as possible.
    d. Encouraging unlimited visits by members of the patient's family.

31. Which of the following side effects is unlikely in a patient who has radiation to the abdomen?

    a. Nausea and vomiting
    b. Diarrhea
    c. Skin reactions
    d. Alopecia (hair loss) of the head

32. Which of the following may be applied to the skin after radiation therapy?

    a. Deodorants
    b. Petroleum jelly
    c. Water-soluble lotions and cream
    d. Cornstarch to control perspiration

CHAPTER 5

CHEMOTHERAPY

CHAPTER OBJECTIVE

After completing this chapter, the reader will be able to recognize the rationale for cytotoxic chemotherapy and combination chemotherapy regimens in treatment of cancer, specify the major classifications of cancer chemotherapeutic drugs, recognize common side effects of chemotherapy, and indicate proper procedures for safe handling of chemotherapeutic drugs.

LEARNING OBJECTIVES

After studying this chapter, the reader will be able to

1. Specify factors that influence the effectiveness of chemotherapy.

2. Specify side effects associated with use of various chemotherapeutic drugs.

3. Indicate complications common to side effects of chemotherapy.

4. Select interventions commonly used to reduce side effects associated with chemotherapy.

5. Indicate routes of delivery of chemotherapy for various types of cancer.

6. Recognize factors important in the safe preparation and administration of chemotherapeutic drugs.

INTRODUCTION

Drugs and chemicals have been used to treat cancer for thousands of years. In ancient Egypt and Greece, a variety of herbs, natural products, and chemical derivatives were given to reestablish a balance between "humors" or to dissolve the tumor. The role of drugs as a potent weapon in the fight against cancer in modern medicine came about somewhat by accident. During World War I, health care workers noticed that mustard gas, an agent used in chemical warfare, had a deleterious effect on the bone marrow of the soldiers who were exposed to it. Investigators theorized that if uncontrolled exposure to mustard gas could deplete the bone marrow, controlled use of this substance might be useful in treating hematologic tumors, for which the underlying problem was a malfunctioning marrow. In the 1940s, nitrogen mustard became the first chemotherapeutic drug in modern times to be used successfully to treat cancer.

The term chemotherapy merely refers to drug therapy and could be applied to cardiology, endocrinology, or any other medical specialty. However, the connotation, and the understanding of the lay public, is that chemotherapy refers to drugs used to treat cancer, and the word automatically conjures up images of nausea, vomiting, and hair loss. Chemotherapy has become a cornerstone of cancer care. More and more drugs are being developed, and combination drug regimens are constantly being refined and improved. In addition, huge strides have been made in supportive care for control of the signs and symptoms of the toxic side effects associated with many of these drugs. Unlike either surgery or radiation therapy, chemotherapy is generally used as a systemic treatment. It is traditionally the first-line treatment for most hematologic tumors and for cancers that have spread beyond the point of local control. The progress made in chemotherapeutic research has resulted in legitimate cures for some hematologic tumors (e.g., childhood leukemia, Hodgkin's disease) and advanced-stage solid tumors (e.g., testicular cancer).

CELL-CYCLE THEORY

Although clinical practice focuses on the tumor as an entire entity, the rationale for use of cytotoxic, or cell-killing, drugs actually rests on the characteristics of individual tumor cells and cell-cycle kinetics. Both normal and malignant cells undergo a 5-step process of cell growth between mitoses. In Gap 0 (G_0) cells are resting and out of cycle. When activated, the cells enter the cycle at Gap 1 (G_1, or interphase), the period when cells prepare for DNA synthesis and also synthesize RNA and certain proteins. During S-phase (synthesis), DNA replication occurs. The gap between the end of S-phase and mitosis is termed Gap 2 (G_2, or premitotic phase) and is a brief pause in the cycle while the cell readies itself for division. During mitosis (M), the chromosomes and nucleus move through prophase, metaphase, and anaphase to telophase, when the cell actually divides to become two distinct daughter cells.

The length of time a specific cell stays in each phase of the cell cycle may be highly variable. Generally, cells in G_0 and G_1 are considered out of cycle, although many

activities take place during these phases. The average time between mitoses is 1–2 days for most normal cells and 2–3 days for malignant cells. Intermitotic time, however, does not describe the entire picture of tumor growth. For example, the length of the cell cycle of tumor cells in squamous cell carcinoma of the skin is somewhat shorter than that of the tumor cells in acute myelogenous leukemia. Although one might assume that if left untreated, squamous cell cancer would become lethal much more quickly than acute myelogenous leukemia, quite the opposite is true. Also, if cell growth depended only on individual cellular kinetics, a tumor might be expected to double in size every 2–3 days. This assumption is also untrue. The answer lies in cell-cycle kinetics in the context of the entire tissue.

TISSUE GROWTH KINETICS

When an entire tumor is examined, it becomes clear why the cell-cycle kinetics of individual cells cannot be used to predict tissue growth: Not every cell in the tissue is in cycle and poised to proliferate. In fact, most of the cells are not proliferating. These cells may be in Gap 0 or in Gap 1 and differentiated to the point at which they are no longer replicating, or they may be dead as a result of necrosis, lack of nutrients, the basic genetic instability of malignant cells, or other means. A basic property of malignant cells is the inability to check the balance between cell growth and cell loss. Ultimately, the rate of cellular proliferation exceeds the rate of cell death, resulting in tumor growth and progression.

The life cycle of a tumor differs somewhat from the life cycle of a single cell. At first, growth of a tumor is rapid, even exponential. However, as the tissue expands, the rate of growth slows. By the time the tumor has undergone approximately 30 cell divisions, or doublings, it is usually clinically detectable, with a mass of 1 g, or 10^9 cells. At this point, tumor growth has slowed, and the additional 10 doublings required to produce a lethal mass of tumor (approximately 1 kg, or 10^{12} cells) occur at a significantly slower rate than the initial growth did. As previously noted, in larger tumors, this slowing of growth may be due to hypoxia, necrosis, lack of nutrients and hormones necessary for growth, excess of toxic substances, and cell-to-cell inhibition. Calculations of tumor doubling times that do not take into account the slowing in growth that occurs as the tumor increases in size will be inaccurate. Consequently, estimates that indicate that a tumor began growing 10–20 years before it was detected clinically are generally incorrect.

Because of the tissue growth kinetics of tumor cells, chemotherapy given when tumors have already begun to slow their growth rate will most likely be ineffective. For these tumors, a better approach would be to debulk the tumor first by using surgery or radiation therapy, to minimize the mass of the tumor (lower tumor burden). Cells in the residual tumor that are in Gap 0 will be brought back to the cell cycle, and the growth rate of the tumor will increase. This may be the optimal time to administer chemotherapy. The rationale described is also the justification for adjuvant chemotherapy, giving chemotherapeutic drugs when no clinically detectable tumor is present but the risk of tumor recurrence is high. A shorter cell-cycle time, coupled with a higher percentage of tumor cells that are proliferating at one time (growth fraction), should lead to increases in the number of cells killed by chemotherapeutic agents.

Another factor that influences the number of tumor cells killed is the dose of chemotherapeutic drugs delivered. Generally, it is anticipated that a particular dose of a chemotherapeutic agent will destroy a certain proportion of tumor cells at risk for that drug. This means that each time the full dose of the drug is given, a certain proportion of tumor cells is killed. Between courses of chemotherapy, the tumor will grow (e.g., one log of cell growth). Thus, repeat cycles of treatment must be given to continue to decrease the number of cells that survive treatment. If the dose of the drug were decreased, a larger number of cancer cells would survive.

This description does not take into account the possibility that tumor cells might be resistant to the chemotherapeutic agents from the beginning or become resistant during the course of the treatment. Although no clinical evidence of disease is apparent once the tumor burden decreases to fewer than 10^9 cells, treatment cycles must persist beyond that point to continue the killing of surviving, but undetectable, malignant cells. Modifications of drug dose and schedule can be useful in manipulating the number of cells killed: Higher doses may be able to overcome plateaus in cell killing, and use of multiple agents can compensate for one drug whose major action is during a single phase (e.g., S-phase) of the cell cycle.

The final characteristic of tumor cells that affects their response to chemotherapeutic agents is the concept of drug resistance. Theoretically, according to cell-cycle kinetics, as tumor burden decreases and rate of proliferation increases, tumors in which cells were killed by a particular chemotherapeutic regimen would become even more sensitive to the same therapy over time. If this situation were true, then any drug intervention that initially leads to a response would automatically lead to a cure. Certainly, this is not the case most of the time. Many tumors respond at the beginning of chemotherapy and then recur and progress even though the same therapy is continued.

One possible explanation for tumor recurrence is that tumor cells can hide in the central nervous system and a few other sites where chemotherapeutic drugs cannot go; cancer chemotherapeutic agents usually cannot cross the blood-brain barrier in the central nervous system. A more common reason is the genetic, biochemical, and molecular composition of the tumor cells. As is the case with bacteria exposed to antibiotics, spontaneous mutations to drug-resistant cells readily occur in malignant tumors. The Goldie-Coldman model predicts that as tumor burden increases, the probability that significant numbers of resistant cancer cells will develop increases as well. Thus, the optimal time to treat cancers is as soon as possible after diagnosis and when the tumor burden is the lowest obtainable. Simultaneously, the model indicates that regimens that use multiple, non–cross-resistant drugs would be beneficial. If non–cross-resistant agents are used, they should be alternated rather than given sequentially, to reduce the possibility of multidrug resistance. Even when this approach is used, however, multidrug resistance may occur, and a gene for such resistance has been identified oin some tumor cells.

Last, because of the diversity and various degrees of differentiation present in tumor cells, chemotherapy may be ineffective. The genetic instability of tumor cells makes them prime subjects for further mutations caused by the chemotherapeutic agents themselves, which are known mutagens. Clearly, the relationships between malignant cells, tumor tissue, and chemotherapeutic drugs and the problem of drug resistance are complex issues. Resolution of these problems will increase the effectiveness of chemotherapeutic agents and eventually affect the mortality and morbidity associated with cancers that require systemic therapy.

COMMON CHEMOTHERAPEUTIC DRUGS

Many chemotherapeutic drugs are currently available and in use for many types of cancer (Table 5-1). Newer analogues of several drugs have been developed in an attempt to maintain or increase efficacy while decreasing associated toxic effects. Combinations of drugs are used for specific types of cancer.

Chemotherapeutic drugs are classified according to the mechanism of action or derivation of the drug group:

- **Alkylating agents:** Alkylating agents cause breakage of DNA and incorrect pairing of purine and pyrimidine bases. Because they can act at any time during the cell cycle, these agents are called cell cycle–nonspecific. Common side effects associated with their use are hematologic (bone marrow suppression) and gastrointestinal problems.

- **Nitrosoureas:** A subclassification of alkylating agents, nitrosoureas are also cell cycle–nonspecific. They disrupt DNA repair and duplication. Because they are non–cross-resis-

tant with each other, nitrosoureas and alkylating agents may be combined in multidrug regimens. Nitrosoureas are lipid soluble and so can cross the blood-brain barrier; they are used to treat tumors of the central nervous system. Major side effects include myelosuppression and gastrointestinal reactions.

- **Antimetabolites:** Antimetabolites inhibit both protein and DNA synthesis. Because they are most effective during the S-phase of the cell cycle, they are called cell cycle–specific. Their major toxic effects are hematologic and gastrointestinal side effects. A subclass of this group is the purine analogues, including analogues of guanine and adenosine. These analogues are similar in structure and activity, and resistance to one analogue may be predictive of resistance to another.

- **Antitumor antibiotics:** Antitumor antibiotics inhibit both RNA and DNA synthesis. They are cell cycle–nonspecific. The most common side effects are hematopoietic and gastrointestinal problems and cardiac changes after significant cumulative doses of certain of the agents.

- **Plant alkaloids:** Plant alkaloids include the established vinca alkaloids and the newer taxol. Vinca alkaloids bind with microtubule proteins to stop the cell in metaphase and thereby inhibit RNA and protein synthesis. Taxol, produced from the Western Yew tree, stabilizes the mitotic spindle, causing disruption of cell division. These chemotherapeutic drugs are known for neurotoxic effects, primarily peripheral, and effects on the hematopoietic, skin, and reproductive systems.

- **Hormones:** A variety of hormones, although not specifically classed as cytotoxic chemotherapeutic agents, are often used as single agents or in combination as cancer chemotherapy. The effect of each hormone is related

Table 5-1
Common Chemotherapeutic Agents

Classification	Drug Name	Common Name	Indication	Toxic Effects
Alkylating agent	Mechlorethamine	Nitrogen mustard	Hodgkin's disease	GI, BM
	Cyclophosphamide	Cytoxan, CTX	Breast, lung, leukemia	Hemorrhagic cystitis
	Thiotepa		Breast, Hodgkin's disease	BM, reproductive system
	Ifosfamide	IFEX	Testicular	BM, CNS
	Busulfan	Myleran	CML, bone marrow transplant	BM, GI
	Chlorambucil	Leukeran	CLL, NHL	BM, GI
	Melphalan	Alkeran	Multiple myeloma	BM, GI
	Dacarbazine	DTIC	Melanoma	GI, BM
Nitrosourea	Carmustine	BCNU	CNS	GI, BM
	Lomustine	CCNU	Hodgkin's disease	GI, BM
Antimetabolite	Methotrexate	MTX	Breast, GI	GI, BM
	5-Fluorouracil	5-FU	Breast, GI	Skin, GI
	Cytosine arabinoside	Ara-C, cytarabine	Leukemia	BM
Purine analogue	6-Thioguanine	6-TG	Leukemia	BM, GI
	6-Mercaptopurine	6-MP	Leukemia	BM, GI
	Pentostatin		Hairy cell leukemia	BM
	Fludarabine	Fludara	CLL	BM, CNS
Antitumor antibiotic	Doxorubicin	Adriamycin, Adria	Breast, GI, Hodgkin's disease	Cardiac, BM
	Daunorubicin	Cerubidine	Leukemia	BM, cardiac
	Mitoxantrone	Novantrone	Leukemia	Cardiac
	Bleomycin	Blenoxane, Bleo	Hodgkin's disease, testicular	Pulmonary fibrosis
	Mitomycin C	Mutamycin	Gastric, pancreatic	BM, GI
	Dactinomycin	Actinomycin D	Wilms' tumor, sarcoma	Skin, GI
Plant alkaloid	Vincristine	Oncovin	Hodgkin's disease, NHL	Neurologic
	Vinblastine	Velban	Breast, testicular	Neurologic, skin
	Etoposide	VP-16	Lung, testicular	Neurologic, cardiovascular
	Teniposide	VM-26	Leukemia	Neurologic
	Taxol	Paclitaxel	Ovarian, breast	BM, neurologic
Hormone	Antiestrogen	Tamoxifen, Nolvadex	Breast	Reproductive system
	Antiandrogen	Diethylstilbestrol, flutamide	Prostatic	Endocrine, impotency
	Steroids	Prednisone	NHL, leukemia	Endocrine
	Fluoxymesterone	Halotestin	Breast	Endocrine
	Medroxyprogesterone	Provera	Endometrial	Endocrine
	Megestrol acetate	Megace	Breast, endometrial, prostatic	cardiovascular

Table 5-1
Common Chemotherapeutic Agents (cont.)

Classification	Drug Name	Common Name	Indication	Toxic Effects
Miscellaneous	Cisplatin	Platinum, CDDP, Platinol	Ovarian, bladder, testicular	Renal
	Carboplatin	Carbo, CBDCA, Paraplatin	Lung, ovarian	BM, neurologic
	Hydroxyurea	Hydrea	CML, head and neck	BM, GI
	Procarbazine	Matulane	Hodgkin's disease	Skin, GI
	Bacille Calmette-Guérin	BCG	Bladder, melanoma	GU, GI
	Leucovorin	Leucovorin rescue after MTX, potentiator for 5-FU	GI, lung, with MTX	Allergy
	L-Asparaginase	Elspar	Leukemia	Cardiovascular, GI
	Levamisole	Ergamisol	Colon	GI

Note: GI = gastrointestinal, BM = bone marrow suppression, CNS = central nervous system, CML = chronic myelogenous leukemia, CLL = chronic lymphocytic leukemia, NHL = non-Hodgkin's lymphoma, GU = genitourinary.

to its particular mode of action. Treatment ranges from administration of antiestrogens and antiandrogens to exogenous addition of other hormones. Side effects depend on the type of agent used.

- **Miscellaneous agents:** Miscellaneous agents include drugs that are highly effective and widely used, but whose mechanism of action is not well understood.

COMMON SIDE EFFECTS OF CHEMOTHERAPY

Toxic side effects are common in patients receiving cytotoxic chemotherapy, and the types can be predicted on the basis of the drug or multidrug combination prescribed. In general, toxic effects occur because the chemotherapeutic agents used target rapidly proliferating cells. In addition to tumor cells, many normal cells are dividing at high rates and are also affected by chemotherapy.

Myelosuppression

The hematopoietic system is a prime target for the cytotoxic drugs used in chemotherapy because of the frequent generation of cells by the bone marrow. Myelosuppression can cause neutropenia, anemia, and thrombocytopenia. Neutropenia and granulocytopenia occur most often and lead to the most serious consequences of chemotherapy. Febrile neutropenia and infection in patients with neutropenia may necessitate hospitalization for intravenous administration of antibiotics and careful monitoring for possible sepsis. Although periods of neutropenia and bone marrow suppression are usually relatively brief, alkylating agents can produce prolonged myelosuppression or even failure of the bone marrow to recover. The widespread use of hematopoietic growth factors (e.g., granulocyte-macrophage colony-stimulating factor or granulocyte colony-stimulating factor) has helped address the problem of febrile neutropenia and acute infection in myelosuppressed patients. Patients should be cautioned to limit their exposure to known or suspected environmental sources of infection (e.g., crowded public settings, raw foods or foods high in bacteria, persons with infectious diseases). However, some patients can take this precaution to extreme limits. Therefore, health care providers should remind patients also that hospitals are sites of far greater exposure to infectious agents than most public settings. The best method to reduce exposure is strict handwashing for all visitors and health care workers.

Anemia associated with cancer therapy is not usually a severe problem, although for some patients and with certain regimens, the prevalence of anemia is increased. Transfusion of red cells or use of the growth factor erythropoietin can diminish the anemia. The fatigue reported by many patients undergoing chemotherapy may be correlated with the degree of anemia as well as with other factors. Patients at risk for or experiencing anemia should be instructed in ways to decrease fatigue, including exercise, diet, and nutritional supplements.

Thrombocytopenia continues to be a complication both of underlying cancerous conditions and of the chemotherapy used to treat them. Currently, investigational growth factors reported to stimulate the manufacture of platelets are undergoing clinical trials. Transfusions of platelets may be used in cases in which thrombocytopenia or the associated signs and symptoms are severe. Indications of thrombocytopenia include petechiae, easy bruising, oozing from gums or other tissues, and frank bleeding (e.g., gastrointestinal or rectal bleeding). Patients should be advised to avoid activities in which trauma could occur, including falling out of bed or in their room. Trauma to the head, particularly when the number of platelets is low, can be serious and lead to intracranial bleeding or subdural hematoma. Patients also should avoid activities in which cuts or bruises can occur (e.g., using a straight razor or a hard toothbrush or even filing fingernails or toenails).

Gastrointestinal Effects

Gastrointestinal side effects are common with many types of cancer chemotherapy and are well known to the public, who automatically associate all chemotherapy with nausea and vomiting and consequently fear it. The fear of these side effects can be so pronounced that a patient may have them even in the absence of the chemotherapeutic drug. Sights, sounds, smells, or sim-

ply the thought of chemotherapy can be enough to stimulate the effects. This anticipatory nausea, vomiting, or both can be activated by the trip to the outpatient clinic; the paging system in the hospital; or the sight of the chemotherapy nurse, even in a different context (e.g., at the grocery store). Considerable progress has been made in the prevention and control of chemotherapy-induced nausea and vomiting, even with chemotherapeutic drugs that have high emetic potential. Control can be achieved by giving antiemetics intravenously or orally and by judicious use of amnesics, tranquilizers, and psychotropic medications.

Another common gastrointestinal side effect is mucositis. This toxic effect may be manifested as reddened, irritated areas in the oral mucosa (stomatitis), particularly in the mouth and throat. Mucositis may also progress to severe ulceration, inability to swallow, and constant pain. Topical therapy ("magic mouthwash"), pain control, and avoidance of food that is difficult to eat or irritating to the mucosa may help relieve signs and symptoms. This complication often leads to impaired nutrition, which can be a serious problem in patients who may already be experiencing anorexia or altered sense of taste. Like myelosuppression, mucositis is due to the effect of chemotherapeutic drugs on rapidly proliferating cells, in this case, the gastrointestinal mucosa. Mucositis and stomatitis, although uncomfortable, are usually self-limiting, and the mucosa will heal between cycles of chemotherapy or when use of the drug causing the condition is stopped.

Although diarrhea and constipation can occur with cytotoxic chemotherapy, they can also be caused by drugs (e.g., narcotics) given for control of signs and symptoms. If severe, these conditions can be quite debilitating, further compromising patients' nutritional status and quality of life. Loss of electrolytes through severe and chronic diarrhea should be carefully monitored in order to assess for other metabolic or functional changes, such as alteration in heart rhythms. Constipation may be due to chemotherapy, lack of exercise, or insufficient nutrition. However, it can also herald an intestinal obstruction or ileus. In patients treated with chemotherapeutic drugs with potential neurotoxic effects, constipation may be a sign of ileus due to severe *ototoxic ?*

neurotoxic effects. In these cases, intervention and discontinuation of the drug are necessary.

Toxic hepatic reactions and jaundice can be due to direct effects of chemotherapy, metabolism of the chemotherapeutic drug, the cancer itself or hepatic metastases, or use of concomitant medications. Attention should be paid to clinical manifestations of hepatic changes as well as to laboratory values indicating liver dysfunction. Because the liver is frequently a major source of drug clearance, changes in its ability to function can have severe adverse effects.

Genitourinary Effects

Several cancer drugs with important therapeutic efficacy also have side effects associated with renal dysfunction or bladder complications. Because drug clearance is often mediated by the kidneys, changes in renal function can lead to drug retention and prolonged toxic effects. Cisplatin is well known for its potential for renal compromise, and determinations of serum levels of creatinine and of creatinine clearance can be useful if baseline values are obtained before treatment and compared with values obtained over the course of the chemotherapy. Adequate hydration and the use of other drugs that can enhance renal clearance are essential.

Cyclophosphamide and ifosfamide can affect the bladder, causing hemorrhagic cystitis, which can be severe. Hydration before, during, and after therapy to promote high urine output can help prevent this complication. In addition, the bladder should be irrigated continuously when cyclophosphamide is used at very high doses. The use of mesna as a uroprotector with ifosfamide has allowed administration of full or higher doses of ifosfamide.

Cardiac Effects

The two main cardiac side effects due to chemotherapy are arrhythmias and a decrease in left ventricular ejection fraction. Electrocardiograms obtained before and after therapy can be used to track any changes in heart rhythm. Similarly, echocardiograms or nuclear medicine scans of the myocardium obtained before and after therapy can be used to assess adequacy of ejection fraction. Anthracycline drugs (e.g., doxorubicin, idarubicin,

and mitoxantrone) affect heart function through a cumulative effect, and total doses given of these drugs must be accurately documented.

Neurologic Effects

Toxic neurologic effects related to chemotherapy can occur in both in the peripheral and the central nervous systems. Peripheral effects include numbness or tingling in the distal parts of the extremities, which can worsen over the course of treatment until a loss of function or mobility (e.g., footdrop) occurs. If innervation of the bowels becomes compromised, ileus can occur. If the central nervous system is affected, patients can experience changes in level of consciousness, mood changes, ototoxic effects, and alteration in smell and taste.

Neurologic complications can be more dangerous than some other changes associated with chemotherapy because interventions depend on accurate, regular, and thorough assessment of a patient's neurologic status rather than review of a laboratory test. Neurologic changes can be subtle and slow or dramatic and rapid, and both patients and their families and the health care team should be aware of what changes are possible. For some drugs, neurologic side effects are the dose-limiting toxic effects. Neurotoxic effects that progress while the drug continues to be given may be irreversible. Signs and symptoms of neurologic side effects often cannot be relieved by routine pharmaceutical interventions, so usually the chemotherapeutic drug must be stopped or the dose reduced to accommodate these changes.

Skin Effects

Chemotherapy-induced side effects involving the skin can range from redness, irritation, and mild rash to severe sloughing and scaling of the skin. Pruritus, ophthalmic irritation, and dermatitis can occur. One of the least dangerous but most feared side effects of chemotherapy is hair loss (alopecia), which is possible with many drugs and treatment regimens. Often, the scalp is the only area affected; thinning, falling off in patches, or loss of all scalp hair may occur. Depending on the type of chemotherapeutic drug given, and the doses, total loss of all body hair can also occur; the hair of the eyebrows, lashes, extremities, genitals, and scalp are lost.

Alopecia in nearly every form can be devastating to patients, both male and female. Hair generally grows back after use of the offending drug or drugs is stopped, but it may be a different shade, curly rather than straight, or a different texture than before. In the interim, use of wigs, hairpieces, scarfs, hats, and makeup may be critical to helping a patient deal with hair loss.

Pulmonary Effects

A few chemotherapeutic drugs can affect the pulmonary system, causing dyspnea and, especially, pulmonary fibrosis, which can affect overall pulmonary function. Patients considered at risk who will be receiving these drugs should have pulmonary function measured before and after chemotherapy to assess any changes in status over time. Often changes in pulmonary function are cumulative and may be irreversible.

Effects on the Reproductive System

Like the cells of the hematopoietic, gastrointestinal, and integumentary systems, some cells of the reproductive system are rapidly proliferating and therefore are prime targets of cytotoxic chemotherapeutic drugs. Temporary or permanent amenorrhea in women and oligospermia and azoospermia in men can lead to sterility. Patients who will be receiving drugs with known permanent effects on ferility, such as standard therapy for Hodgkin's disease, should be carefully counseled in this regard. Sperm banking before chemotherapy starts may be an option for male patients. Various hormones as well as cytotoxic chemotherapeutic drugs can affect sexual functioning, causing premature menopause or menopauselike signs and symptoms, loss of lubrication, impotence or inability to sustain an erection, or loss of libido.

METHODS OF DRUG DELIVERY

Chemotherapeutic agents can be administered by a wide variety of routes and schedules. Some drugs are given orally only, which, although convenient, can be a problem if a patient is experiencing nausea or difficulty swallowing because of mucositis. If some of the drugs used in a regimen are given at home, the patient's compliance with oral medication must be carefully assessed and documented. Examples of drugs given by mouth are tamoxifen and leucovorin.

Self-injection and injection by health care personnel are options for some drugs given subcutaneously or intramuscularly. Care must be taken in immunocompromised or thrombocytopenic patients that injections do not increase risk of infection and bleeding. Examples of drugs given by injection are various growth factors and L-asparaginase.

Most chemotherapeutic drugs are given as intravenous infusions, ranging from brief bolus injections to slower, limited delivery to long-term continuous infusions. Long-term intravenous delivery of chemotherapeutic drugs can result in sclerosing of veins and loss of peripheral venous access, often necessitating insertion of a central venous access device. For drugs that are considered vesicants (i.e., those that cause necrosis and tissue damage if they leak out of the vein into the adjacent tissue), perfect patency of the vein is essential. For this reason, a central venous access device may be warranted if a patient is receiving vesicants and there is any question about the adequacy of peripheral access. Examples of vesicants are doxorubicin and vincristine.

Intrathecal administration of chemotherapeutic drugs may be used prophylactically or therapeutically for tumors (e.g., acute leukemia) that tend to spread to the central nervous system. An example of a drug given intrathecally is methotrexate. Intrathecal administration requires a lumbar puncture or surgical implantation of a device such as an Omaya reservoir to distribute the drug directly to the central nervous system.

Tumors that occur in body cavities, such as the peritoneal cavity, may be amenable to a "body bath" approach, with drugs given intraperitoneally. Cisplatin has been given in this way for ovarian cancer. This type of delivery requires frequent change in the patient's position, both to allow adequate coverage of all organs and tissue sites in the peritoneal cavity while the drug is instilled, and to facilitate drainage of the drug after the treatment is complete. Sometimes intraperitoneal drugs are left in the cavity to be reabsorbed over time. Theoretically, the localized focus of intraperitoneal chemotherapy, compared with drugs given intravenously, should enhance the efficacy of a drug on residual tumors left in the cavity after debulking.

Occasionally, intraarterial infusion may be used to perfuse limbs or concentrate chemotherapeutic drugs in local or regional areas. Catheters for administration of the drug must be surgically placed, and placement of the catheters must be confirmed radiographically. An example of this method of delivery is administration of 5-fluorouracil via a pump inserted in the hepatic artery. Bleeding and embolism are possible complications of intraarterial infusion.

Bladder cancer may be treated by intravesicular instillation of a chemotherapeutic agent directly into the bladder. Bacille Calmette-Guérin is an example of a drug that may be given this way. A Foley catheter is used, and cystitis and infection are possible complications.

Intrapleural administration of cytotoxic or other types of chemotherapeutic agents may be used in attempts to prevent recurrence of malignant pleural effusions. Bleomycin and some antibiotics may be delivered by this route by using a thoracotomy tube and thoracentesis.

Regardless of the route of delivery used, nurses who administer chemotherapeutic agents must be thoroughly familiar with the anticipated side effects, potential problems associated with administration (e.g., if the drug is a vesicant), and institutional policies that address these problems if they should occur. Technical skills in venous access or familiarity with venous access devices is also essential. Proper precautions must be taken to protect the person who prepares the chemotherapeutic agent for administration as well as the person who administers it.

VENOUS ACCESS DEVICES

A variety of venous access devices are available, and the product line is constantly changing. Most require surgical implantation of a type of catheter that feeds into the superior vena cava or other large cardiac vein and has an exit port or a line for access from the chest. Both external-access and totally implanted ports are used for central venous access. Peripherally inserted catheters provide another approach to venous access. Central-access devices often have more than one port or line available to allow concomitant administration of noncompatible intravenous solutions and provide access to obtain blood samples. For venous access devices with external access (e.g., Hickman catheter), the exit site on the chest is dressed, the entry ports are easily visualized, and access is simple. For devices with totally implanted ports (e.g., Portacath), the port must be palpated under the skin and a specialized needle used for access.

Institutional policies determine how venous access devices are dressed; how often the dressing is changed; whether or how often ports are flushed; and if flushed, whether heparin or saline is used. If heparin is used, care must taken to discard heparin-containing specimens in order to avoid inaccurate laboratory results, especially for coagulation studies. Before patients are discharged from the hospital, they or their caregivers should be given instructions on how to care for the venous access device at home.

BASIC CONCEPTS IN ADMINISTRATION OF CHEMOTHERAPY

Administration of cancer chemotherapy is a specialized nursing function and generally should be done only by nurses with training in this function. Chemotherapy nurses should be familiar with the specific drugs and combination regimens, anticipated immediate and short- and long-term side effects so they can teach patients and patients' families about the effects, technical aspects of venous access and drug-delivery systems, characteristics unique to the drugs being administered, safe handling and disposal of chemotherapeutic drugs, and medication regimens used before and after chemotherapy to prevent or reduce anticipated side effects. All this information must be applied throughout the course of chemotherapy administration.

Nurses who administer chemotherapeutic agents must know the properties of the drugs to be given in order to prepare for possible extravasation and choose appropriate sites for administration. If the chance of anaphylaxis is high, emergency equipment, including a crash cart if necessary, should be available. Before chemotherapy, patients may need medications as prophylaxis for allergic reaction, as antiemetics, as amnesics, or for other reasons. Appropriate supplies and equipment, including saline boluses, heparin flushes, infusion pumps, and so forth should be available before treatment begins. Patients should be adequately informed about potential side effects and the rationale for the administration of each drug, the dose, the route, and the schedule for the specific type and stage of cancer. Often, informed consent for administration of chemotherapy will be required to ensure that patients receive the needed education and information.

If a venous access device is used, the nurse giving the chemotherapy prepares the device for access, secures access to the device appropriately, and obtains any required specimens for laboratory tests. If peripheral veins are to be used, the nurse carefully assesses the location and patency of veins and chooses the site of access according to what drugs are to be given. Usually, more distal sites are selected first, and care is taken not to interfere with venous access for obtaining blood samples and to avoid extremities on the side of a previous mastectomy or sites of recent venipuncture or other invasive procedures. The order of drug delivery is usually established. Usually, vesicants are given first, when the vein is considered optimally patent, although this approach may vary from institution to institution and according to the nurse's preference. Regardless of the order, regular and frequent assessment of the intravenous site for patency, flow, signs of infiltration or irritation, and blood return is essential. About 5–10 ml of saline should be instilled before chemotherapy begins to test for patency and after the drug is given to flush all residual chemotherapeutic agent into the system and out of the vein.

Nurses who administer chemotherapeutic agents must be familiar with which drugs require monitoring of vital signs throughout infusion (e.g., etoposide, which can cause hypotension if administered too quickly, and taxol, which has been associated with allergic reactions manifested by shortness of breath, hypotension, tightness in the chest, and frank anaphylaxis). Patients can assist in drug delivery by advising the nurse when or if the vein feels irritated or painful or if they are experiencing other adverse reactions. As is the case with any other medication, the nurse must validate that the correct drug and schedule are being used. Because many doses of chemotherapeutic drugs are calculated on the basis of body surface area (measured in square meters, m^2), the patient's weight should be measured before the dose of drug is prepared. If the patient has had previous cycles of treatment, the nurse should also assess the patient for evidence of toxic effects that might necessitate modifying the dose for the current cycle.

SAFE HANDLING OF CHEMOTHERAPEUTIC DRUGS AND EQUIPMENT

Depending on the work setting, nurses may be responsible for both preparing and administering chemotherapeutic drugs. They must be familiar with both institutional and federal (Occupational Safety and Health Administration [OSHA]) guidelines for the safe handling and disposal of antineoplastic drugs and the equipment used with these drugs. When medical oncology was still a developing specialty, many nurses and other health care personnel handled cytotoxic chemotherapeutic agents without any recognition of the health risks associated with occupational contact with these agents. These workers included nurses; pharmacists; and housekeeping, laundry, and other employees. Over the past two decades, more attention has been paid to short- and long-term effects attributed to exposure to antineoplastic drugs, including possible mutagenic changes and an increased risk for cancer.

Regardless of the work site, nurses must have a clear understanding of institutional policies for implementing OSHA guidelines for the safe handling and disposal of antineoplastic drugs. Home health care may necessitate use and transport of portable disposal systems and pre-mixing of chemotherapeutic products to accommodate a lack of protective environment in a patient's home. Nurses should also be aware of how compliance with standards is evaluated, to be sure that they are not unnecessarily exposed to chemotherapeutic drugs because of a lack of compliance on the part of other staff members.

Drug Preparation

An appropriate work environment is necessary for safe preparation of chemotherapeutic agents. Use of a class II, type B biosafety cabinet (drug-preparation hood) with adequate ventilation and space for the amount of drug preparation that will be performed is essential. The person who prepares the drugs should be knowledge-

able about operation of the hood and make sure that the hood is properly maintained, or its use will be ineffective. The work area in the hood should be protected with disposable, absorbent, waterproof pads, commercially available for use with antineoplastic drugs. The pads should be changed at regular intervals and whenever any contamination occurs.

The person preparing the drugs should be properly attired according to institutional standards. Generally, this involves wearing a closed-front, disposable gown; latex, nonpowdered gloves; and a mask or protective goggles. The goal of all protective garb, equipment, and procedures is to minimize or remove entirely exposure to antineoplastic agents by direct or indirect contact, inhalation, or any other means. Careful hand-washing and use and disposal of gloves are essential for both drug preparation and administration.

Drug Administration

Events during drug administration that may expose the nurse to hazardous material (i.e., chemotherapeutic agent) include the following:

- Priming of intravenous tubing.

- Spiking with intravenous set of the bag containing the chemotherapeutic drug.

- Injection of the antineoplastic agent into the side arm of a set-up in which an intravenous solution is flowing.

- Making connections between intravenous sets and the solution of chemotherapeutic agent.

- Contact with body fluids (e.g., emesis, urine) from the patient that may contain chemotherapeutic agents.

- Frank spills from defective or broken bags, bottles, or syringes containing chemotherapeutic drugs.

Exposures should be handled by following institutional guidelines. Minimum steps include washing exposed areas with large volumes of water and soap, or using an eyewash for eye involvement, and completing an accident report. Accidental spills, if large, should be cleaned up by using commercial "spill kits" for hazardous substances or specifically for chemotherapeutic drugs. Protection of nurses, patients, and other health care workers should be paramount during clean-up of a spill.

Disposal of Drugs and Equipment

Most outpatient and inpatient health care settings are equipped with commercially available waste containers for proper disposal of antineoplastic drugs and the equipment and tubing used to administer the drugs. Material to be disposed of may include vials with or without residual chemotherapeutic drug inside, used intravenous bags and tubing, spill pads, gowns, gloves, and so forth. In lieu of such containers, biohazard bags or boxes that are clearly labeled "Chemotherapy Waste" should be used. Sharp objects, such as needles or glass, should always be disposed of in a puncture-proof, leak-proof container that is plainly marked. Linen or hospital gowns that are definitely contaminated with body fluids from a patient receiving chemotherapy, or with antineoplastic drugs, should be sent to the laundry in special bags clearly labeled as "Cytotoxic Waste" or "Chemotherapy." If chemotherapy is given in a home care setting, a plan should be in place for proper collection and subsequent disposal of equipment used to administer the drug, contaminated materials, and sharp objects.

STUDY QUESTIONS

Chapter 5

Questions 33–43

33. One reason chemotherapeutic drugs are often ineffective in treating brain tumors is the:

    a. Resistance of brain tumor cells
    b. Blood-brain barrier
    c. Increased tumor burden in the brain
    d. Frequency of spontaneous mutations in brain tumors

34. Neurotoxic effects are commonly associated with what class of chemotherapeutic drugs?

    a. Alkylating agents
    b. Antimetabolites
    c. Antitumor antibiotics
    d. Plant alkaloids

35. A potential toxic side effect in a patient receiving bleomycin is:

    a. Cardiac arrhythmia
    b. Pulmonary fibrosis
    c. Rash
    d. Hemorrhagic cystitis

36. One sign of neurotoxic effects associated with chemotherapeutic drugs is:

    a. Constipation
    b. Anemia
    c. Cystitis
    d. Facial flushing

37. The most serious potential complication due to chemotherapy-related myelosuppression is:

    a. Vomiting and dehydration
    b. Severe mucositis
    c. Sepsis
    d. Flulike syndrome

38. Patients who fall when thrombocytopenic should be carefully assessed for what possible serious complication?

    a. Reduced cardiac output
    b. Bacteremia
    c. Febrile neutropenia
    d. Subdural hematoma

39. Which of the following is used to reduce the risk of hemorrhagic cystitis associated with chemotherapy?

    a. Hydration
    b. Blood transfusions
    c. Nutritional supplements
    d. Hematopoietic growth factors

40. What is/are the most serious toxic effect or effects associated with use of anthracycline chemotherapeutic drugs?

    a. Renal failure
    b. Ileus
    c. Cardiac effects
    d. Gastrointestinal effects

41. Which of the following routes is sometimes used for delivery of chemotherapeutic drugs for treatment of ovarian cancer?

    a. Intrathecal
    b. Intraperitoneal
    c. Intramuscular
    d. Intraarterial

42. Minimal protection for the preparation of chemotherapeutic drugs for administration should include:

    a. Drug preparation hood, gloves, protective eyewear
    b. Spill kit, labeled disposal containers, gloves
    c. Preprimed intravenous sets, gown, mask
    d. Absorbent pads, mask, spill kit

43. Items that may expose a nurse to chemotherapeutic drugs during administration of the drugs include:

    a. Laundry soiled with the patient's body fluids
    b. The patient's food trays
    c. Intravenous fluids for hydration
    d. The patient's sneezes

CHAPTER 6

INNOVATIVE METHODS OF CANCER THERAPY

CHAPTER OBJECTIVES

After completing this chapter, the reader will be able to discuss innovative cancer treatments such as biotherapy and bone marrow transplantation, list the techniques and approaches used in these treatments, and specify nursing care of patients who have these treatments.

LEARNING OBJECTIVES

After studying this chapter, the reader will be able to

1. Recognize the synonym for biotherapy.

2. List the various types of biological response modifiers used in cancer therapy.

3. Recognize side effects of biotherapy.

4. Specify the types of treatment for which bone marrow transplantation is used.

5. Specify the types of bone marrow transplantation.

6. Describe the process used for harvesting and administering bone marrow.

7. List complications associated with bone marrow transplantation.

BIOTHERAPY

For most of this century, surgery, radiation, and chemotherapy have been used to fight cancer. For the past three decades, scientists have explored immunologic approaches as a fourth method of cancer treatment (Groenwald, Frogge, Goodman, & Yarbro, 1990). These technologic advances, referred to as biotherapy, are becoming common in cancer therapy.

Biotherapy is defined as treatment with agents that are derived from biological sources or that can affect biological responses (Clark & McGee, 1992). The term *biological response modifiers* (BRMs) is often used as a synonym for biotherapy. Biological response modifiers refer to agents or methods that change the relationship between the tumor and the host by modifying the biological response of the host to tumor cells to produce a therapeutic effect (Baird, McCorkle, & Grant, 1991; Clark & McGee, 1992; Wittes, 1990). The term *immunotherapy* has often been considered synonymous with biotherapy and BRMs. However, biotherapy and BRMs can influence tumor growth by both immunologic and nonimmunologic mechanisms (Groenwald et al., 1990; Wittes, 1990).

Biotherapy combines knowledge from several disciplines, including biology, genetics, immunology, pharmacology, medicine, and nursing. It is used in two distinct areas of cancer care: diagnosis and treatment. New biotherapeutic techniques and approaches are being developed all the time. Because of the advances in recombinant DNA technology, BRMs can now be produced in large quantities (Dudjak & Fleck, 1991; Yasko & Dudjak, 1990).

Biological response modifiers are unique in their ability to regulate or enhance the bodys immune system. The cytotoxic effects of chemotherapy and radiation therapy are primarily a result of the direct effects these treatments have on cancer cells. In contrast, BRMs can activate the body's own natural defenses. Consequently, BRMs have potentially greater antineoplastic activity and fewer toxic side effects (Yasko & Dudjak, 1990).

Biotherapy or BRMs can be classified into three major categories (Clark & McGee, 1992; Groenwald et al., 1990; Rumsey & Rieger, 1992; Wittes, 1990):

1. Agents that augment, modify, or restore the host's immune response.

2. Agents that have direct antitumor activity.

3. Agents that have other biological effects, such as affecting the differentiation or maturation of cells or the ability of tumor cells to metastasize or survive.

The body's immune system recognizes cancer cells as material that should be eradicated. However, the body often does not have the ability to kill the cells. Biological response modifiers, which are natural body proteins, act as self-guided missiles targeted at the cancer cells. Attached to chemotherapeutic agents or radioisotopes, BRMS can give the body the weapons it needs to seek out and destroy a tumor.

The mechanism of action of BRMs is not entirely understood. In some cases, more than one mechanism is involved (Wittes, 1990). The following sections review BRMs currently used in cancer care. Some of these agents are investigational; others have been approved by the Food and Drug Administration (FDA) for use in cancer treatment.

Interferon

Interferon was identified in 1957 as a substance capable of protecting cells from attack by viruses. The biological properties of interferon are not entirely understood, but it is known to have antiviral, antiproliferative, and potent immunomodulatory effects. Each of these effects alone or in combination with others may be responsible for the anticancer actions of interferon (Rumsey & Rieger, 1992). Interferon is used alone or in combination with chemotherapy. Three types of interferon are used: α, β, and γ (Yasko & Dudjak, 1990). Each type originates from a different kind of cell and has distinct biological and chemical properties (Groenwald et al., 1990). α,-Interferon has been approved by the FDA for treatment of hairy cell leukemia, Kaposi's sarcoma in patients with acquired immune deficiency syndrome (AIDS), and condyloma acuminata. In clinical trials, the interferons have been effective in treatment of hematologic tumors, renal cell carcinoma, melanoma, and superficial bladder cancers (Clark & McGee, 1992).

Interleukins

Interleukins are among the most important regulatory substances produced by lymphocytes and monocytes. Seven types of interleukins have been isolated and identified. Currently, only interleukin-2 and interleukin-3 are being actively studied in clinical trials (Groenwald et al., 1990). Interleukin-2 supports growth and maturation of subpopulations of T cells (Clark & McGee, 1992) and was initially called *T-cell growth factor* (Rumsey & Rieger, 1992).

Tumor Necrosis Factor

Tumor necrosis factor is a nonspecific macrophage product that acts by infiltrating and causing hemorrhagic necrosis in the tumor itself (Ashwanden, Belcher, Mattson, Moskowitz, and Riese, 1990). This agent can destroy malignant cells without destroying normal cells

(Rumsey & Rieger, 1992). Tumor necrosis factor is a potent anticancer agent in animals. However, results of trials in patients have been disappointing. Current trials are focusing on combining tumor necrosis factor with other BRMs and chemotherapy (Rumsey & Rieger, 1992). The factor has not been approved by the FDA for use in humans (Clark & McGee, 1992).

Monoclonal Antibodies

Monoclonal antibodies have been described as biologic tracers because of their target-specific nature (Ashwanden et al., 1990). Monoclonal antibodies are proteins produced by B cells in response to nonself antigens (Yasko & Dudjak, 1990). Hybridoma technology has made it possible to mass-produce or clone specific monoclonal antibodies, which can be created to bind with almost any antigen (Ashwanden et al., 1990; Yasko & Dudjak, 1990). The antibodies can be used alone or bound to radioisotopes, toxins, chemotherapeutic agents, or other BRMs. Monoclonal antibodies appear to seek out and bind to tumor cells (Ashwanden et al., 1990; Yasko & Dudjak, 1990). For this reason, the antibodies have wide applications for both treatment and diagnosis (Rumsey & Rieger, 1992). In cancer treatment, monoclonal antibodies are targeted to the cancer, which they find and destroy. In diagnosis, monoclonal antibodies may be used to locate tumor cells (American Cancer Society [ACS], 1990; Ashwanden et al., 1990). For example, monoclonal antibodies may be attached to low-dose radioisotopes. This combination can seek out cancer cells and make the cells visible. Therapy can then be targeted to the specific areas visualized by using the antibodies. In clinical trials, monoclonal antibodies have shown activity against leukemia; lymphoma; metastatic breast cancer; metastatic

colorectal carcinoma; and ovarian, renal, bladder, and prostatic cancers (Yasko & Dudjak, 1990).

Colony-Stimulating Factors

A class of proteins known as colony-stimulating factors (CSFs) can stimulate and induce proliferation in specific hematologic cell lines (Baird et al., 1991; Rumsey & Rieger, 1992). Because these factors induce proliferation in hematopoietic cells, they can counteract the bone marrow suppression usually observed after cancer treatment (ACS, 1990). Each of the CSFs has been named for the major cell lineage it affects (see below) (Groenwald et al., 1990; Yasko & Dudjak, 1990):

Colony-stimulating factors are not directly tumoricidal. They are useful in cancer treatment because of their ability to decrease bone marrow suppression, neutropenia, and infection. Because of their ability to decrease myelosuppression, CSFs may make it possible to use higher doses of other cancer treatments (Yasko & Dudjak, 1990).

Erythropoietin

Erythropoietin, the first growth factor discovered (in 1906), is a hormone produced by the kidney. This factor regulates the production and maturation of red blood cells. Erythropoietin was approved by the FDA in 1986 for treatment of anemia in end-stage renal disease. Erythropoietin replacement provides a 35% increase in hematocrit levels without additional blood transfusions (Baird et al., 1991). The hormone is often given intravenously three times a week, and hematocrit levels become normal in almost all patients treated (Rumsey & Rieger, 1992). Erythropoietin is currently being investi-

Factor	Targets
Granulocyte-macrophage colony-stimulating factor (GM-CSF)	Granulocyte and macrophage lineage
Granulocyte colony-stimulating factor (G-CSF)	Granulocyte lineage only
Macrophage colony-stimulating factor (M-CSF)	Macrophage lineage only
Pleuripoietin interleukin-3 or multi-CSF	Early cell lineages
Erythropoietin	Erythrocyte lineage only

gated for clinical use in anemia related to chemotherapy of cancer.

Nursing Care of Patients Receiving Biotherapy

Because many of the biological agents used in cancer treatment are investigational or newly approved, nurses should be aware of the potential implications of biotherapy. The side effects of all the biological agents are similar. Flulike illness, with fever, chills, headache, and fatigue, is common. Cardiovascular, pulmonary, and neurologic side effects also occur (Baird et al., 1990; Rumsey & Rieger, 1992; Yasko & Dudjak, 1990).

Educating patients about side effects and how to manage the signs and symptoms is essential. Fever and headaches can be controlled by using acetaminophen or nonsteroidal antiinflammatory agents or both. Neurologic side effects can be the most alarming for patients and patients' families. Because they often play a key role in early detection of slight neurologic changes in a patient, family members or significant others should be included in discussions about these effects (Rumsey & Rieger, 1992).

Future Directions for Biotherapy

In a relatively brief period, the field of biotherapy has grown tremendously. Treatments that seemed beyond comprehension 15 years ago are now common practice (Ashwanden et al., 1990). Although much is left to discover about biotherapy in cancer treatment, successful use of this therapy promises to provide new information on how to battle this disease.

BONE MARROW TRANSPLANTATION

Bone marrow transplantation has been described as both intensive investigational therapy and standard curative treatment. Both descriptions are accurate (Whedon,

1991). Given the wide variety of malignant and nonmalignant conditions and the many types of bone marrow transplants, this form of treatment may be standard for one condition and investigational for another. One clear finding is that the implications for bone marrow transplants are growing rapidly.

The first bone marrow transplants in humans were attempted in the 1950s in patients with end-stage leukemia. These transplants were unsuccessful; all the patients had relapses (Baird et al., 1991). The first successful transplants occurred in 1968. In 1970, fewer than 100 bone marrow transplants had been done at fewer than 10 centers. In 1988, a total of 10,000 bone marrow transplants were done at more than 100 centers (Ashwanden et al., 1990). Today, thousands of bone marrow transplants are done annually at more than 250 centers worldwide (Whedon, 1991).

Whether bone marrow transplantation is used as an investigational procedure or as standard treatment of a disease, skilled nursing care is essential. Nurses must be knowledgeable about the treatment, indications for it, and prognoses and be able to serve as patients' advocates, educators, and expert clinicians (Whedon, 1991).

Goal of Therapy

The goal of bone marrow transplantation is to provide patients with well functioning bone marrow to sustain life, carry out essential bodily functions, and provide defense mechanisms. The ability of bone marrow to function properly can be altered by disease as well as by treatment. Many diseases, such as leukemia, can affect the bone marrow and so cause immunosuppression. The same effects can be caused by procedures used to treat disease. The disease itself may not affect the bone marrow, but high-dose chemotherapy or radiation may leave the patient severely immunosuppressed. In both of these situations, bone marrow transplantation may be necessary. The rationale for bone marrow transplantation thus includes both rescue and replacement (Ashwanden et al., 1990).

Rescue is necessary when disease does not affect the bone marrow but treatment will. Rescue begins with obtaining and preserving a quantity of the patient's func-

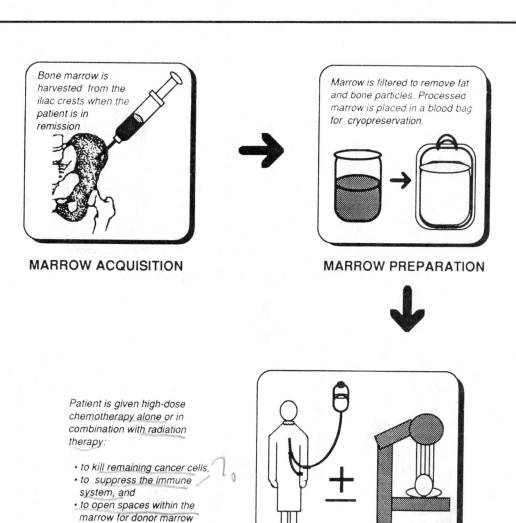

MARROW ACQUISITION

Bone marrow is harvested from the iliac crests when the patient is in remission

MARROW PREPARATION

Marrow is filtered to remove fat and bone particles. Processed marrow is placed in a blood bag for cryopreservation.

Patient is given high-dose chemotherapy alone or in combination with radiation therapy:

• to kill remaining cancer cells,
• to suppress the immune system, and
• to open spaces within the marrow for donor marrow engraftment.

PREPARATION OF MARROW RECIPIENT

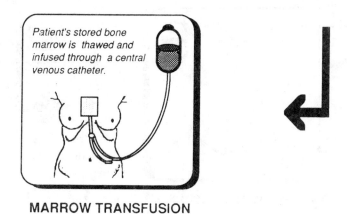

Patient's stored bone marrow is thawed and infused through a central venous catheter.

MARROW TRANSFUSION

Figure 6-1. Process for autologous bone marrow transplantation. Reprinted with permission from Clark, J. C., and McGee, R. F. (1992). *Oncology Nursing Society core curriculum for oncology nursing* (2nd ed., p. 361). Philadelphia: Saunders.

Recipient is given high-dose
chemotherapy alone or in
combination with radiation
therapy:

- to kill remaining cancer cells,
- to suppress the immune
  system, and
- to open spaces within the
  marrow for donor marrow
  engraftment.

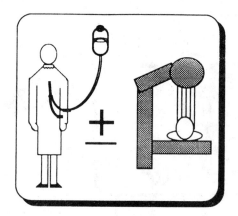

PREPARATION OF MARROW RECIPIENT

Bone marrow is
harvested from the
iliac crests of the
donor.

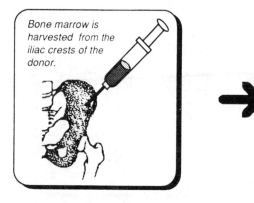

Bone marrow is filtered to remove
fat and bone particles.
Processed marrow is placed in a
blood bag for transfusion.

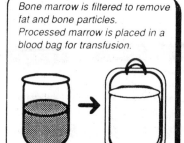

MARROW ACQUISITION   **MARROW PREPARATION**

Donor bone marrow is
infused through a central
venous catheter.

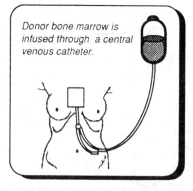
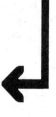

MARROW TRANSFUSION

Figure 6-2. Process for allogeneic bone marrow transplantation. Reprinted with permission from Clark, J. C., and McGee, R. F. (1992). *Oncology Nursing Society core curriculum for oncology nursing* (2nd ed., p. 362). Philadelphia: Saunders.

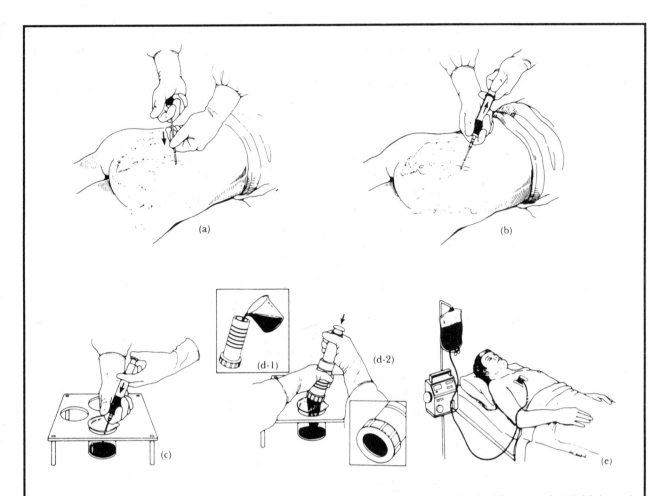

Figure 6-3. Collection and infusion of bone marrow. a) Large-bore needle placed in the iliac crest. b) Multiple aspirations. c) Marrow drawn up in large syringe. d-1) Marrow placed in collection beaker. d-2) Marrow strained. e) Marrow placed in a blood administration bag and administered through a multilumen catheter. Reprinted with permission from Groenwald, S. L., Frogge, M. H., Goodman, M., & Yarbro, C. H. (Eds.). (1990). *Cancer nursing: Principles and practice* (2nd ed., p. 313). Boston: Jones and Bartlett.

tioning bone marrow. Then the patient has high-dose chemotherapy or radiation, which destroys most of the remaining bone marrow. The preserved bone marrow is returned to the patient to rejuvenate the immune system.

Replacement is used when a disease affects the functioning of bone marrow. Functioning, disease-free marrow is obtained from a donor. The patient then has chemotherapy, radiation, and other treatment to eradicate the disease. When treatment is complete, the donated marrow is given to the patient.

Types of Bone Marrow Transplantation

There are three types of bone marrow transplants: autologous, syngeneic, and allogeneic. An autologous

(self) transplant (Figure 6-1) uses the patient's own bone marrow. Autologous transplants are often used for patients who have malignant diseases such as acute lymphocytic leukemia, acute myelogenous leukemia, lymphoma, neuroblastoma, melanoma, breast cancer, testicular cancer, and other solid tumors (Groenwald et al., 1990; Thomas, 1988; Wittes, 1990).

The goal of autologous transplantation is to remove disease-free bone marrow from the patient and preserve it while the patient undergoes high-dose chemotherapy or radiation. Cryopreservation, the method for freezing and storing bone marrow, has been well established for 25 years (Ashwanden et al., 1990; Thomas, 1988). After treatment, the preserved marrow is returned to the patient by infusion. For patients with leukemia, the marrow is usually collected during a period of remission and may be preserved until the patient has a relapse. At that time, the patient may receive high-dose chemotherapy or radiation or both and then receive the autologous bone marrow (Thomas, 1988).

In syngeneic bone marrow transplantation, the donor and recipient are identical twins. The bone marrow of the donor is genetically identical and a perfect histocompatible match to that of the recipient (Ashwanden, et al., 1990). Both autologous and syngeneic bone marrow transplantation eliminate the complications of graftversus-host disease, a side effect in which the cells in the graft recognize the body as foreign tissue, and rejection occurs (Ashwanden et al., 1990; Thomas, 1988). Graft-versus-host disease is discussed later in this chapter.

Allogeneic bone marrow transplantation (Figure 6-2) uses compatible donor bone marrow that is not genetically identical to the recipient's (Ashwanden et al., 1990). The patient is given high-dose chemotherapy or radiation or both. This treatment kills the cancer cells but also suppresses the immune system. Donor marrow is obtained and administered to the patient to rejuvenate the immune system. Allogeneic bone marrow transplantation depends on the availability of a donor whose HLA profile matches that of the patient or recipient. About on-third of patients seeking an allogeneic transplant will find an HLA match in a sibling. The other two-thirds must seek a compatible match in more distant family members or unrelated persons (Whedon, 1991). Unrelated histocompatible donors can be located through volunteer blood donor programs (Ashwanden et al., 1990). Graft-versus-host disease is a complication unique to allogeneic bone marrow transplantation. It is the major obstacle in successful transplantation.

Collection and Infusion of Bone Marrow

Bone marrow is obtained from the patient (autologous transplant) or donor (syngeneic or allogeneic transplant) in the operating room under sterile conditions (Figure 6-3). General or spinal anesthesia is used. Multiple samples of bone marrow are collected from the posterior and anterior iliac crests. Occasionally, the sternum is

used to obtain bone marrow stem cells. Collection can require 1–4 hr, depending on the number of bone marrow cells needed and the ease of aspiration (Clark & McGee, 1992; Groenwald et al., 1990; Schaefer & Beelen, 1991; Whedon, 1991).

The bone marrow is filtered or strained and then processed for infusion. Bone marrow should be infused within 3 hr of collection or should be cryopreserved to be transported or used later (Whedon, 1991).

Complications of Bone Marrow Transplantation

Bone marrow transplantation potentially can cure a number of diseases. However, complications associated with this treatment often interfere with the successful accomplishment of this goal. Complications can be divided into three categories (Groenwald et al., 1990):

1. Complications associated with high-dose chemotherapy and radiation.

2. Graft-versus-host disease (allogeneic transplants only).

3. Problems associated with the original disease.

Most complications occur as a result of chemotherapy and radiation treatment. However, if infusion of bone marrow were not used for rescue, the chemotherapy or radiation therapy would be fatal (Groenwald et al., 1990). Common complications include the following (Baird et al., 1991; Groenwald et al., 1990):

- Gastrointestinal mucositis (often involving oral, esophageal, gastric, and intestinal mucosa).

- Hemorrhage.

- Graft-versus-host disease.

- Renal insufficiency.

- Veno-occlusive disease.

CHAPTER 6 —
INNOVATIVE METHODS OF CANCER THERAPY

69

- Infections (bacterial, viral, and fungal).

Most of these complications are acute and usually occur during the first 100 days after transplantation (Baird et al., 1991).

Mucositis. Mucositis is a side effect all transplant patients experience. It may start on the day of transplantation with dryness of the mouth, sore throat, and thickening saliva. These are followed by an increase in secretions of the oral mucosa and development of pain. Narcotics are often necessary. Mucositis does not subside until the bone marrow graft begins to function (Baird et al., 1991).

Hemorrhage. Hemorrhage and thrombocytopenia can occur any time after treatment but are most likely the first month after transplantation (Baird et al., 1991; Whedon, 1991). The patient must be given red blood cells and platelets until the bone marrow becomes fully functional. All blood products should be irradiated to destroy the T lymphocytes that cause graft-versus-host disease in recipients of allogeneic bone marrow (Groenwald et al., 1990).

Graft-versus-host disease. The major complication of allogeneic bone marrow transplantation is graft-versus-host disease (Ashwanden et al., 1990; Whedon, 1991). In this syndrome, the cells in the donated marrow, particularly the T lymphocytes, recognize the recipient's body tissue as foreign and attack it. Graft-versus-host disease develops in about half of the recipients of allogeneic bone marrow (Groenwald et al., 1990).

Graft-versus-host disease primarily affects the liver, skin, and gastrointestinal tract (Baird et al., 1991; Whedon, 1991). Skin manifestations are usually the first indications. They may range from a mild rash to generalized erythroderma with peeling that may be as severe as a third-degree burn (Ashwanden et al., 1990). Gastrointestinal effects may include abdominal cramping, diarrhea, and bleeding. Involvement of the liver may occur, causing degeneration of the small bile ducts (Ashwanden et al., 1990).

Graft-versus-host disease is a significant obstacle to successful bone marrow transplantation. Treatment of this complication historically has not been promising, so generally efforts have focused on prevention. These include limiting transplant donors to identical HLA matches, infusing T cell–depleted bone marrow, and irradiation of all blood products (Ashwanden et al., 1990; Whedon, 1991).

Veno-occlusive disease. The major task of the liver is to maintain the quality of the blood by clearing waste and drugs from the body. Veno-occlusive disease is a disease of the liver that can occur after bone marrow transplantation (Whedon, 1991). It is rarely seen in other patients. It occurs during the first 3 weeks after transplantation. Signs and symptoms include weight gain, ascites, pain in the upper right quadrant, and increased levels of bilirubin and serum glutamic-oxaloacetic transaminase (SGOT; aspartate aminotransferase [AST]). The only treatment is to decrease stress on the liver (Baird et al., 1991).

Infections. Infections pose an enormous threat to the recipients of bone marrow transplants. No population of patients is more immunosuppressed. Some type of infection develops in almost all recipients of bone marrow transplants (Baird et al., 1991; Wittes, 1990). Infections caused by bacteria, viruses, or fungi occur alone or in combination. Infections are often the major cause of death in transplant patients (Baird et al., 1991).

Prevention of infection is a major focus of medical and nursing protocols. All recipients of bone marrow transplants must have protective isolation in private rooms. Many units that care for these patients have laminar-airflow rooms. Handwashing is essential for everyone coming in contact with the patients. Strict handwashing guidelines should include all health care personnel and all visitors.

The Future for Bone Marrow Transplantation

Bone marrow transplantation, once highly experimental, is now becoming standard in many health care centers (Ashwanden et al., 1990). The procedure evolves daily. Bone marrow transplantation is now a specialty in nursing. The success of this type of transplantation is greatly influenced by the skills, knowledge, and abilities of the nurses who assess and care for transplant patients. As the number of patients undergoing bone marrow transplantation increases, the demand for nurses educated in this procedure will increase.

OTHER NEW THERAPIES

One of the exciting challenges in oncology nursing is the ever-changing developments in the discipline. New approaches are discovered and refined continuously. Other new therapies in cancer treatment include the following.

Photodynamic Therapy

Photodynamic therapy involves the use of a photosensitizing agent, a special type of laser light, and oxygen. The interaction of these three components produces a localized fluorescence for detection and treatment of tumor cells. This therapy is an experimental approach used to treat recurrent breast cancer, head and neck cancer, endobronchial tumors, bladder cancer, skin tumors, and early-stage gynecologic cancers (Ashwanden et al., 1990).

Gene Replacement Therapy

Malfunctions in specific genes in the body can produce molecular disease and cause neoplasms. Replacement of these malfunctioning genes with functional genes is currently being studied (Ashwanden et al., 1990; Thomas, 1988). Gene manipulation is reflected in other molecules that have been cloned or identified. They include colony-stimulating factors, interleukins, interferons, tumor necrosis factor, and oncogenes. The implications of gene replacement therapy in biotherapy are limitless and exciting (Ashwanden et al., 1990).

Oncogenes, first discovered in the 1970s, are genes that may be linked to specific cancers. They may be activated by exposure to chemical carcinogens, radiation, viruses, familial genetic predisposition, or spontaneous mutations (Jenkins, 1992; Weinberg, 1994). With the discovery of oncogenes, it may be possible to determine which persons are at high risk for cancer and make prevention and monitoring of potential oncologic diseases specific to each person.

NURSE'S ROLE IN CLINICAL TRIALS

This chapter explores many innovative oncologic treatments, some of which are still investigational. A clear understanding of nurse's role in clinical trials is important. Nurses must be educators and advocates for the patients. This can be accomplished only if the nurses have a clear understanding of the clinical protocol being used in the trial. This information may be in writing as well as gathered through discussions with other members of the health care team.

It is the nurse's role to be sure that patients in the trial have a clear understanding of all the information known related to the potential treatment. Patient's education in clinical trials relies heavily on open and ongoing communication between the patients and health care providers and researchers (Ashwanden et al., 1990).

BIBLIOGRAPHY

American Cancer Society, Massachusetts Division. (1990). *Cancer manual* (8th ed., pp. 85–98). Boston: Author.

Ashwanden, P., Belcher, A. E., Mattson, E. A., Moskowitz, R., & Riese, N. (1990). *Oncology nursing: Advances, treatments and trends into the 21st century.* Rockville, MD: Aspen.

Baird, S. B., McCorkle, R., & Grant, M. (1991). *Cancer nursing: A comprehensive textbook* (pp. 246–290). Philadelphia: Saunders.

Bockheim, C. M., & Jassak, P. F. (1993). The expanding world of colony stimulating factors. *Cancer Practice, 1*(3):205–216.

Clark, J. C., & McGee, R. F. (1992). *Oncology Nursing Society core curriculum for oncology nursing* (2nd ed., pp. 319–328). Philadelphia: Saunders.

Dudjak, L., & Fleck, A. (1991). BRMs: New drug therapy comes of age. *RN, 54*(10): 42–48.

Groenwald, S. L., Frogge, M. H., Goodman, M., & Yarbro, C. H. (Eds.). (1990). *Cancer nursing: Principles and practice* (2nd ed., pp. 200–283). Boston: Jones and Bartlett.

Jenkins, J. (1992). Biology of cancer: Current issues and future prospects. *Seminars in Oncology Nursing, 8*(1):63–69.

Rumsey, K. A., & Rieger, P. T. (1992). *Biological response modifiers.* Chicago: Precept Press.

Schaefer, U. W., & Beelen, D. W. (1991). *Bone marrow transplantation.* Basel: Karger.

Thomas, E. D. (1988). *Bone marrow transplantation.* New York: American Cancer Society.

Weinberg, R. A. (1994). Oncogenes and tumor suppressor genes. *CA—A Cancer Journal for Clinicians, 44*(3):160–170.

Whedon, M. B. (1991). *Bone marrow transplantation: Principles, practice, and nursing insights.* Boston: Jones and Bartlett.

Wittes, R. E. (1990). *Manual of oncologic therapeutics* (pp. 60–65). Philadelphia: Lippincott.

Yasko, J. M. , & Dudjak, L. A. (1990). *Biological response modifier therapy: Symptom management.* Emeryville, CA: Cetus Corp.; Park Row Publishers.

STUDY QUESTIONS

Chapter 6

Questions 44–51

44. Biotherapy is often used as a synonym for which of these terms?

    a. Teletherapy
    b. Chemotherapy
    c. Biological response modifiers
    d. Bone marrow transplantation

45. Erythropoietin is a biological response modifier that may eliminate the need for which of the following in cancer patients?

    a. Blood transfusions
    b. Radiation
    c. Chemotherapy
    d. Pain management

46. Side effects related to treatment with biological response modifiers include:

    a. Flulike illness
    b. Hepatic side effects
    c. Hematologic side effects
    d. Graft-versus-host disease

47. Bone marrow transplantation is characterized as which of the following?

    a. Investigational treatment only
    b. Standard treatment only
    c. Neither investigational nor standard treatment
    d. Both investigational and standard treatment

48. Which of the following is *not* a type of bone marrow transplantation?

    a. Autologous
    b. Allogeneic
    c. Parageneic
    d. Syngeneic

49. Within 3 hr after collection, bone marrow should be used or:

    a. Discarded
    b. Frozen
    c. Dried
    d. Rejected

50. Graft-versus-host disease is a common complication of which type of bone marrow transplantation?

    a. Autologous
    b. Allogeneic
    c. Parageneic
    d. Syngeneic

51. What is usually the first indication of graft-versus-host disease?

    a. Liver problems
    b. Memory loss
    c. Hemorrhage
    d. Skin manifestations

CHAPTER 7

UNPROVEN METHODS OF CANCER TREATMENT

CHAPTER OBJECTIVE

After completing this chapter, the reader will be able to recognize common types of unproven methods of cancer treatment and the possible rationale for their pursuit by cancer patients and patients' families.

LEARNING OBJECTIVES

After studying this chapter, the reader will be able to

1. Recognize the hallmarks of unproven methods of cancer therapy.

2. Select nursing interventions to objectively help patients and their families make decisions about using unproven methods of cancer treatment.

INTRODUCTION

During treatment of cancer, it is not unusual for patients and their families to wish to pursue some aspect of an unproven method of therapy. The range of needs and the type of methods pursued vary greatly, and nurses who provide care for these patients may be responsible for seeing that such needs are recognized and met satisfactorily. Some clients only want reassurance that everything possible, plausible, and reasonable is being, or has been, pursued. Others may actually desire alternative sources of medical care, resent the medical model as the sole approach to care, or know about a particular method of care from publicity or from articles in the popular press.

TYPES OF UNPROVEN METHODS

Unproven methods of cancer treatment frequently fit into four general categories:

1. Nutritional interventions.

2. Therapy involving immune stimulation to fight off the cancer.

3. Psychologic interventions as cancer therapy.

4. Drugs or "natural products."

As more information is gained about carcinogenesis and tumor biology and immunology, the theory behind some of these unproven methods does not seem unreasonable. The role of nutrition in cancer etiology and prevention has been widely studied and appears to be a critical one for many types of cancer. Immunotherapy is an accepted treatment in certain cancers. Psychoneuroimmunology is a growing field of legitimate research as investigators try to determine the reality of a "mind-body link" and what effect that link might have on cancer initiation and therapeutic response. And certainly most systemic cancer therapy is built on drug treatments, all of which were new and investigational at some point in their development. Unfortunately, the response rates associated with some approved therapies is dismal and surely not guaranteed to produce a response, much less a cure.

HALLMARKS OF UNPROVEN METHODS

On first look, then, the differences between unproven methods of cancer treatment and accepted or standard therapy appear rather small. However, unproven methods, sometimes referred to as cancer quackery, have some hallmarks that health care professionals, patients, and the general public can use to judge carefully the claims of certain approaches to cancer therapy:

Lack of Reports in Peer-Reviewed Journals

The scientific method calls for careful scrutiny of research through peer-reviewed publications. Evaluation of a treatment requires data on what exactly the treatment entails, the toxic effects experienced, numbers and types of subjects treated, and subjects' responses. Proponents of unproven methods frequently avoid submitting their research findings to peer-reviewed journals. Instead, they publicize their therapy through the mass media, which often present the information in a skewed fashion and play on the hopes and fears of those who are dealing with a diagnosis of cancer. Unproven methods may also be presented as a book in the popular press, but again the scientific data necessary for careful evaluation of the treatment are missing. What information is presented tends to be in the form of anecdotes, a few unique cases, glowing tributes from persons who have experienced the benefits of the treatment, and data that often are nonreproducible.

Lack of Training or Credentials by the "Author" of the Treatment

Often the promoter of the therapy, which may be named for this person, is not a scientist or a physician. Although classic scientific or medical training does not guarantee rigid adherence to scientific principles, promoters of unproven methods frequently have "generic" backgrounds, referring to themselves as "natural healers" or by similar titles. The division between the medical model of health care and other models (e.g., chiropractic and homeopathic medicine) tends to support the argument of these promoters of alternative methods, who may state that MDs are attempting to establish a monopoly on health care and not allow competition.

Focus on Personal Control and the "Natural" Approach

When cancer patients undergo traditional surgery, radiation therapy, chemotherapy, or immunotherapy for their disease, often the first loss they experience is the loss of personal control. They are told what their treatment will involve, what the schedule will be, what they need to do. Although these therapies may include some informed choices, patients often feel as if medicine is doing all this to them and that they are peripheral to the therapy, certainly not partners in their care. Unproven methods tend to be marketed as a way for patients to regain that sense of control. Complex diet plans (e.g., macrobiotic diet, megavitamins), intricate treatments for which the patient has considerable responsibility (e.g., coffee enemas), and psychologic interventions that are intended as therapy (e.g., Simonton method, faith healing) give back much control to the patient.

Unavailability of the Drug Therapy in the United States

Although the Food and Drug Administration carefully regulates the import of drugs manufactured outside the United States, as well as approval and distribution of drugs produced in this country, a number of unproven methods are available only in other countries. Examples are laetrile in Mexico, or immune-augmentative therapy in the Bahamas. Patients not only must deal with the expense of purchasing products that have shown no benefit therapeutically, they also must bear the cost of travel to international locations to obtain the desired treatment.

NURSING INTERVENTIONS FOR UNPROVEN METHODS

To plan an effective intervention regarding unproven methods of cancer treatment, the health care team must first know that a patient is participating, or planning to participate, in such an approach. Often it is the nurse who assesses this situation. Patients may be reluctant to discuss these activities with their physicians because of fear of disapproval, abandonment, or lack of support.

Patients often become involved in unproven methods because of a perceived loss of control, perhaps combined with a lack of a sense of hope. Thus, it is important for nurses and other health care providers to ascertain how a patient can acquire a greater sense of control in approved therapy and how to reinstill hope in the patient. Some unproven methods that focus on diet or nutritional supplements can be modified to make the method benign or even a helpful adjunct to standard therapy. Psychologic approaches that give patients emotional support and enhanced ability to cope with diagnosis, prognosis, and therapy should be encouraged and recognized as a legitimate need of patients and their family members. Nurses may need to clarify misinformation about unproven methods; present the known, scientific data on that approach; and suggest alternatives that the patient could pursue that would meet the patient's needs but not be considered dangerous or manipulative.

To be valuable resources to patients and their families in this area, nurses and other health care providers must be familiar with safe alternative therapies, be knowledgeable about unproven methods, and even be able to design alternative approaches (e.g., psychologic methods, relaxation techniques, support groups) in which patients and patients' families can participate. Referrals to appropriate health care professionals or agencies (e.g., counselors who specialize in cancer patients or the American Cancer Society's data base on unproven methods) may be effective interventions for patients who have been pursuing unproven methods.

STUDY QUESTIONS

Chapter 7

Questions 52–53

52. What is one hallmark of unproven cancer methods?

    a. Publication in peer-reviewed journals
    b. The investigator's training in osteopathic medicine
    c. Use of investigational drugs
    d. Lack of controlled clinical trials

53. Nursing interventions to address use of unproven methods of cancer therapy may include which of the following?

    a. Keeping the health care team in control
    b. Reinstilling hope in the patient
    c. Dismissing all unproven methods as worthless
    d. Increasing the dose of chemotherapy

CHAPTER 8

PROBLEMS RELATED TO CANCER AND ITS TREATMENT

CHAPTER OBJECTIVE

After completing this chapter, the reader will be able to describe the most common problems associated with cancer and its treatment and suggest appropriate nursing interventions for patients with these problems.

LEARNING OBJECTIVES

After studying this chapter, the reader will be able to

1. Recognize the various types of nausea and vomiting associated with cancer and cancer treatments.

2. Calculate an absolute granulocyte count.

3. Select appropriate interventions for patients with complications due to myelosuppression.

4. Recognize signs and symptoms of gastrointestinal effects due to cancer or cancer treatments.

5. Indicate appropriate drugs to include in various pain management programs for patients with cancer.

6. Recognize appropriate interventions for patients with gastrointestinal effects due to cancer or cancer treatments.

7. Recognize appropriate interventions for patients with cutaneous changes due to cancer or cancer treatments.

8. Select the most common cause of infections of the oral cavity in patients with stomatitis.

9. Indicate the pathophysiology of vomiting.

10. Specify the signs and symptoms of thrombocytopenia.

INTRODUCTION

Patients with cancer generally experience side effects caused by the disease or its treatment. Problems can develop because of the cancer, by-products from destruction of tumor cells, and cancer treatments. Side effects can occur in any body organ; however, those related to treatment usually are due to the effects of the treatment on rapidly dividing cells. Unlike side effects due to chemotherapy and biotherapy, those due to radiation usually are limited to the tissues and organs within the field of treatment. Side effects can be acute or chronic and mild to severe. The type and severity of side effects related to cancer treatment are affected by the intensity of the treatment regimen. Compliance with therapy is often influenced by the severity of side effects. Therefore, patients' ability to cope with the associated side effects is an important factor in compliance.

Management of patients' problems related to cancer and its treatment is an important role of nurses. The role includes anticipating, preventing, and assessing side effects; intervening as appropriate; and educating patients and their families about side effects. Written instructions and booklets should be given to patients to reinforce teaching. Mutual goals need to be developed with patients to prevent or minimize side effects. It is important that signs and symptoms be treated appropriately. Whenever a sign or symptom becomes unacceptable or intolerable, patients consider stopping, and may stop, potentially life-saving treatments.

GASTROINTESTINAL SIDE EFFECTS

The gastrointestinal tract is particularly sensitive to the toxic effects of cancer and cancer treatments because it is composed of rapidly dividing cells. Gastrointestinal side effects include stomatitis, nausea and vomiting, alterations in nutrition, and diarrhea. These effects often cause the most distress for patients.

Stomatitis

The mucous membranes are constantly being renewed and therefore are vulnerable to the effects of cancer, cancer treatments, and the side effects of treatments (e.g., anorexia). The cells of the epithelial layer of the mucous membranes are generally replaced every 7–14

days. Mucosal thinning or ulcerations occur when the rate of cell loss (by sloughing off) is greater than the rate of cell renewal. Regeneration can be slowed for a variety of reasons, including age and the effects of cancer treatments. Because the mucous membranes serve as a barrier to the invasion of microorganisms, any alteration in the integrity of the membranes provides an entrance for organisms and increases the risk of infection.

The terms *mucositis* and *stomatitis* are often used interchangeably. Mucositis is defined as a generalized inflammation of the mucous membranes of the body that can progress to ulcerations. Stomatitis, the most common type of mucositis, occurs in the oral cavity. Stomatitis is an uncomfortable side effect. It can lead to alterations in nutrition, cause sleep disturbance, and directly affect patients' quality of life.

The degree of stomatitis varies from mild to severe (Table 8-1). It is influenced by the type of cancer; the treatment regimen; and the patient's age, nutritional status, and dental hygiene practices. Stomatitis can be severe enough to be a dose-limiting toxic effect, resulting in delay, modification, or discontinuation of treatment.

Stomatitis develops in cancer patients for a myriad of reasons. The effects of this abnormality often can be prevented or minimized by appropriate pretreatment and aggressive preventive measures. Nurses need to determine which patients are at risk for stomatitis and then implement interventions designed to minimize the signs and symptoms associated with it.

Causes and Contributing Factors. Stomatitis is more common in patients with head and neck cancer than in patients with other types of cancer, and the prevalence is higher in patients with hematologic tumors (e.g., leukemia) than in those with solid tumors. Immunosuppression and myelosuppression increase the risk of complications associated with stomatitis, such as infections and bleeding. The stomatitis usually resolves when the white blood cell (WBC) count returns to normal.

Stomatitis may occur in patients who have biotherapy, especially those who are treated with interleukin-2. Administration of chemotherapeutic agents that damage

Table 8-1
Evaluation of Stomatitis

Grade	Stage of Stomatitis	Characteristics
0	No evidence of stomatitis	Mucosa moist and pink No lesions No inflammation No report of discomfort
1	Mild	Mild erythema redness Mild discomfort or soreness
2	Mild to moderate	Moderate erythema Small isolated ulcers Mild to moderate discomfort requiring topical and, sometimes, systemic analgesics Able to eat and drink normally
3	Moderate to severe	Confluent ulceration Moderate discomfort requiring topical and systemic analgesics Liquid intake only
4	Severe	Severe erythema Ulcerations with bleeding Severe discomfort requiring systemic analgesics Difficulty swallowing Unable to eat or drink

Source: Baird, S. B., McCorkle, R., & Grant, M. (Eds.). (1991). Cancer nursing: A comprehensive textbook. Philadelphia: Saunders, pp. 742-758, and National Institutes of Health. (1994, January). Protomechanics: A guide to preparing and conducting a clinical research study at the Warren Magnuson Clinical Center (2nd ed.). Bethesda: Author, p. 86.

the mucous membranes often causes this side effect. These include antitumor antibiotics (e.g., doxorubicin, bleomycin) and antimetabolites (e.g., 5-fluorouracil, methotrexate, cytarabine, 6-mercaptopurine). The degree of stomatitis depends on the drug, dose, schedule of administration, drug metabolism, and severity of myelosuppression associated with the drug (e.g., intensity and duration). Stomatitis usually begins 3–5 days after treatment, peaks around 7–10 days, and begins to resolve over the next week.

Radiation therapy involving the head and neck and total-body irradiation place a patient at risk for stomatitis. The severity of the stomatitis is affected by the type of radiation, fraction per dose, total dose, time between fractions, type of tissues irradiated, size of the treatment field, and the anatomic structures exposed to radiation. Signs and symptoms usually resolve within 2–3 weeks after therapy is completed. Stomatitis is common in patients who have surgery of the head and neck for treatment of cancer and in those whose therapy includes more than one type of treatment (e.g., radiation and chemotherapy).

Alterations in nutritional status (e.g., malnutrition, cachexia, anorexia, nutritional deficiencies) can affect mucosal integrity and increase a patient's risk for stomatitis. Other factors that increase risk are poor oral hygiene (e.g., preexisting periodontal disease), irritating dentures, and use of alcohol and tobacco, which aggravate the mucosa.

Younger patients are at greater risk than older patients because of the more rapid cell turnover in younger persons. Older patients may experience prolonged side effects because of slower regeneration of mucous membranes.

Signs and Symptoms. Signs and symptoms of stomatitis include dry, rough, cracked, ulcerated, and bleeding lips. Drying of the mucosa, edema, erythema, swelling, and ulceration may occur in the oral cavity. The saliva may be profuse and watery in the early stages and then become thick and ropy and finally be lacking. Patients may experience tenderness, a burning sensation, pain, an increased sensitivity to acidic and spicy substances, difficulty swallowing, and a decrease in oral intake.

Maintaining a patent airway may be difficult if the stomatitis is severe. In extreme cases, intubation may be necessary to protect the airway until mucosal recovery occurs.

Complications. Complications associated with stomatitis include anorexia, weight loss, dehydration, and infection. Infection occurs most often in myelosuppressed patients who are receiving antibiotics. Colonization can result in local infection or provide an entry for systemic infection. Infections with *Candida albicans* and herpes simplex virus are the most common. Patients with stomatitis may also have gingival bleeding and pain.

Nursing Management. The goal of nursing management in stomatitis is prevention and minimization of the effects. For these, a comprehensive nursing assessment is essential.

The first step in assessment is to determine which patients are at risk. Patients should be examined by a dentist before treatment of cancer begins. After treatment starts, the oral cavity should be examined at least twice a day. The appearance of the mucosa, the quality of the voice, and the ability to swallow should be determined. A variety of guidelines are available to facilitate consistent assessment among practitioners.

Other factors that should be assessed include the patient's oral hygiene practices, ability to control secretions and maintain a patent airway, and hydration and nutritional status. The complete blood cell count should be monitored, because myelosuppression is associated with severity of stomatitis and onset of recovery.

The cornerstone of prevention is a meticulous oral care program that is simple and easy for patients to follow. Although many products are available for preventing and treating the signs and symptoms associated with stomatitis (Table 8-2), the frequency and consistency of oral care are more important than the actual products used. The optimum frequency depends on the severity of the stomatitis. For example, patients with mild stomatitis should perform oral care every 4 hr while awake; patients with moderate stomatitis, every 2 hr while awake and every 4 hr during the night; and patients with severe stomatitis, every 2 hr while awake

Table 8-2
Mouth Care Products

Type of Product	Product or Agent

Cleansing	Tools
	  Soft toothbrush
	  Toothettes
	
	Rinses
	  Normal saline
	  Sodium bicarbonate
	  Chlorhexidine (Peridex)
	  Perox-a-mint

Lip lubricants	A & D Ointment Moisture Balm Mouth Moisturizer Petroleum jelly
Artificial saliva	MoiStir Salivart XeroLube

Pain relievers	Topical
	  Benzocaine 15-20% (Hurricaine, Oratect)
	  Dyclonine hydrochloride 0.5% (Dyclone)
	  Kaopectate
	  Lidocaine (Xylocaine) viscous 2%
	  Ulcerase
	
	Systemic
	  Opioids

Antifungals	Local
	  Clotrimazole troches
	  Nystatin suspension
	  Nystatin popsicles
	
	Systemic
	  Ketoconazole
	  Fluconazole
	  Amphotericin

Source: Gross, J., & Johnson, L. (Eds.). (1994). *Handbook of oncology nursing.* Boston: Jones and Bartlett, pp. 416-419, and Pizzo, P., & Poplack, D. (Eds.). (1993). *Principles and practice of pediatric oncology* (2nd ed.). New York: Lippincott, p. 1067.

and every 2–4 hr during the night. Patients with no stomatitis or mild stomatitis should be encouraged to perform mouth care after meals and at bedtime.

Rigorous use of mouth rinses may decrease or control stomatitis. Patients should avoid using commercial mouthwashes, which often contain alcohol. Other steps patients can take include applying lip lubricants and avoiding irritants to the oral cavity (e.g., tobacco, alcohol, poorly fitting dentures).

Because of the possibility of infections in patients with stomatitis, material should be collected from any suspicious lesions on the lips or in the oral cavity and cultured for microorganisms. Local antifungals are often prescribed prophylactically for patients at risk and are administered orally. Patients should not eat or drink anything for 30 min after using an oral antifungal. A commonly prescribed antifungal is clotrimazole, which is administered as a troche five times per day. To be effective, the troche must be dissolved completely in the mouth, a requirement that can make this agent inappropriate for patients with severe stomatitis. Nystatin suspension is swished and swallowed, but for patients unable to swallow, it can be swished and spit. Intravenous antifungals such as fluconazole or amphotericin are used for more severe cases or when systemic infection is suspected. Antivirals should be used as prescribed. Patients receiving bone marrow transplants may take acyclovir prophylactically.

Dietary consultation should be requested for patients with stomatitis. Patients can be encouraged to do the following:

- Eat bland, soft foods.

- Eat cool foods (e.g., yogurt, ice cream), which may be soothing.

- Avoid very hot foods.

- Avoid acidic foods and beverages.

Nurses should encourage oral intake and administer enteral or parenteral nutrition as ordered.

Nursing interventions to increase patients' comfort include the following:

- Offer ice chips and popsicles, which may be soothing.

- Use topical anesthetics as indicated; overuse can result in a decreased or absent gag reflex.

- Administer systemic opioids in conjunction with topical anesthetics or when topical anesthetics are ineffective.

- Apply antifibrolytics and administer platelets as ordered to control bleeding.

- Encourage use of yankeur suction to assist in controlling secretions.

- Provide patients with emotional support.

Any changes noted during inspection of the oral cavity should be recorded in the patient's chart. A variety of grading systems have been developed to describe the effects of stomatitis (Table 8-1).

Patients should be taught how to inspect the oral cavity and should be instructed to inspect it daily. They should report persistent signs and symptoms, especially changes in oral sensation, taste, and appearance of lesions. Patients should also be instructed about the importance of meticulous oral care. Nurses should review oral care products and the purpose of each product and provide patients with written instructions. Patients should also be taught about sleeping positions that minimize the risk of aspiration.

Nausea and Vomiting

Nausea and vomiting are among the most challenging side effects associated with cancer and its treatment. Most patients associate these two effects with cancer treatments and think their occurrence is inevitable. However, not every patient treated for cancer experiences nausea and vomiting. Each patient has his or her own threshold for the development of nausea and vomiting, and the threshold is influenced by the disease process and treatment regimen. Patients tolerate the same treatment regimens differently, and some may experience more or less nausea and vomiting than would be expected.

The severity of nausea and vomiting can vary from mild to severe, and the duration may be protracted. Prolonged vomiting can lead to other complications, such as anorexia, dehydration, malnutrition, metabolic imbalances, depression, and poor compliance with treatment. Inadequate management can directly affect patients' quality of life. When nausea and vomiting become intolerable, patients may decide to stop treatment. It is therefore important for nurses to have a basic knowledge of the types, causes, and management of nausea and vomiting. To plan and implement appropriate interventions, nurses need to be familiar with each patient's (1) medical condition, (2) predisposing factors that may increase his or her risk, and (3) anticipated severity of nausea and vomiting associated with the treatment regimen. The goals should be treatment of the nausea and vomiting and promotion of the patient's comfort.

Pathophysiology. Cancer patients can experience nausea, vomiting, and retching during the course of their disease and its treatment. Nausea is an unpleasant sensation experienced when a person feels as if he or she must vomit. Vomiting is an involuntary reflex that results in the forceful expulsion of gastric contents. Retching occurs when the stomach contains no gastric contents to expel. Vomiting is generally preceded by nausea and several physiologic changes, such as an increase in respirations, increased heart rate, dilated pupils, and pallor. Patients may also have decreased gastric motility. The feeling of nausea may persist even after the patient vomits, although many patients feel relief after vomiting.

Vomiting is coordinated by the vomiting center, which is stimulated by input from a variety of pathways through neurotransmitters such as acetylcholine, dopamine, histamine, serotonin, and norepinephrine. The vomiting center is located in the medulla and is composed of two parts: the chemoreceptor trigger zone and the true vomiting center.

The chemoreceptor trigger zone is located on the floor of the fourth ventricle. This zone contains receptors for a variety of neurotransmitters (e.g., dopamine, histamine, prostaglandin, and serotonin) and is sensitive to chemicals in blood and cerebrospinal fluid. Impulses sent from the chemoreceptor trigger zone to the true vomiting center often lead to vomiting. The true vomiting center receives stimuli from a variety of pathways and initiates vomiting.

Other pathways involved in the mechanism of nausea and vomiting include vagal visceral afferents, midbrain afferents, sympathetic visceral afferents, and the cerebral cortex. Irritation of the gastrointestinal tract (e.g., distension, obstruction, delayed gastric emptying) results in vomiting via vagal visceral afferents. In addition, neuroreceptors in the gastrointestinal tract play a role in triggering the vomiting center. Midbrain afferents are stimulated by increased intracranial pressure. Sympathetic visceral afferents are stimulated by a variety of conditions (e.g., obstruction, irritation), and they receive stimuli from the gastrointestinal tract. The cerebral cortex is affected by noxious stimuli (e.g., odor, taste) and is responsible for anticipatory nausea and vomiting.

Types of Nausea and Vomiting. Three different types of nausea and vomiting occur: acute, delayed, and anticipatory. Acute nausea and vomiting generally begin a few hours after treatment and last approximately 24 hr. The occurrence and severity are influenced by the treatment agent, route of administration, dose, frequency, and, for radiation therapy, the treatment field irradiated. Acute nausea and vomiting associated with chemotherapy with cyclophosphamide and cisplatin begin approximately 4–8 hr after administration of the drugs.

Delayed nausea and vomiting occur most often in patients who receive chemotherapy. The onset is 24 hr after treatment, and the average duration is 5–7 days. The nausea and vomiting are most severe 48–72 hr after chemotherapy. Generally, delayed nausea and vomiting are less severe than the acute type.

Anticipatory nausea and vomiting are a learned or conditioned response. The nausea and vomiting begin before treatment is administered, sometimes as early as the day before. The reaction can be triggered by the hospital environment; the sight of the nurse who administers the therapy; and sounds, tastes, and odors associated with treatment. Just the thought of receiving another treatment can trigger a response.

Patients with poor emesis control are at greatest risk for anticipatory nausea and vomiting, and patients who achieve effective emesis control during the first 24 hr after treatment are less likely to experience this type of nausea and vomiting. Therefore, it is important that patients' first cancer treatment includes measures to prevent or minimize nausea and vomiting. Treatment of anticipatory nausea and vomiting may include administration of lorazepam to decrease anxiety and steps to induce relaxation, which provides a sense of control.

Causes and Contributing Factors. Nausea and vomiting may occur in patients who receive biotherapy, especially interleukin-2. Nausea and vomiting are more common with chemotherapy than other cancer treatments; however, not every chemotherapeutic agent causes vomiting. Each agent has a different emetic potential, which can be affected by the dose of the drug administered and the route and schedule of administration. Nausea and vomiting associated with radiation therapy depend on the dose of radiation and the area treated. Vomiting is uncommon; however, patients with treatment fields involving the brain, large portions of the abdomen, the pelvic area, the epigastrium, and the whole body are at risk. When vomiting occurs, it usually begins within 6 hr after treatment and lasts up to 3–6 hr.

Nausea and vomiting are more common in patients who have metastases to the central nervous system or liver or who have intestinal inflammatory disease. Medical conditions that increase the risk for these side effects include fluid and electrolyte imbalances (e.g., hypercalcemia), intestinal obstruction (e.g., ileus), infections, sepsis, and uremia. Antibiotics, analgesics, and long-acting bronchodilators also may cause nausea and vomiting.

Management of Nausea and Vomiting. Younger patients (less than 30 years old) appear to be more susceptible to the development of dystonic reactions due to antiemetics such as butyrophenones, phenothiazines, and substituted benzamides. Patients who have a history of alcohol abuse or chronic heavy alcohol use are less likely to experience problems with nausea and vomiting. These patients generally respond better to antiemetic treatments and achieve better control of emesis. Patients who have a history of motion sickness are more likely to have problems with nausea and vomiting. Patients who have had poor control of emesis often have anticipatory nausea and vomiting.

A variety of pharmacologic and nonpharmacologic interventions are used to manage nausea and vomiting. Antiemetics are often administered to patients receiving cancer treatments to prevent or minimize nausea and vomiting (Table 8-3). Effective antiemetic coverage is important, especially during the first cancer treatment a patient receives.

An effective antiemetic regimen generally incorporates more than one agent and involves combining agents with different actions and side effects. Diphenhydramine is often used to decrease or treat dystonic reactions associated with the administration of certain antiemetics. Dexamethasone has been combined with ondansetron for increased effectiveness. The emetogenic potential of the treatment regimen is an important factor in choosing an antiemetic regimen. Antiemetics are generally administered 30–60 min before the treatment, and, depending on the emetogenic potential of the treatment, they may be administered around the clock for the next 24 hr. Antiemetics may also be used to decrease nausea, which many patients experience for several days after treatment.

Nonpharmacologic interventions may be behavioral, dietary, or environmental. Behavioral interventions are especially helpful in the treatment of patients with anticipatory nausea and vomiting. Examples are biofeedback, deconditioning or desensitization, distraction or diversion, guided imagery, hypnosis, and relaxation. Dietary interventions include eating small, frequent meals and easily digested foods (e.g., toast, crackers, rice) and avoiding fatty and spicy foods. Patients should also avoid drinking or eating their favorite foods; some patients develop aversions to foods they associate with periods of nausea and vomiting.

[handwritten margin notes: "CTZ ?", "Anxiolytics → sedation", "Dystonic Rx ?", "Dystonic Rx Blocks CTZ"]

Table 3
Pharmacologic Agents for treatment of Nausea and Vomiting in Cancer Patients

Drug Classification	Generic Name	Trade Name	Pharmacologic Actions	Side Effects
Antihistamine	Diphenhydramine	Benadryl	Inhibits histamine Depresses cerebral cortex Depresses vestibular stimuli	Drowsiness Dry mouth Sedation
Benzodiazepines	Diazepam Lorazepam	Valium Ativan	Anxiolytic effects Sedation Amnesic effects Depress CNS and cerebral cortex	Sedation Amnesia Confusion Dizziness
Butyrophenones	Droperidol Haloperidol	Inapsine Haldol	Dopamine antagonists Block CTZ stimuli Anxiolytics	Dystonic reactions Agitation and restlessness Sedation Orthostatic hypotension
Cannabinoid	Dronabinol (THC)	Marinol	Anticholinergic activity Depresses cerebral cortex	Dizziness Ataxia Sedation Dry mouth Orthostatic hypotension Euphoria and dysphoria Hallucinations and confusion
Corticosteroids	Dexamethasone Methylprednisolone	Decadron Solu-Medrol	Unknown; hypothesized to inhibit prostaglandin synthesis	Euphoria Insomnia Hyperglycemia
Phenothiazines	Chlorpromazine Perphenazine Prochlorperazine Promethazine Thiethylperazine	Thorazine Trilafon Compazine Phenergan Torecan	Dopamine antagonists Block CTZ stimuli Some also block VC	Dystonic reactions Drowsiness Dizziness Hypotension Dry mouth
Serotonin antagonists	Granisetron Ondansetron	Kytril Zofran	Block serotonin (5-HT$_3$) receptors Block CTZ Block stimuli from peripheral nervous system	Headache Dry mouth Transient elevation of serum transaminase levels
Substituted benzamide	Metoclopramide	Reglan	Dopamine antagonist Blocks CTZ Blocks stimuli from peripheral nervous system Affects gastrointestinal tract Increases gastric motility	Dystonic reactions Restlessness Sedation Diarrhea

Note: CNS = central nervous system, CTZ = chemoreceptor trigger zone, VC = true vomiting center.

Patients should maintain fluid intake to prevent dehydration. They can begin by drinking clear liquids and then, if these are tolerated, try soups and broths as tolerated. Flat carbonated beverages, popsicles, and gelatin are often tolerated well.

Environmental interventions include creating a conducive environment, avoiding food odors that enhance the potential for nausea and vomiting, and avoiding unpleasant sights and smells (e.g., perfumes, hair spray).

Nursing Management. Nursing care should be designed to educate patients about the causes, expected duration, and management of nausea and vomiting. The cornerstone of nursing management should be psychologic support of the patient. Nursing management includes assessment, interventions, documentation, and education of patients.

Assessment begins by determining characteristics of the patient that may affect emetogenic potential (e.g., anxiety, alcohol use, history of motion sickness) and the emetogenic potential of the scheduled treatment. Other factors to be considered include the patient's previous experience with cancer treatment and his or her expectations about side effects of treatment. If nausea and vomiting do occur, the nurse should assess the frequency, severity, and duration of the side effects and determine the precipitating factors, aggravating factors, and measures most effective in alleviating the problem. Patients should be monitored for complications of prolonged nausea and vomiting (e.g., dehydration, fluid and electrolyte imbalances, anorexia), and the effectiveness of pharmacologic and nonpharmacologic interventions should be determined.

Possible nursing interventions include the following:

- Place emesis basin within easy reach of the patient.

- Offer the patient mouth rinses to cleanse the oral cavity after each vomiting episode.

- Administer antiemetics as prescribed.

- Monitor intake and output.

- Monitor electrolyte balance.

- Modify the environment to eliminate noxious stimuli.

- Provide the patient with emotional support during vomiting.

Nurses should make a record of the outcome of interventions, so that ones that were effective can be used when the patient receives his or her next treatment. The amount of material vomited during each episode of vomiting should be noted in the patient's chart.

As part of each patient's education, the nurse should assess the patient's knowledge of causes of nausea and vomiting and provide information as needed. After reviewing the treatment regimen and determining the potential for nausea and vomiting, he or she should inform the patient about interventions that will be used to prevent, minimize, and treat nausea and vomiting. Patients should be instructed to record episodes of vomiting, including any precipitating or aggravating factors and measures that are effective in managing the problem. Patients should also be taught which signs and symptoms should be reported to the nurse or other caregiver.

Alterations in Nutrition

Alterations in nutrition can be due to physiologic or psychologic factors. Alterations in taste, anorexia, cachexia, and weight loss are examples of common manifestations observed in cancer patients. These manifestations are often intertwined and can result in a self-perpetuating cycle. Alterations in nutrition can be severe enough to cause debilitating effects that have a profound impact on a patient's quality of life.

Alterations in taste occur frequently and can contribute to the development of anorexia or cachexia by affecting appetite. The ability to taste is influenced by sensations created by the taste buds, production of saliva, and smell. The tongue is covered with taste buds, which are responsible for creating variations in taste sensations. Taste buds located on the tip and anterior part of the tongue are responsible for sweet tastes; those located on

Anorexia — loss of appetite

Cachexia — loss of body wt, fat, lean musc. mass

the sides, for sour and salty tastes; and those located posteriorly, for bitter tastes.

Anorexia or loss of appetite is a vague symptom that can lead to weight loss, weakness, and fatigue. Cachexia, the most severe form of malnutrition observed in cancer patients, is characterized by progressive loss of body weight, fat, and lean muscle mass. The rate of wasting associated with cachexia does not appear to be related to the stage of disease, histologic features of the tumor, size of tumor, or site of involvement. Anorexia further complicates cachexia. Patients with cachexia are thought to have altered metabolism. They often have increased basal metabolic rates despite decreased food intake, and fat and muscle are used as sources of energy. Because patients cannot survive a 30% loss in body protein, one goal in their treatment is to decrease the loss of protein. *Imp ↓ loss of protein*

Most cancer patients have anorexia, cachexia, or both at some time during the course of their disease. It is not unusual for patients to report feelings of anorexia at the time cancer is diagnosed. Although rarer, patients may also be cachectic at the time of diagnosis. The prevalence and severity of cachexia increase as cancer progresses, and this abnormality is the major cause of death in patients with advanced stages of cancer. Patients with severe cachexia appear emaciated.

Causes and Contributing Factors. A number of factors related to cancer contribute to alterations in nutrition. Anorexia is often an initial indication of cancer and may be a sign of cancer recurrence. Gastrointestinal obstruction due to cancer can cause alterations in nutrition, and alterations are more common in patients with head and neck cancer than in patients with other types of cancer. Metabolic changes related to the tumor and wastes from breakdown of tumor cells are also contributing factors. *Metabolic changes related to the tumor*

Treatment with interferon can cause foods to taste metallic or bitter, and biotherapy with interleukin-2 is associated with a decrease in appetite. Changes in taste are associated with treatment with the chemotherapeutic agents cisplatin, cyclophosphamide, dactinomycin, 5-fluorouracil, methotrexate, and mechlorethamine. Radiation therapy to the head and neck destroys taste buds

and the cells responsible for production of saliva. Taste buds can regenerate, so the effects are generally temporary; however, permanent changes can occur. Patients often report that food tastes like cardboard. Surgery of the oral cavity, tongue, nasal area, olfactory nerve, and inner ear may alter taste perception.

Side effects of cancer or cancer treatments can result in appetite suppression and development of food aversions. Alterations in taste perception (e.g., decrease in perception, loss of perception, distorted perception) are common and can lead to altered dietary habits, disinterest in food, and development of food aversions. Patients often experience a decreased tolerance for bitter foods; these include foods such as meats, which have a high protein content. Patients also often have difficulty tasting sweet foods unless the foods are overly sweet. Changes in taste are usually temporary; taste may return to normal when the tumor responds to treatment or may persist for several months after treatment. *generally temp Tx*

↓ in taste temp

Patients may develop food aversions and avoid eating because they fear they may vomit. Other factors that may contribute to alterations in nutrition include stomatitis, changes in the ability to ingest and digest food, anemia, constipation, fatigue, and infection. Deficiencies in copper, nickel, niacin, vitamin A, and zinc are associated with changes in taste. Other contributing factors are inactivity and immobility; physical discomfort (e.g., pain); and psychologic factors such as anxiety, depression, and discouragement.

Signs and Symptoms. Signs and symptoms of anorexia are malaise, pallor, weakness, and weight loss. Cachexia is characterized by anorexia, anemia, edema, hypoalbuminemia, hypoglycemia and glucose intolerance, and lactic acidosis. Patients with cachexia may also have mouth lesions, muscle and tissue wasting, dull sunken eyes, sparse and thinning hair, weight loss, and temporal wasting. Progressive weight loss is associated with poor prognosis. *temporal wasting* ?

Nursing Management. The main goal of assessment of patients who have anorexia or cachexia is to determine the cause, if possible. Interventions are designed to prevent and alleviate the cause when feasible and to treat the signs and symptoms.

Anthropometric measurement — ht, wt, skinfold

The first step in assessment is to determine which patients are at risk. Other components in assessment are obtaining a diet history, including pattern of intake, food preferences, and mealtime routines; determining any contributory factors; and assessing the patient's motivation to eat. Anthropometric measurements (e.g., height, weight, skin fold measurements) should be obtained and albumin and transferrin levels monitored.

levels of albumin + transferrin

Interventions should be simple and easy for the patient. Megestrol acetate administered once a day may be prescribed to stimulate appetite in patients who have cachexia. Consultation with a dietitian, nutritional counseling, and dietary modifications may be used. Enteral and parenteral nutrition may be used to prevent severe nutritional deficiencies.

Patients can be encouraged to do the following:

- Use smaller plates.

- Eat small, frequent meals (six to eight per day).

- Eat favorite foods.

- Eat protein and foods high in calories (e.g., cheese, peanut butter).

- Drink high-protein shakes and eat high-calorie snacks (e.g., ice cream).

- Experiment with new recipes.

- Avoid drinking fluids before and during meals. Fluids are filling and can create a feeling of satiety.

- Avoid fatty foods.

- Increase activity level, which may stimulate appetite.

- Drink a glass of wine, if permitted, to stimulate appetite.

- Monitor and record weight.

- Count calories.

- Use nutritional supplements.

- Marinate meats (e.g., teriyaki sauce, soy sauce, or sweet marinades).

- Experiment with seasonings and different foods.

- Eat foods that are cold or at room temperature; they may be more palatable than hot foods.

- Eat acidic foods, pickled foods, citrus foods, citrus drinks, and lemon to stimulate taste buds.

- Create a conducive environment for eating.

- Eat with family and friends.

- Change settings for mealtime. For example, eat at a friend's house or at a restaurant.

Besides providing emotional support, the nurse should teach patients about the importance of maintaining adequate nutrition, emphasizing ways to make the most of nutrients and calories, especially protein; record their daily food intake; and instruct them on which signs and symptoms to report to caregivers. Education on administration of enteral or parenteral feedings should be provided as needed.

Diarrhea

Diarrhea is the frequent passage of stools of soft or liquid consistency with or without discomfort. Normal bowel function varies tremendously from person to person. The normal pattern may be elimination as often as three times per day or as infrequent as three times per week. The mucosal layer of the gastrointestinal tract is constantly being damaged by the digestion of food, absorption of nutrients, and the passage of stool through the colon. Because the tract is composed of rapidly dividing cells, the mucosa is continually renewed. However, when cancer or cancer treatments interrupt the normal process of renewal, inflammation and edema

↑ motility = ↓ nutrient, electrolytes + H₂O

can occur. As a result, the production of mucus may increase, which increases the motility of contents through the intestines and allows insufficient time for absorption of nutrients, electrolytes, and water. The resultant phenomenon is diarrhea.

The severity of diarrhea is variable and is affected by many factors. It can be severe enough to necessitate a temporary cessation of therapy to allow bowel recovery, and it can be a dose-limiting toxic effect of therapy. Profound diarrhea often leaves patients feeling weak and exhausted. Skin integrity may become compromised, and the perianal area may become painful. Patients may express feelings of embarrassment and disruption of lifestyle.

Causes. Causes of diarrhea include cancer itself (e.g., cancers impinging on the gastrointestinal tract causing obstruction, pancreatic tumors) and cancer treatments. The latter include biotherapy and use of chemotherapeutic agents such as 5-fluorouracil, cytarabine, 5-azacytidine, hydroxyurea, mithramycin, and mitotane. With radiation therapy to the abdomen or pelvis, diarrhea usually begins once 2000 cGy has been administered.

Resections of the gastrointestinal tract can result in dumping syndrome or malabsorption. Patients who have allogeneic bone marrow transplantation may have diarrhea due to the effects of graft-versus-host disease on the gut. Other causes of diarrhea in cancer patients include use of antibiotics, use of supplemental feedings, fecal impaction, increased stress and anxiety, bowel infections (e.g., *Clostridium difficile* infection), and malabsorption.

Signs and Symptoms. The signs and symptoms of diarrhea are loose watery stools, hyperactive bowel sounds, cramping and bloating, flatus, and pain.

Nursing Management. A thorough assessment is necessary to determine the nature and severity of the diarrhea. Assessment of elimination includes evaluating the patient's bowel habits to determine his or her usual pattern of elimination; auscultating bowel sounds; noting onset, duration, character, color, amount, and frequency of diarrhea; determining any precipitating factors and

Bowel sounds

measures used to alleviate them; and inspecting the patient for signs of perianal skin breakdown. Other aspects are assessment of the patient's nutritional status and determination of nutritional needs; assessment of fluid intake, with particular attention to hydration and electrolyte levels (especially potassium); and a review of the patient's dietary and medication history. Patients should be asked about abdominal cramping, abdominal distension, and flatus, and the perirectal area should be examined for erythema, excoriation, and tenderness and pain. Patients' ability to care for themselves, their energy levels (e.g., fatigue) and tolerance, and the impact of diarrhea on their lifestyle should also be assessed.

electrolyte ✱ K⁺

Nursing interventions for patients with diarrhea are designed to promote healing and comfort. Interventions are based on information obtained from the assessment and can include the following:

- Monitor intake and output.

- Monitor electrolyte levels.

- Weigh the patient.

- Maintain an accurate record of episodes of diarrhea.

- Test the stool for occult blood.

- Send stool samples for culture as ordered.

- Gently cleanse the patient's rectal area. Use warm water, rinse well, and pat dry.

- Apply barrier-type creams, ointments, or skin sealants (e.g., A & D Ointment, Soothe and Cool, Bard protective barrier) to protect skin and mucous membranes and promote healing.

- Administer total parenteral nutrition or fluids for hydration as necessary for treatment of severe and persistent diarrhea.

- Apply local anesthetics as needed (e.g., Tucks).

- Administer systemic medications for pain relief as needed.

- Administer antidiarrheals as ordered. Antidiarrheals are usually given every 4–6 hr around the clock or after each liquid bowel movement. The medication should be discontinued within 12 hr once the diarrhea subsides. Examples of antidiarrheals are opium derivatives (e.g., paregoric, tincture of opium), diphenoxylate hydrochloride (Lomotil), and loperamide hydrochloride (Imoduim).

- Support the patient psychologically.

Patients should be encouraged to do the following:

- Eliminate foods that irritate or stimulate the gastrointestinal tract.

- Eat small, frequent meals.

- Eat slowly and chew thoroughly.

- Eat a low-residue diet, which increases absorption and decreases bowel irritation. Low-residue foods include bananas, applesauce, white rice, noodles, broth, bouillon, consomme, gelatin, and white bread. A nutritionist can provide a list of low-residue foods and beverages.

- Avoid milk and milk products.

- Avoid foods that are too hot or too cold. Extreme temperatures may stimulate gastrointestinal activity or aggravate diarrhea.

- Drink at least 3,000 ml of fluid each day. Gatorade; weak, tepid tea; gelatin; caffeine-free drinks; and flat carbonated beverages are usually well tolerated. If the diarrhea is severe, clear liquids may be necessary until the diarrhea resolves.

- Apply heat to the abdomen to relieve cramping.

- Take sitz baths.

- Wear loose-fitting clothes that allow the rectal area to be exposed to air.

- Schedule and use rest periods.

- Engage in relaxed activities.

- Decrease stress, because stress increases gastrointestinal motility.

The frequency, amount, and appearance of stools and the effectiveness of interventions used to control diarrhea should be recorded in the patient's chart. Educational interventions should include discussions with the patient about dietary changes and the importance of good rectal care. Patients should be instructed in the use of sitz baths and asked to report changes in bowel movements.

MYELOSUPPRESSION

Proliferation, differentiation, and functional activation of blood cells are regulated by a complex set of hierarchical steps referred to as the hematopoietic cascade. Hematopoiesis (Figure 8-1) is initiated in the bone marrow. The most primitive blood-forming cells in the bone marrow, the pluripotent stem cells, are capable of self-renewal and give rise to myeloid and lymphoid stem cells. Myeloid stem cells differentiate and give rise to the precursors for thrombocytes, erythrocytes, and leukocytes (e.g., neutrophils, basophils, eosinophils, monocytes). Lymphoid stem cells differentiate and give rise to the precursors for lymphocytes (e.g., T and B lymphocytes). Precursors are the earliest recognizable cells of the various blood cell lineages. Factors that can affect the production of blood cells include infection, bleeding, anemia, certain diseases (e.g., hematologic tumors), and medical treatments (e.g., chemotherapy).

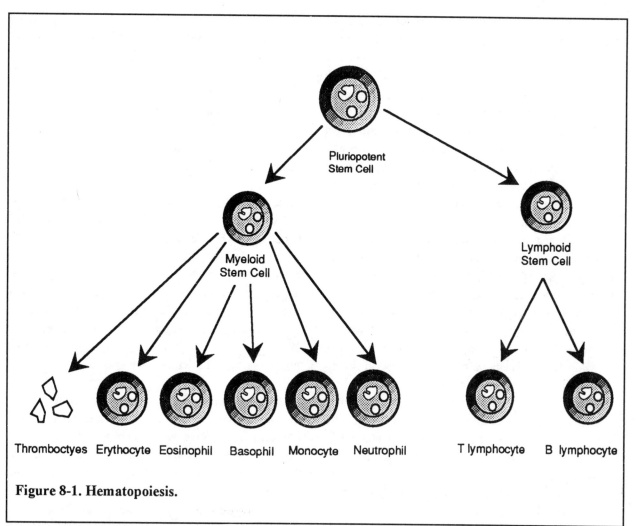

Figure 8-1. Hematopoiesis.

Myelosuppression or bone marrow depression results in a decrease in the number of circulating WBCs (leukocytes), red blood cells (erythrocytes), and platelets (thrombocytes). A variety of reasons account for the occurrence of myelosuppression.

Cancer itself is one cause of myelosuppression. Hematologic tumors (e.g., leukemia, lymphoma) often crowd out normal bone marrow and result in the release of immature blood cells into the circulation. Solid tumors (e.g., breast and lung cancer) that metastasize to the bone marrow can cause replacement of normal marrow cells by cancer cells. Poor nutrition and debilitated health in cancer patients can affect the severity and recovery of bone marrow. Other factors related to cancer include increased sequestration of platelets in the spleen; acute infection; shock; and disseminated intravascular coagulation, which causes increased consumption of platelets.

Chemotherapy and biotherapy that affect rapidly dividing cells can cause bone marrow suppression. The severity of suppression depends on the drug or agent, dose, schedule, and route of administration. Other causes of myelosuppression include radiation therapy that involves a treatment field containing large amounts of bone marrow (e.g., pelvis, sternum, vertebral bodies, craniospinal area) and pharmacologic agents that interfere with the production or function of platelets.

The duration and severity of myelosuppression are influenced by the treatment regimen. The more intensive the therapy, the longer is the period of myelosuppression and recovery. The longer the duration and the depth of myelosuppression, the greater is the risk that a

[handwritten: Normal WBC – 5,000–10,000 cells/mm³]

life-threatening complication such as sepsis will develop. The toxicity of therapy related to myelosuppression is graded according to established criteria on a scale of 0 to 4, with 0 = no toxic effect and 4 = severe toxic effects (Table 8-4). When treatment causes myelosuppression, bone marrow recovery is generally required before additional treatment is given. Prolonged myelosuppression can be a dose-limiting toxic effect resulting in delays, modifications, or cessation of therapy. Prolonged delays of therapy can result in inadequate therapy and recurrence of the cancer.

The signs and symptoms and potential complications associated with myelosuppression depend on the blood cell line affected, the depth of the nadir (maximum point of bone marrow depression), and the length of time until the bone marrow recovers. Most nadirs and the recovery period associated with treatment can be predicted. Nurses should have a basic understanding of hematopoiesis and be familiar with the expected side effects of various cancer treatments and recovery from treatment side effects in order to plan appropriate interventions. Education of patients is the most effective strategy for preventing and minimizing potentially life-threatening complications associated with myelosuppression. Patients and their families should be taught what to observe and report. Written instruction sheets should be used to reinforce teaching.

Neutropenia

The normal WBC count is 5,000–10,000 cells/mm³. A decrease in the total number of circulating leukocytes or WBCs is called leukopenia. Leukopenia can affect humoral and cellular immunity. The leukocytes responsible for fighting infections are called granulocytes. Examples of granulocytes are neutrophils, basophils, and eosinophils. Neutrophils account for the majority of granulocytes and constitute approximately 50–60% of the WBCs. Neutrophils are also called polys, polymorphonuclear cells, and segs.

A patient's ability to fight infections is directly related to the patient's absolute granulocyte count (AGC), which is also referred to as absolute neutrophil count. The AGC is used to determine a patient's risk for infection. When the number of neutrophils is less than

1,500/mm³, the patient is neutropenic and at increased risk for infections. When the AGC is less than 500/mm³ (severe neutropenia), infections can flourish and lead to sepsis.

[handwritten: → or Neutrophils]
[handwritten: AGC <1,500 neutropenic   <500 – severe → sepsis]

The following formula is used to calculate the AGC:

AGC = Total WBC count × %Granulocytes (polys + bands)

For example, the results of Mrs. Smith's complete blood cell count are WBCs = 1,000/mm³, polys = 20%, and bands = 10%. Her AGC is 1,000 × (20% + 10%) = 300.

[handwritten: 30% =]

Neutropenia is the most serious form of myelosuppression. When infection occurs in patients who are neutropenic, the usual manifestations of infection may not be present. For example, in a patient with a decreased WBC count, pus may not form; as a result, a localized infection may be difficult to diagnose.

Signs and symptoms of infection may include fever; redness, tenderness, or pain; malaise; decreased level of alertness; and a nonproductive cough. The most common infections observed in cancer patients are due to Gram-negative bacteria (e.g., *Escherichia coli, Klebsiella, Pseudomonas*). Infections with Gram-positive bacteria (e.g., *Staphylococcus aureus, Staphylococcus epidermidis*) also occur. Fungi such as *Candida* and *Aspergillus* cause the second most common type of infections. Fungal infections are most often observed in patients with severe and prolonged neutropenia. The treatment of choice for systemic fungal infections has been amphotericin B. Although it is an effective agent, many side effects are associated with use of this drug (e.g., hypokalemia, fever, chills, and nephrotoxic effects). Currently, several antifungal agents are being investigated. These include ambisome and amphotericin B lipid complex.

Viral infections in cancer patients may be due to varicella-zoster virus, herpes zoster virus, herpes simplex virus, or cytomegalovirus. Infections caused by herpesviruses are often the most serious of the viral infections. Acyclovir is used for treatment, and in certain situations (e.g., bone marrow transplantation), it is prescribed prophylactically.

[handwritten left margin: Leukocytes fight infect — Neutrophils – 50 60 80% granulocytes – polys/polymorphonuclear & segs]

*[handwritten: *Gram – Bacteria]*

[handwritten: infect – nonprod cough]

Table 8-4
Toxicity Criteria for Myelosuppression

Criteria	Grade				
	0	**1**	**2**	**3**	**4**
White blood cells Total count (cells/mm^3)	^{3}4000	3000-3900	2000-2900	1000-1900	<1000
Neutrophils/bands (cells/mm^3)	^{3}2000	1500-1900	1000-1400	500-900	<500
Lymphocytes (cells/mm^3)	^{3}2000	1500-1900	1000-1400	500-900	<500
Infection	None	Mild	Moderate	Severe	Life-threatening
Hemoglobin (g/dl)	Within normal limits	Normal to 10.0	8-10.0	6.5-7.9	<6.5
Hemorrhage	None	Mild No transfusions	Gross Transfusion 1-2 units per episode	Gross Transfusion 3-4 units per episode	Massive Transfusion >4 units per episode
Platelets (cells/mm^3)	Within normal limits	Normal to 75, 000	50,000-74,999	25,000-49, 999	<25,000

Reprinted from National Institutes of Health. (1994, January). *Protomechanics: A guide to preparing and conducting a clinical research study at the Warren Magnuson Clinical Center* (2nd ed.). Bethesda: Author, p. 86.

The most common protozoal infection in cancer patients is due to *Pneumocystis carinii*. Cancer patients who are receiving treatment that increases their risk for *P. carinii* infection often are given oral Bactrim (trimethoprim and sulfamethoxazole) or aerosolized pentamidine prophylactically.

Common sites of infection are blood, skin, perineal or perianal area, bladder, kidneys, oral cavity, and lungs. Most infections are due to endogenous sources. Often the source of infection cannot be determined. Any patient who is neutropenic in whom a fever develops should be examined for signs of infection. Diagnostic tests should include blood cultures, cultures of specimens obtained from any areas that may be infected, and chest radiographs. Treatment usually consists of broad-spectrum antibiotics, which are administered as soon as possible, usually within 1 hr. The antibiotics chosen depend on the patient's signs and symptoms and institutional guidelines. If a patient remains febrile for 7 days while receiving antibiotics, an antifungal agent such as amphotericin is usually started. Vancomycin is often administered to patients with suspected infections of central venous lines.

Nursing Management. Assessment of patients who are neutropenic includes monitoring their WBC count and AGC, monitoring vital signs, and assessing sites of invasive procedures (e.g., lumbar puncture, venipuncture, intravenous insertion sites, central venous catheters) for evidence of infection. Assessment of dental hygiene is usually completed before therapy begins.

Protective isolation of the patient and the wearing of masks by anyone who entered the patient's room were once the standard for any hospitalized neutropenic patient. However, research has shown that meticulous handwashing before contact with patients is the most effective intervention. Nursing interventions include instituting neutropenia precautions and administering antibiotics and colony-stimulating factor as prescribed.

Patients should be encouraged to take the following precautions to prevent or minimize the risk of infection:

- Practice good handwashing (i.e., meticulous handwashing for at least 15 sec).

- Practice good daily hygiene.

- Have dental prophylaxis as recommended.

- Avoid crowds (e.g., shopping centers and church during peak times).

- Avoid anyone who has an infection.

- Monitor body temperature every 4 hr. Interventions are required if the temperature is 38.5°C or if body temperature is more than 38.0°C three times within a 24-hr period.

- Do not take antipyretics (e.g., aspirin, acetaminophen, ibuprofen).

- Avoid activities that require inserting anything into the rectum (e.g., use of rectal thermometers or suppositories, enemas, rectal intercourse).

- Report signs and symptoms of infection (e.g., fever, cough, sore throat) to a health care provider immediately.

Patients' education should include review of the importance of monitoring body temperature, instructions on the significance of blood counts, information on neutropenic precautions and when to initiate them, and a review of what to report and to whom.

Sepsis. Sepsis is a potentially life-threatening complication associated with neutropenia. It occurs as the result of an overwhelming infection in the blood. Gram-negative organisms are the most common cause. The mortality rate for patients who are septic is high, because sepsis often leads to circulatory failure, inadequate tissue perfusion, and hypotension. The patient's condition, underlying disease, and state of neutropenia (i.e., depth of nadir and point of recovery) influence outcome. Determining which patients are at risk, monitoring of patients at risk, early detection of indications of sepsis, and immediate interventions are important. The risk of sepsis increases with prolonged neutropenia.

Platelets Normal 150,000–350,000

Thrombocytopenia

Platelets play an important role in thrombus formation, blood coagulation, and hemostasis. The normal number of platelets in the blood is 150,000–350,000/mm^3. The average life span of a platelet is 10 days. Thrombocytopenia is a decrease in the number of circulating platelets. This decrease increases the risk of bleeding.

The risk of bleeding increases when the number of platelets is less than 50,000/mm^3. Bleeding can occur spontaneously in patients with platelet counts less than 20,000/mm^3. The risk of life-threatening hemorrhage increases when the platelet count is less than 10,000/mm^3. Intracranial, gastrointestinal, and pulmonary bleeding are of particular concern.

Life-threatening Hemorrhage <10,000

Depending on institutional guidelines, platelet transfusions are started when a patient's platelet count is less than 20,000/mm^3 or less than 10,000/mm^3, unless the patient is bleeding. The threshold for transfusion may be higher for patients with certain diseases (e.g., brain tumors) or for patients with a history of bleeding. Invasive procedures (e.g., lumbar puncture) should not be done if the platelet count is less than 50,000/mm^3. Platelet transfusions may be necessary to raise the platelet count before such procedures are done. Platelet counts are obtained after transfusion to monitor the patient's response to the transfusion.

Signs and Symptoms. Signs and symptoms of thrombocytopenia include petechiae, bruising, gingival bleeding, epistaxis, and ecchymosis. Patients may also have tarry stools, bloody urine, coffee-ground emesis, and hypermenorrhea.

Nursing Management. Assessment of patients with thrombocytopenia includes examining the skin for evidence of increases in petechiae, bruising, and purpura; monitoring blood counts; and assessing patients' bowel habits and pattern of elimination. Possible nursing interventions include the following:

- Institute thrombocytopenia precautions.

- Heme test all body excreta.

- Apply direct pressure to the affected site after venipunctures, fingersticks, and injections.

- Institute measures to decrease constipation (e.g., encourage fluid intake, administer laxatives, encourage roughage in diet).

- Transfuse platelets as prescribed.

Patients of both sexes should be encouraged to do the following:

- Use a soft toothbrush and avoid gingival trauma. Toothettes may be needed.

- Avoid shaving with a straightedge razor. Use electric razors only.

- Apply pressure to areas of bleeding, if possible, for 5 min or until bleeding stops. On sites that continue to ooze, use thrombin (Thrombostat) or absorbable gelatin (Gelfoam) to stop the bleeding. Nose bleeds are common. If bleeding does not stop with direct pressure, the nose may need to be packed. Cocaine-soaked gauze has been used in uncontrolled nose bleeds.

- Avoid excessive or forceful nose blowing. Patients should be taught how to control epistaxis.

- Avoid trauma and falling.

- Do not participate in contact sports, activities with potential for injury, or strenuous activity.

purpura

- Follow a bowel program to prevent constipation. Do not strain when having a bowel movement.

- Do not take over-the-counter medications containing aspirin, which may interfere with platelet function.

- During sexual intercourse, use water-based lubricants to prevent tearing of mucous membranes.

- Avoid rectal intercourse.

- Report signs of bleeding (e.g., gingival bleeding, increased bruising, petechiae, purpura, hypermenorrhea, tarry stools, blood in urine, coffee-ground emesis) to a health care provider immediately.

Women should be encouraged to do the following:

- Avoid using vaginal suppositories and douches.

- If menstruating, do not use tampons, and keep an accurate pad count.

- Report any vaginal bleeding or spotting that occurs between periods.

- If postmenopausal, report immediately any vaginal bleeding.

Patients should be instructed on the significance of blood counts and taught how to examine the skin daily for signs of low platelet count and for bleeding (e.g., presence of petechiae and bruising). In addition, they should be given information about thrombocytopenia precautions, when to initiate the precautions, and what to report and to whom.

Anemia

Red blood cells or erythrocytes carry oxygen to the tissues. Production of these cells is affected by a variety of factors, including diseases and treatment regimens. Anemia occurs as the result of a decrease in the number of circulating erythrocytes and is manifested as decreases in hemoglobin level, hematocrit, and red blood cell count. Dehydration may mask anemia.

Hemorrhage can result in anemia. A rapid drop in the hemoglobin level may indicate hemorrhage. Bleeding can occur anywhere. If no external site of bleeding is detected, the hemorrhage may be internal.

Signs and Symptoms. Signs and symptoms of anemia may include pallor; feeling cold or chilly; headache; dizziness, faintness, or light-headedness; weakness; fatigue; irritability; and becoming easily upset. Patients may also have tachycardia, palpitations, tachypnea, and dyspnea or shortness of breath. When signs and symptoms are severe, activities of daily living are affected. For example, a patient may find it difficult to eat, and walking up stairs may be an effort.

Nursing Management. Assessment of patients with anemia includes monitoring blood counts and vital signs and examining the patients for signs or symptoms of anemia or blood loss (e.g., emesis, melena, epistaxis). Respiratory status and activity tolerance should also be assessed.

Possible nursing interventions include the following:

- Encourage rest periods. Naps may be necessary to conserve energy.

- Encourage quiet activities.

- Determine nadir and anticipated recovery time.

- Transfuse packed red blood cells. The circumstances under which a patient is given a transfusion depend on the signs and symptoms and on the transfusion guidelines established by the institution or organization. Many cancer patients are transfused when their hemoglobin is less than 8 mg/dl or their hematocrit is less than 25.

- For patients who are thrombocytopenic, implement bleeding precautions.

- Encourage a diet high in protein and vitamins (including iron).

Patients should be informed about the significance of blood counts and taught how to examine the skin daily for signs of bleeding. They should know the signs and symptoms of anemia and appropriate interventions, including what to report and to whom. Nurses can also help patients determine ways to conserve energy during episodes of anemia.

CUTANEOUS CHANGES

Skin Reactions

The skin covers the entire body and serves as a barrier against infection. Skin folds are particularly vulnerable to breakdown and the development of infection. These areas include the axilla, tissue under the breast, the groin, and the gluteal fold. Special care should be taken to inspect these areas frequently and to make sure they are cleansed thoroughly each day. Changes in the skin can range from mild (e.g., dryness, slight erythema) to severe (e.g., complete breakdown, sloughing, localized pain). Additionally, rashes or pruritus may develop. The type and degree of skin changes a patient experiences are influenced by many factors, including the patient's underlying disease, treatment regimen, age, and nutritional status.

Types of Skin Reactions. A number of cutaneous reactions have been associated with cancer treatments (Table 8-5). Hyperpigmentation can occur as the result of the administration of chemotherapeutic agents or radiation therapy. Some chemotherapeutic agents (e.g., mechlorethamine, bleomycin, 5-fluorouracil) cause darkening along the veins. Nails can also become hyperpigmented, and their growth may be retarded. There is no treatment for hyperpigmentation. It is generally permanent. Because of the greater amount of melanin in their skin, dark-skinned patients who receive radiation generally have more hyperpigmentation than lighter skinned patients.

Many patients with cancer have photosensitivity, an increased sensitivity to exposure to sunlight. Patients should limit their exposure and be instructed to stay out of the sun whenever possible during the hours of 10 a.m. to 2 p.m., the hottest part of the day. Protective clothing such as long-sleeved garments, pants, and hats that protect the head and face can be worn. Patients should use a sunscreen with an SPF factor of 15 or greater.

Radiation recall is an uncommon side effect that can occur several weeks after radiation therapy. It is precipitated by the administration of chemotherapeutic agents such as doxorubicin, daunorubicin, and dactinomycin. Most treatment regimens involving radiation are designed to minimize the risk of radiation recall. When radiation therapy is required in patients who have spinal cord compression at the time of diagnosis, administration of chemotherapeutic agents associated with radiation recall may be delayed for several weeks.

Radiation recall is confined to the skin and tissue of the area (treatment field) that was irradiated. It often begins as erythema and can develop into blisters and progress to wet desquamation. It causes permanent hyperpigmentation of skin. If radiation recall occurs, patients should be instructed to wear loose-fitting clothing and avoid the use of perfumes and powders. Patients should also avoid exposure to sunlight, which can exacerbate the condition.

Nursing Management. Assessment of the skin in cancer patients who are having cutaneous reactions should include determining the onset of changes, the pattern and location of changes, and the severity of change. The skin should be examined for any signs of breakdown. Factors that aggravate and alleviate signs and symptoms of skin changes should also be assessed.

Nursing interventions for patients with problems in skin integrity should include measures to restore integrity by promoting healing. Patients who have severe skin reactions while receiving radiation therapy usually have their treatments stopped temporarily. Patients should be encouraged to do the following:

- Use mild soaps (e.g., Aveeno, Dove, Neutrogena) to bathe, rinse the skin thoroughly, and pat dry.

Table 8-5
Cutaneous Changes Associated with Cancer Treatment

Biotherapy	Chemotherapy	Radiation
Alopecia (rare)	Alopecia	Alopecia
Dry desquamation	Acne	Photosensitivity
Dry skin	Acral erythema	Radiation recall
Erythema	Delayed wound healing	
Exfoliative dermatitis	Drug extravasation	Acute reactions
Flushing	Hyperpigmentation	Erythema
Rash	Hypersensitivity	Hyperpigmentation
Pruritus	Nail changes	Dry desquamation
Urticaria *wheals*	Photosensitivity	Moist desquamation
	Rash/pruritus	Pruritus
	Transient erythema	
	Urticaria	Chronic reactions
	Vein darkening	Atrophy
		Hyperpigmentation
		Hypopigmentation
		Depigmentation
		Fibrosis
		Telangiectasia
		Ulceration
		Necrosis

Source: Gross, J., & Johnson, L. (Eds.). (1994). *Handbook of oncology nursing.* Boston: Jones and Bartlett, pp. 421-463.

- Avoid hot baths, hot showers, and products containing alcohol, because they may be drying to the skin.

- Avoid using powders and perfumed lotions on the skin.

- Use water-soluble lotions (e.g., Lubriderm, Aquaphor, Soothe and Cool lotion). Patients receiving radiation therapy must remove all lotions before daily treatment. *Ø lotions*

- Avoid scratching the skin. Hydrocortisone 1% cream may be helpful for pruritus.

- Avoid exposure to sunlight, especially between 10 a.m. and 2 p.m.

- Wear protective clothing (e.g., long-sleeved shirts, hats) when exposed to sunlight.

- Apply sunscreen to all exposed areas, especially the face, neck, and ears. Use a sunscreen with an SPF of 15 or greater.

If receiving radiation therapy, avoid temperature extremes (e.g., hot, cold), do not use perfumed lotions on the skin, and do not use tape over the treatment area.

Alopecia

Alopecia, the loss of hair anywhere on the body, can have a profound impact on a patient's body image. Alopecia occurs because the hair follicles are rapidly dividing cells. These cells are affected by the cancer treatment in one of two ways: (1) atrophy of the hair bulb or (2) constriction of the hair shaft and breakage. The degree of hair loss varies from thinning to complete loss. In general, alopecia is temporary; however, in some cases it may be permanent. Regrowth of hair often occurs while the patient is receiving therapy; however, the new hair is fragile and breaks off easily. Many patients report that their hair is a different color, lighter or darker, and has a different texture when it regrows.

Most patients receiving chemotherapy lose their hair completely or experience thinning. The amount of hair loss is affected by the chemotherapeutic agents received, the dosage administered, and the intensity of the therapy. Nurses should inform patients which agents are more likely to cause alopecia. In patients who receive radiation, temporary alopecia develops in the treatment area only. High doses of radiation such as those used to treat brain tumors may cause permanent alopecia. Patients receiving biotherapy may also experience alopecia, although this is a rare occurrence.

Rare ī biotherapy

Nursing Management. Many patients ask about methods to decrease hair loss. Scalp tourniquets or scalp hypothermia (e.g., ice turban) have been used in patients receiving chemotherapy in an attempt to minimize or prevent alopecia. However, the effectiveness and safety of these methods are questionable. The goal of these measures is to minimize alopecia by preventing damage to the hair follicles. This is accomplished by decreasing blood flow to the follicles and thus the amount of drug that reaches the scalp. However, cancer cells may be spared along with the hair follicles. These methods are not recommended for patients with hematologic tumors (e.g., leukemia, lymphoma) or patients with cancers that metastasize to the brain.

hematologic tumors leukemia, lymphoma

The best strategy for preparing patients for alopecia is education. They should be informed about why, how, and when alopecia is likely to occur. Patients should be made aware of the anticipated duration of alopecia. They should be provided with information on head coverings such as wigs, scarves, and hats. Ideally, wigs should be selected before alopecia occurs so that the patient's hair coloring and hair style can be matched. It is important that patients find wigs that make the patients feel good. Most insurance companies pay for wigs for cancer patients. Nurses and other patients can teach the patient how to tie scarves and bandanas in a variety of ways to cover the head. Head coverings serve two purposes: They provide protection for the head, and they generally increase the patient's self-esteem.

In preparing for alopecia, patients should decide what will make them most comfortable as their hair begins to fall out. Because long hair puts tension on the hair follicles and often increases the rate of hair loss, patients with long hair may find cutting their hair shorter helpful. Other patients have found that shaving the head is helpful during the time of rapid hair loss. Patients should be instructed on how to care for their hair once alopecia begins, how to care for the scalp, and how to care for new hair once it appears.

Patients should be encouraged to do the following:

- Use gentle shampoos.

- Use soft brushes and combs with wide teeth.

- Avoid the use of items that are damaging to the hair, such as curling irons, hair dryers, electric curlers, permanents, and hair coloring.

- Minimize trauma to the hair and scalp by avoiding use of items that place tension on the hair, such as hair bows, ponytail holders, and hair clips.

- Protect the scalp from sunburn by applying sunscreen and wearing a protective covering (e.g., hat) when out in the sun.

- Minimize heat loss from the scalp in cold weather by wearing a protective covering such as a scarf or a cap.

- Express concern and feelings related to changes in body image.

PAIN

Pain is one of the cancer-related problems that patients and their families fear. Feelings of pain are subjective and depend on a person's perception and response. Physical, psychologic, and environmental factors influence the perception of pain. Pain can vary from mild to severe and from tolerable to intolerable. Adequate and effective pain relief can be achieved in most cases when pharmacologic and nonpharmacologic interventions are used appropriately. Nurses play a key role in pain relief and should be familiar with concepts of pain management. The clinical practice guidelines on management of cancer pain published by the federal Agency for Health Care Policy and Research are helpful in educating health care workers about concepts of pain management.

Pain has many definitions. For example, McCaffery states that pain is "whatever the patient says it is and exists whenever and wherever he/she says it does." This definition is simple and easy to apply to the clinical situation. It assumes that each patient, not some clinician, is the authority in assessing the patient's level of pain. Nurses should heed both what a patient says about pain and his or her nonverbal behaviors, which can provide additional information.

Types and Causes of Pain in Cancer Patients

Pain due to cancer is often categorized as acute or chronic. Because the pain may have multiple causes, a patient may experience acute and chronic pain simultaneously.

Acute pain has a definite beginning and an end. Thus, its pattern of onset can usually be determined. Acute pain is often associated with physiologic changes (e.g., changes in heart rate or blood pressure) and visible expressions (e.g., facial grimaces, knotted forehead, anxious appearance). Verbal expressions such as crying are common.

Acute pain is often a symptom that prompts patients to seek medical assistance. In cancer patients, acute pain may be due to invasion of the tumor into areas such as bone, bone marrow, and soft tissue or compression by the tumor of nerves in the central or peripheral nervous system. Cancer treatments can cause changes that are painful. These include myalgia or arthralgia related to biotherapy; stomatitis or extravasation related to chemotherapy; skin breakdown, dermatitis, or skin burn related to radiation therapy; and postoperative pain related to resection for staging or resection of tumor. In addition, many procedures associated with cancer treatment (e.g., bone marrow biopsy and aspiration, lumbar punctures, venipunctures, dressing changes) are painful.

Chronic pain has no beginning or end and lasts more than 6 months. Patients learn to adapt to the pain, so generally it is not associated with any physiologic changes or visible expressions. Chronic pain can affect a patient's personality, activities of daily living, and quality of life.

One cause of chronic pain is tumor progression. This includes metastasis to bone and tumor invasion and infiltration of bone, nervous tissue, and other soft-tissue structures. The final or end stages of cancer are painful, and increasing pain may be a sign of tumor progression. Other causes are cancer treatments. Examples of chronic pain due to treatments are peripheral neuropathies associated with chemotherapy; pain of fibrosis and demyelination associated with radiation therapy; phantom limb pain after amputation; and postoperative pain associated with mastectomy and thoracotomy. Cancer patients may also have chronic pain due to other diseases they have, such as arthritis or migraine headaches.

Obstacles to Treatment of Pain

fibrosis

One obstacle to the treatment of pain is lack of knowledge about pain. This includes lack of understanding of the pathophysiology and the causes of pain and the belief that signs and symptoms of pain will be manifested overtly when in reality they often are not. Some caregivers may not know the appropriate drugs, doses, routes, schedules, and use of adjuvant agents. Many patients and their families, and some caregivers, fear addiction and respiratory depression will occur if drugs are used to control pain. Sometimes, knowledge of the side effects of medications and appropriate interventions is inadequate, as is knowledge about nonpharmacologic interventions and their role in managing pain.

Other obstacles are inadequate assessment and evaluation of interventions; inadequate reporting by patients; beliefs that pain is inevitable or is difficult or impossible to control in cancer patients; and sociocultural values, such as the belief that pain must be tolerated. Occasionally, patients decide to stop pain medications because of the side effects of the drugs.

Pain Management

A successful pain management plan incorporates interventions that are easy for the patient, are effective in controlling pain, and have minimal or acceptable side effects that do not interfere with the patient's quality of life. The plan also includes continual reassessment of pain. Depending on the cause of the pain, a combination of pharmacologic and nonpharmacologic interventions may be used. Management of acute pain is directed at the cause of the pain. In contrast, management of chronic pain is often directed at control of signs and symptoms, because the cause may not be detectable. Disease-related pain often decreases as the cancer responds to treatment.

Pharmacologic Interventions. A variety of pharmacologic agents are used to treat pain associated with cancer (Table 8-6). When choosing pharmacologic interventions, the clinician should consider the type, cause, and level of pain. A combination of short, intermediate, and long-acting medications may be necessary to achieve adequate control. Nurses should be familiar with dosing, schedule, duration of action, routes, and side effects.

Titration of opioid doses involves increases of 25–50% over the previous dose. Because patients may experience pain between doses, a plan to provide treatment of breakthrough pain should be considered. The usual rescue dose is 33–50% of the scheduled dose.

For intermittent administration, an around-the-clock schedule is more effective than an as-needed schedule in providing consistent pain relief. Pain medications can be administered by oral, rectal, subcutaneous, intramuscular, intravenous, intraspinal (e.g., intrathecal, epidural), and intraventricular (through an Ommaya reservoir) routes. The route chosen depends on the pain assessment and the determined needs of the patient. Nurses should be familiar with the side effects associated with the pharmacologic agents being administered and the appropriate management of signs and symptoms.

A stepwise approach is used to decide which pharmacologic interventions are appropriate. The goal is effective pain relief. Management begins with nonopioids. Progression through stronger drugs is based on the results of pain assessment and the patient's response. The usual order is (1) nonopioids or nonsteroidal antiinflammatory drugs, (2) nonopioids and weak opioids, (3) moderate-strength opioids, and (4) opioids and others.

Nonopioids and nonsteroidal antiinflammatory drugs are used to treat mild pain and may be beneficial in treatment of bone pain. Their primary effect is on the peripheral nervous system. They do not produce tolerance or dependence. Many have antiinflammatory and antipyretic effects (may mask fevers). The side effects are minimal. All nonsteroidal antiinflammatory drugs except choline magnesium trisalicylate affect platelets, so these drugs may not be appropriate for patients who are thrombocytopenic. Patients may experience gastrointestinal side effects. Nonopioids and nonsteroidal antiinflammatory drugs are combined with opioids to enhance analgesic effect, decrease potential side effects, and provide more effective coverage.

Opioids primarily affect the central nervous system. A wide variety are available, and they can be administered by several different routes. Side effects can be a problem. Respiratory depression is a rare side effect and is

Table 8-6
Pharmacologic Agents for Mnagement of Pain in Cancer Patients

Drug Classification	Pharmacologic Agent
Nonopioids *Acetylated salicylates*	Aspirin (acetylsalicylic acid)
Nonacetylated salicylates	Choline magnesium trisalicylates (Trialisate) Diflunsial (Dolobid) Salsalate (Disalcid, Salsitab)
Para-aminophenol derivatives	Acetaminophen (e.g., Tylenol)
Proprionic acid derivatives	Fenoprofen (Nalfon) Ibuprofen (e.g., Advil, Motrin, Nuprin) Ketoprofen (Orudis) Naproxen (Naprosyn) Naproxen sodium (Anaprox)
Indole acetic acid derivatives	Indomethacin (Indocin) Sulindac (Clinoril) Tolmetin (Tolectin)
Oxicam	Piroxicam (Feldene)
Pyrrolopyrrole	Ketorolac (Toradol)
Opioids (weak)	Codeine Oxycodone + acetaminophen (Percocet, Tylox) Oxycodone + aspirin (Percodan) Propoxyphene hydrochloride (Darvon)
Opioids (strong)	Fentanyl (Sublimaze, Duragesic transdermal) Hydromorphone (Dilaudid,) Levorphanol tartrate (Levo-Dromoran), Methadone (Dolophine), Morphine sulfate (MS Contin, Roxanol), Oxymorphone (Numorphan)
Adjuvant drugs *Anticonvulsants*	Carbamzepine (Tegretol) Clonazepam (Klonopin) Phenytoin (Dilantin)
Tricyclic antidepressants	Amitriptyline (Elavil) Doxepin (Sinequan) Imipramine (Tofranil)
Anxiolytics	Alprazolam (Xanax) Lorazepam (Ativan) Oxazepam (Serax)
Corticosteriods	Dexamethasone (Decadron) Methylprednisolone (Medrol)
Skeletal muscle relaxants	Baclofen (Atrofen, Lioresal) Carisoprodol (Soma) Cyclobenzaprine (Flexeril) Methocarbamol (Robaxin)
Stimulants	Dextroamphetamine (Dexedrine) Methylphenidate (Ritalin)

generally more pronounced in patients who have not been receiving opioids. Tolerance to opioids develops rapidly. Respiratory depression may also occur in patients with severe pain whose opioid doses are increased rapidly. Resting respiratory rates of 8 breaths/min are common. Nurses should assess the pattern and depth of the respirations and intervene according to institutional guidelines. Naloxone (Narcan) is used to reverse opioid-induced respiratory depression or arrest. The drug is diluted (0.4 mg in 10 ml of normal saline) and administered over 2–4 min by intravenous push, with titration to the desired effect. It is important to titrate naloxone to restore respiratory rate yet still maintain the analgesic effect of opioids and prevent withdrawal signs and symptoms.

Some patients experience nausea when receiving opioids; however, it usually resolves within 3–4 days. Use of antiemetics may be helpful but, depending on the agent selected, can increase the sedation. If nausea is related to delayed gastric emptying, low doses of metoclopramide (Reglan) may be helpful. Another gastrointestinal side effect associated with use of opioids is constipation, which does not resolve over time. Therefore, patients receiving opioids should be given stool softeners and laxatives prophylactically.

Urinary retention is a common side effect associated with use of opioids. This problem is more common with some opioids (e.g., morphine) than with others. Sedation may occur with the initial doses of opioids. This is an expected side effect and usually resolves in 3–5 days. Sedation may also occur in patients with severe pain who have rapid increases in the dose of opioid. Patients receiving large doses of opioids may experience sedation due to a variety of reasons. Changes in the dosing schedule and use of stimulants (e.g., caffeine, amphetamines) may be helpful in reducing sedative effects.

Tolerance and physical and psychologic dependence to opioids can develop. Tolerance is an involuntary change in the body that necessitates increasing amounts of medication to achieve pain relief for the same level of pain. In most situations, increasing requirements for pain relievers can be attributed to progression of disease.

Physical dependence (withdrawal) is an involuntary change in the body that is manifested as signs and symptoms of withdrawal when use of an opioid is abruptly discontinued without tapering off. Physical dependence often develops in patients who have been receiving opioids for 3 weeks; however, signs and symptoms of withdrawal have been observed in patients who have been receiving opioids for as few as 6 days. This phenomenon is often confused with addiction. If the use of opioids is slowly tapered off, signs and symptoms of withdrawal are minimal to nonexistent. The signs and symptoms include agitation, irritability, abdominal pain, "gooseflesh," and itching.

Psychological dependence (addiction) is a behavioral pattern in which a patient seeks drugs to relieve signs and symptoms other than pain and for the psychic or euphoric effects gained. Although addiction is a possibility for cancer patients, the occurrence is rare.

Several medications are used as adjuvants in the management of pain. Antidepressants (e.g., amitriptyline [Elavil]) are used to treat sleep disturbances (e.g., insomnia) and to reduce depression. They are also useful in the treatment of neuropathic pain (e.g., neuropathy from herpes zoster) It takes approximately 2 weeks of treatment before a response occurs.

Anticonvulsants are used to increase sleep and decrease neuropathic pain. Phenytoin (Dilantin) and carbamazepine (Tegretol) are examples. Corticosteroids are used to help relieve the pain of rheumatoid diseases during flare-ups in bone pain due to cancer. They are also useful in management of spinal cord compression, increased intracranial pressure, and bone pain. Skeletal muscle relaxants are used for treatment of muscle spasms, anxiolytics are used to decrease anxiety, and stimulants (e.g., methylphenidate [Ritalin] and dextroamphetamine [Dexedrine]) are used to reduce sedative effects.

Nonpharmacologic Interventions. Nonpharmacologic interventions for relief of pain include behavioral interventions, cutaneous stimulation, radiotherapy, and surgery. Examples of behavioral methods are use of distraction, focused breathing, guided imagery, music therapy, positioning, and relaxation. Cutaneous stimulation includes acupressure, acupuncture, massage, use of heat and cold, and transcutaneous electrical nerve stimulation. For the last method, electrodes attached to a battery-operated device are placed on the skin near the painful area. Continuous mild electrical stimulation is provided to interfere with the perception of pain.

Radiation may be administered to the tumor or sites of metastasis to provide relief of pain due to the tumor. Patients may experience relief within 3–4 days of treatment. The primary goal of surgery to relieve pain is palliation. Temporary nerve blocks may be used for diagnostic purposes or for treatment of intractable neuropathic pain. Peripheral neurotomy, rhizotomy, cordotomy, and myelotomy are used in patients with end-stage disease who are experiencing intractable pain that is not controlled with pharmacologic or nonpharmacologic interventions.

Nursing Management. Nurses are responsible for obtaining a comprehensive assessment of patients' pain. A variety of assessment tools are available, such as the McGill pain questionnaire and visual analogue scales. It is imperative that pain be assessed on a systematic and ongoing basis.

The assessment should include determining if a patient has characteristics that may affect pain. For example, does the patient or any member of the patient's family have a history of substance abuse? What is the patient's previous experience with pain? Will the patient's sociocultural values affect the perception or treatment of pain? The characteristics of the pain should be determined. These include the onset, location, duration, intensity or severity, quality, pattern (if a pattern exists, how the pain begins and progresses), frequency, precipitating and aggravating factors, and guarding behaviors and changes in posture. Other factors to be assessed are the effectiveness of interventions used to alleviate signs and symptoms, the patient's coping behaviors, the meaning and perception of pain to the patient, the patient's normal lifestyle and how the pain interferes with the activities of daily living, and the patient's temperament and any changes in mood.

Possible nursing interventions include the following:

- Provide emotional support to the patient.

- Administer medications to treat pain as prescribed. Encourage use of around-the-clock administration for pain not related to procedures. Titrate the medication until the patient experiences pain relief.

- Monitor the patient for side effects related to pharmacologic interventions (e.g., pruritus, sedation, constipation, respiratory depression).

- Encourage patients to use interventions before pain becomes severe. If a patient waits until pain is severe or intolerable, the intervention will take longer to work, and it may be less effective or ineffective.

- Apply heat or cold compresses.

- Use air mattresses and specialty beds (e.g., Clinitron, Flexicare) to promote comfort.

- Reposition the patient. This may alleviate some types of pain.

Patients and their families should be taught about the cause of the patients' pain and its expected duration, if known. They also should receive information about the pain medications, including why, when, and how to take the medications, and about potential side effects associated with pain medications and interventions for treatment. Patients should be encouraged to report side effects. Other components of patients' education are information about nonpharmacologic interventions and instructions on what signs and symptoms should be reported and to whom.

Nurses often act as liaison between patients and physicians regarding pain and the effectiveness of pharmacologic and nonpharmacologic interventions. It may take some time for an intervention to be effective or to find the intervention or interventions that adequately control a patient's pain and minimize the side effects associated with the treatment. It is important to continually assess pain and to keep exploring options for effective pain relief.

BIBLIOGRAPHY

Clark, R., Tyson, L., Gralla, R., & Kris, M. (1989). Antiemetic therapy: Management of chemotherapy induced nausea and vomiting. *Seminars in Oncology Nursing, 5*(2), 53–57.

Foley, G., Fochtman, D., & Mooney, K. (Eds.). (1993). *Nursing care of the child with cancer.* Philadelphia: Saunders.

Foley, K. (1986). The treatment of pain in the patient with cancer. *CA—A Journal for Clinicians, 36,* 194–215.

Goodman, M. (1989). Managing the side effects of chemotherapy. *Seminars in Oncology Nursing, 5*(2), 29–52.

Gross, J., & Johnson, L. (Eds.). (1994). *Handbook of oncology nursing.* Boston: Jones and Bartlett.

Jacox, A., Carr, D., Payne, R., et al. (1994). *Clinical practice guideline number 9: Management of cancer pain* (AHCPR Publication No. 94-0592). Washington, DC: Department of Health and Human Services, Agency for Health Care Policy and Research.

Lindley, C., Dalton, J., & Fields, S. (1990). Narcotic analgesics: Clinical pharmacology and therapeutics. *Cancer Nursing, 13*(1), 28–38.

McCaffery, M., & Beebe, A. (1986). *Pain: Clinical manual for nursing practice.* St. Louis: Mosby.

McCaffery, M., Ferrell, B., O' Neil-Page, E., Lester, M., & Ferrell, B. (1990). Nurses' knowledge of opioid analgesic drugs and psychological dependence. *Cancer Nursing, 13*(1), 21–27.

Otto, S. (Ed.). (1994). *Oncology nursing* (2nd ed). St. Louis: Mosby.

Pizzo, P., & Poplack, D. (Eds.). (1993). *Principles and practice of pediatric oncology.* New York: Lippincott.

Tait, N., & Aisner, J. (1989). Nutritional concerns in cancer patients. *Seminars in Oncology Nursing, 5*(2), 58–62.

STUDY QUESTIONS

Chapter 8

Questions 54–67

54. Mr. Jones has been receiving cancer treatment for approximately 4 months. He arrives at the clinic to begin his next cycle of chemotherapy. His wife informs you he is anxious about his treatment and has had two episodes of vomiting on the way to the clinic. What type of nausea and vomiting is he experiencing?

    a. Acute
    b. Anticipatory
    c. Delayed
    d. Chronic

Questions 55–58: Mrs. Smith, a 45-year-old with breast cancer, received doxorubicin and cyclophosphamide approximately 7 days ago. She has come to the clinic today for blood tests. The results are WBC count = 1500 cells/mm^3, neutrophils = 20%, bands = 10%, hemoglobin = 7.8 g/dl, and platelet count = 75,000 cells/mm^3.

55. What is her absolute granulocyte count (AGC)?

    a. 20%
    b. 10%
    c. 300
    d. 450

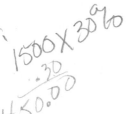

56. On the basis of the results of the blood tests, which of the following interventions would be appropriate for Mrs. Smith?

    a. Admit her to the hospital for monitoring.
    b. Start antibiotics immediately.
    c. Institute neutropenia precautions.
    d. Administer platelets.

57. Mrs. Smith is having difficulty and pain on swallowing. Which of the following is most likely the reason?

    a. Metastasis to the esophagus
    b. Stomatitis
    c. Infection
    d. Local recurrence of tumor

58. Five months later, Mrs. Smith comes to the clinic for a follow-up appointment. She is complaining of leg pain. Workup of the pain indicates she has had a recurrence of her disease and has bone metastasis. Which of the following medications would most likely be used to treat her pain initially?

    a. Nonpioids or nonsteroidal antiinflammatory drugs
    b. Opioids
    c. Opioids and nonsteroidal antiinflammatory drugs
    d. Benzodiazepams

59. Mr. Apple, a patient with an advanced stage of metastatic cancer, is receiving opioids for pain management. He is experiencing insomnia. Which of the following medications most likely would be prescribed to treat his insomnia?

    a. Anticonvulsants
    b. Antidepressants
    c. Anxiolytics
    d. Benzodiazepams

60. Ms. Piggles is experiencing anorexia because of her cancer treatment. Although she knows it is important for her to eat, she informs you she does not have an appetite or a desire to eat. Which of the following recommendations would *not* be appropriate for Ms. Piggles?

    a. Eat small frequent meals.
    b. Eat protein and high-calorie foods.
    c. Eat fatty foods.
    d. Experiment with new recipes.

61. Which of the following statements about alopecia in cancer patients is correct?

    a. Giving chemotherapeutic agents as a continuous infusion over 24 hr decreases the amount of hair lost.
    b. Scalp hyperthermia is an appropriate intervention to prevent alopecia.
    c. Alopecia can be minimized by decreasing the frequency of shampooing.
    d. Shaving the head can be helpful during times of rapid hair loss.

62. Patients with stomatitis who are myelosuppressed and receiving antibiotics are at risk for infections in their oral cavity caused by which of the following organisms?

    a. *Pseudomonas*
    b. *Staphylococcus aureus*
    c. *Candida albicans*
    d. *Pneumocystis carinii*

63. Which of the following statements about the chemoreceptor trigger zone is correct?

    a. It receives impulses from the true vomiting center that lead to vomiting.
    b. It initiates vomiting.
    c. It contains neuroreceptors for dopamine, histamine, and serotonin.
    d. It inhibits vomiting via a feedback mechanism.

64. Which of the following statements about cachexia is correct?

    a. It is characterized by a progressive loss of body weight, fat, and lean muscle mass.
    b. It is observed most often in patients receiving radiation therapy.
    c. It is one of the most common initial indications of cancer.
    d. It is characterized by progressive weight loss only.

65. When or under what circumstances should antidiarrheals be administered to a cancer patient?

    a. Before the patient goes to bed
    b. Every 4–6 hr around-the-clock or after each liquid bowel movement
    c. When abdominal cramping becomes intolerable
    d. Prophylactically to prevent constipation

66. Which of the following is *not* associated with thrombocytopenia?

    a. Petechiae
    b. Amenorrhea
    c. Epistaxis
    d. Bruising

67. Cancer patients who have photosensitivity associated with cancer therapy should be instructed to do which of the following?

   a. Limit their exposure to sunlight, especially between 10 a.m. and 2 p.m.
   b. Use a sunscreen with an SPF of at least 8. *Lens 15*
   c. Stay inside during the day and go outside at night only.
   d. Wear sunglasses.

CHAPTER 9

ONCOLOGIC EMERGENCIES

CHAPTER OBJECTIVE

After completing this chapter, the reader will be able to recognize the signs and symptoms of five types of oncologic emergencies and indicate the primary interventions important for each type.

LEARNING OBJECTIVES

After studying this chapter, the reader will be able to

1. Specify tumors associated with various oncologic emergencies.

2. Specify the underlying pathophysiology of selected oncologic emergencies.

3. Recognize signs and symptoms associated with each kind of oncologic emergency described.

4. Specify interventions appropriate for each oncologic emergency.

INTRODUCTION

In the overall context of oncologic care, most conditions do not meet the definition of a true emergency. At the time of diagnosis, cancer itself is not usually life threatening, and patients are allowed, even encouraged, to consider various treatment options over a reasonable time. Exceptions include acute leukemias, for which rapid initiation of cytotoxic chemotherapy or apheresis to clear the system of huge numbers of circulating white cells would be the usual goal of treatment.

In addition to specific diagnoses, certain conditions exist as a result of an underlying malignant tumor or are related to cancer therapy itself. In many instances, treatment of the underlying tumor resolves the accompanying emergency. Sometimes, however, interventions must deal with the oncologic emergency itself. In any event, clinical decision making must involve not only the manifestation of the immediate condition but also the entire clinical picture of the patient. For a patient with cancer in the terminal stage who is receiving palliative treatment, a frank discussion with optimally the patient, his or her significant others, and the health care team should be held to determine the best course of action, and whether aggressive treatment to resolve the emergency condition is desired by the patient and his or her family.

The following sections describe common oncologic emergencies, including pertinent pathophysiology and signs and symptoms, and present nursing interventions for dealing with such emergencies.

HYPERCALCEMIA OF CANCER

Abnormally high levels of calcium can occur with other metabolic conditions, but cancer is the primary cause of hypercalcemia among hospitalized patients. Hypercalcemia is the most commonly seen metabolic oncologic emergency. It occurs most often with cancers that tend to have bony metastases, although there is no direct correlation between metastases to the bone and high levels of calcium. Hypercalcemia occurs most often in patients with hypernephroma or malignant tumors of the breast, lung, head and neck, or thyroid.

Pathophysiology

Normally, calcium levels are regulated by the parathyroid glands. The glands produce hormones that promote release of calcium from the bones into the circulation when extracellular levels of calcium are low and increase renal excretion of calcium when levels are abnormally high. Bone metastases may directly or indirectly cause osteoclasts to become activated or may cause increased bone resorption. In multiple myeloma, plasma cells produce a substance called osteoclast-activating factor that leads to hypercalcemia.

Hypernephroma and other conditions that affect the kidneys' ability to excrete calcium also cause serum levels of calcium to increase to more than the high-normal level of 11 mg/dl. An additional factor may be an increase in calcium absorption from the gastrointestinal tract, which is also the site of absorption of vitamin D. In women with breast cancer metastatic to bone, use of hormonal therapy may cause increased bone resorption and production of osteolytic prostaglandin by breast cancer cells. Bone pain as well as serum levels of calcium may increase temporarily; prognostically, this effect is an indication that the patient will have a good response to the hormonal manipulation. Head and neck

and lung cancers may cause a pseudostate of hyperparathyroidism that in turn leads to deregulation of calcium levels.

Signs and Symptoms

Except for multiple myeloma and a few other rare conditions, hypercalcemia is usually not the initial indication of a malignant tumor. Early signs and symptoms of hypercalcemia tend to be general and vague. They include anorexia, fatigue, bradycardia, weakness, nausea and vomiting, polydipsia, polyuria, constipation, and some neurologic indications. Later, muscle weakness, hyporeflexia, lethargy, and confusion occur. If left untreated, these can progress to dramatic changes in mental status and level of consciousness, frank coma, seizures, psychosis, heart block and severe arrhythmias, ileus, renal failure, and death.

Because the early signs and symptoms of hypercalcemia are indicative of many other conditions, including normal responses to cancer therapy, care must be taken to assess patients whose clinical features and underlying malignant conditions are suggestive of hypercalcemia. Measurements of the serum levels of calcium and electrolytes and the results of an electrocardiogram should aid in making a diagnosis. Because cancer patients, particularly those with advanced stages of the disease, often have nutritional deficiencies, calculating a corrected serum calcium level, which takes into account serum levels of albumin, may be important: corrected serum calcium level = serum calcium level + (4.0 − serum albumin level) × 0.8.

In addition to a serum level of calcium greater than 11 ml/dl, decreased serum levels of potassium, sodium, and phosphorus; increased levels of blood urea nitrogen and creatinine; and electrocardiographic changes are relevant data in assessing a patient for hypercalcemia.

Interventions

If hypercalcemia is mild, initial therapy may consist of hydration with intravenous normal saline; measures to increase urinary output; and steps, particularly weight-bearing exercise, to maintain or increase the patient's level of mobility. Avoidance of medications (e.g., estrogen therapy, thiazide diuretics) that promote high serum levels of calcium and a decrease in oral intake of calcium are also helpful. If available, effective cancer therapy should be started. Killing or removal of tumor cells will be reflected by gradual decreases in the serum levels of calcium.

For patients in whom hypercalcemia is more pronounced, aggressive therapy may be indicated. Possible options are (1) rapid hydration (more than 250 ml/hr) plus intravenous doses of furosemide and (2) administration of pharmacologic agents that reduce calcium. Drugs prescribed for hypercalcemia of cancer include mithramycin, calcitonin, etidronate, and prednisone; all interfere with bone resorption. Several types of diphosphonates may also be used to inhibit bone resorption and decrease calcium absorption from the intestine. Any hormonal therapy for treatment of the tumor should be discontinued until the hypercalcemia is resolved. Once severe hypercalcemia is controlled, cytotoxic chemotherapy to address the underlying malignant condition may be the next treatment of choice. Some patients may require multiple treatments to correct the calcium imbalance. Long-term therapy, including dialysis, may be necessary for refractory or serious cases of hypercalcemia.

SUPERIOR VENA CAVA SYNDROME

Superior vena cava syndrome is most often associated with lung cancers (75%) and mediastinal lymphomas (10–15%). Certain nonmalignant conditions, including tuberculosis, aneurysm, and thrombus from central venous catheters, can also cause the syndrome. Some patients have a rapid onset of the syndrome, with the classic signs and symptoms. In others, the onset is more gradual, and the signs and symptoms are less dramatic. If the superior vena cava is compressed slowly over time, collateral circulation can develop that compensates for the ongoing compression.

Pathophysiology

As a mechanical, structural problem, the pathophysiology of superior vena cava syndrome is rather straightforward. Because it is a low-pressure vessel surrounded by a variety of anatomic structures, including the trachea, sternum, mediastinum, vertebrae, and other large vessels, the superior vena cava is easily compressed by a mediastinal mass. Because of its critical role in venous return to the heart, compression of this vessel can impair blood return from the head, the upper extremities, and the upper part of the thorax and cause diminished cardiac output.

Signs and Symptoms

The classic signs and symptoms of superior vena cava syndrome are obvious engorgement of the thoracic and neck veins, facial edema, shortness of breath, and confusion or changes in level of consciousness. If collateral circulation has developed, radiologic evaluation may be necessary. If the syndrome is the initial indication of a malignant condition, a tissue biopsy will be necessary to establish the diagnosis and plan the most appropriate intervention. When radiation therapy is the intervention of choice, additional computed tomography, magnetic resonance imaging, or other radiologic studies are done to plan radiation ports. To avoid possible airway obstruction or organ compromise, previous approaches to the syndrome advocated delaying tissue diagnosis until after radiation therapy was begun. More recently, however, doing the biopsy before starting radiation therapy is suggested, for two reasons: (1) the diagnostic value of tissue obtained after radiation therapy is often limited because of necrosis, and (2) if the diagnosis indicates a tumor type that is highly responsive to chemotherapy, this form of therapy may be used rather than radiation as the primary intervention.

Interventions

Previously, superior vena cava syndrome was considered a life-threatening condition for which immediate radiation therapy was the only effective treatment. This situation is still the case when the upper part of the airway is obstructed by edema, cardiac output is severely compromised, lack of venous return causes brain edema, or the patient has non–small-cell lung cancer or certain types of lymphomas. Rapid resolution and relief of signs and symptoms can be obtained within 2 weeks with high doses of radiation therapy, and somewhat less quickly with more conventional doses.

If a histologic diagnosis indicates a tumor (e.g., small-cell lung cancer) for which cytotoxic chemotherapy would likely be rapidly effective, the tumor is widely disseminated, or mediastinal radiation has been used previously, combination chemotherapy is the treatment of choice. In some cases, chemotherapy plus radiation therapy may be used. Persistence or progression of signs and symptoms after therapy begins may be due to tumor necrosis rather than tumor progression. Treatment with corticosteroids may decrease edema associated with cell death due to the intervention. If superior vena cava syndrome is associated with use of a venous access device, the device may be removed and anticoagulant therapy given to dissolve the thrombus compressing the superior vena cava.

Interventions

Nursing interventions in superior vena cava syndrome should be directed at minimizing exacerbation of the syndrome by avoiding invasive procedures, including obtaining blood pressure, in the upper extremities. Raising the head of the patient's bed can ease difficulties with respiration, and explaining interventions to the patient can decrease anxiety and further respiratory compromise. After therapy begins, patients should be assessed carefully for progression of signs and symptoms that could indicate unresponsiveness to therapy or tumor necrosis necessitating use of corticosteroids.

CARDIAC TAMPONADE

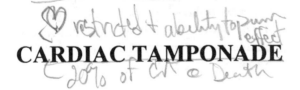

An estimated 20% of cancer patients have tumor involvement of the heart or pericardium at the time of death, either because of tumor extension into adjacent tissue from cancers of the lung or mediastinum or because of metastases from other sites. In cardiac tamponade, the cavity between the two layers of the pericardium fills with malignant pericardial effusions. As intrapericardiac pressure increases, the heart is con-

stricted, and its ability to pump effectively is impaired. Tumor invading the heart tissue or pericarditis due to radiation therapy can have a similar effect on cardiac function.

Pathophysiology

Normally, only about 50 ml of fluid fills the pericardial space between the layers of the pericardium. An increase in the volume of fluid leads to increased intrapericardiac pressure. The pressure compresses the heart, compromising cardiac output, circulation, and the ability of the heart muscle to pump effectively. Increase in intrapericardiac pressure can also be due to direct invasion of cardiac tissue by tumor or to changes in heart function associated with inflammation after radiation therapy. A combination of these factors can increase the severity of tamponade; a small volume of fluid can have a serious effect on cardiac function if tumor invasion or pericarditis is also present. If fluid accumulates gradually, the pericardium may stretch slowly and accommodate the increased volume and pressure. Compensatory tachycardia and peripheral vasoconstriction can occur in an effort to increase cardiac output and blood volume.

Signs and Symptoms

Many patients with tumor involvement of the heart remain asymptomatic. Signs and symptoms of tamponade include dyspnea, tachypnea, tachycardia, cough, hoarseness, retrosternal pain in the chest that increases when the patient is supine, peripheral cyanosis, pulsus paradoxsus, hiccups, and no or weak apical pulse. If impairment of cardiac output becomes severe, reduced urinary output, edema, and decreased cerebral oxygenation resulting in changes in level of consciousness can occur. The diagnostic workup generally includes a chest radiograph; usual findings are mediastinal widening, cardiac enlargement, and hilar adenopathy. An echocardiogram is usually the most accurate test for cardiac tamponade and will show two echoes if this condition is present. Other studies can include computed tomography, electrocardiography, and pericardiocentesis for both cytologic diagnosis and therapeutic management.

Interventions

An emergency pericardiocentesis may be done if a large accumulation of fluid causes severe impairment of cardiac output. Cardiac tamponade can reoccur within 24–48 hr unless reaccumulation of fluid is prevented. Chemicals (e.g., antibiotics or antineoplastics) may be instilled to cause sclerosis: A pericardial catheter is inserted, fluid is drained, and the sclerosing agent is administered. The catheter may be left in place and this process repeated daily for several days if needed.

Surgical approaches to cardiac tamponade may include either formation of a pericardial window to allow draining of fluid or total pericardiectomy, in which the entire pericardial sac is removed. Total pericardiectomy is usually reserved for cardiac tamponade caused by radiation-induced pericarditis. If tumor involvement of the heart is extensive, morbidity and mortality associated with surgical intervention generally exceed the benefits derived. In patients with considerable cardiac metastases, survival is usually limited.

If the tamponade is not a result of previous radiation, radiation therapy may be used if a radiosensitive tumor is the underlying cause of cardiac compromise. Cytotoxic chemotherapy to reduce the size of the tumor may also be given if a fairly rapid response is anticipated. Corticosteroids may be prescribed to reduce the inflammation associated with both tamponade itself and certain procedures, such as pericardial sclerosis, used to treat the tamponade.

COMPRESSION OF THE SPINAL CORD

Unlike many of the other so-called oncologic emergencies for which systemic chemotherapy or interventions with delayed effects may be practical options, compression of the spinal cord is usually a true emergency and requires rapid, definitive therapy. Any serious neurologic deficits, such as paraplegia, that occur are usually permanent. Tumors associated with compression of the spinal cord may originate from breast, prostatic, or lung cancers; multiple myeloma and lymphoma; and primary spinal cord tumors. Locations of tumors that put the patient at risk include epidural, paraspinal, and vertebral.

Pathophysiology

Compression of the spinal cord is usually a mechanical problem. As tumor invades the spinal region from adjacent tissues, or arises from and surrounds the spinal cord itself, increased pressure on the cord and nerve roots develops. Ischemia or hemorrhage caused by this compression can lead to changes in motor, sensory, and autonomic functions. Prolonged or severe compression can cause permanent paralysis. Nonmalignant causes of compression (e.g., herniated disks) can also occur in cancer patients.

Signs and Symptoms

Signs and symptoms of impending compression of the spinal cord vary according to the site of the compression and the severity of the underlying condition. Initially, signs and symptoms may be nonspecific and associated with side effects common to the tumor or to therapies: neck or back pain, loss of sexual functioning, or paresthesias. Other signs and symptoms may be more distinctively neurologic: changes in motor function; progressive, deep back pain; bladder and bowel dysfunction; and loss of sensation for touch, temperature, pain, pressure, and positioning.

A complete physical assessment, including a thorough neurologic examination, will help define the location of the compression and the extent of neurologic impairment. Radiologic studies may include magnetic resonance imaging, computed tomography, myelography, radiography of the spine, and bone scanning. A combination of radiologic techniques may be indicated to determine the exact location of the tumor and the existence or extent of compression of the spinal cord. Magnetic resonance imaging is the procedure of choice for diagnosis of compression. Its specificity, sensitivity, and overall accuracy (about 95%) exceed those of other radiologic techniques in most cases. The primary disadvantage is that patients must lie still for an extended time. If a patient has severe, deep back pain, lying still for so long may be impossible.

Interventions

Once the extent and site or sites of the compression have been determined, a lumbar puncture may be done to obtain a sample of cerebrospinal fluid to ascertain if malignant cells, infection, or other conditions affecting the central nervous system are also present. Immediate consultation with a radiation oncologist and neurosurgeon is required to consider treatment options. If the tumor is radiosensitive, maximum radiation to the spine has not already been given, and the spine is thought to be adequately stable, radiation therapy is started on an emergency basis. Radiation is the primary and most common intervention for spinal cord compression; doses are 30–40 Gy over 2–4 weeks. Recovery of neurologic functioning is usually prompt. However, if neurologic impairment is extensive, including paralysis, prospects for recovery are generally poor.

In cases in which the tumor is known to be radioresistant, maximal doses of radiation have already been given, or the tumor does not respond to radiation therapy, surgery may be an alternative. Decompression of the area by laminectomy often gives prompt, temporary relief, but resection of the tumor is frequently untenable. Consequently, postoperative radiation therapy may be given to relieve signs and symptoms further and to reduce tumor volume. If vertebral bodies have collapsed, surgery may be contraindicated, because it may produce further spinal instability, and alternative approaches should be pursued. If compression of the spinal cord is the initial indication of cancer, laminectomy to relieve compression and simultaneously obtain tissue for pathologic diagnosis is the preferred option. Patients with severe neurologic deficits before therapy rarely show significant improvement after either radiation or surgery.

Pharmacologic interventions may also be appropriate. Corticosteroids can relieve edema and pain, and cytotoxic chemotherapy may be used in addition to radiation therapy or surgery to reduce the size of a tumor. Chemotherapy may be recommended in cases in which the tumor is apt to be responsive to this treatment, such as lymphomas or neuroblastoma. Chemotherapy may be the only option if the patient has previously had radia-

tion (or surgery) at the site of compression or if no response is obtained with primary interventions.

Nurses' role in the evaluation of compression of the spinal cord is critical. A nurse is usually the first health care provider to notice changes in neurologic functioning and to assess changes in patients' neurologic status. Common complaints, including pain, weakness, and changes in bowel and bladder habits, may be the first subtle indications of compression. In the inpatient setting, nurses are responsible for maintaining the stability of the spine and providing feasible approaches to maintain or improve mobility. After treatment of the compression, nurses, often in collaboration with physical therapists or specialists in rehabilitation medicine, are involved in developing strategies to help patients regain loss of function caused by neurologic impairment.

DISSEMINATED INTRAVASCULAR COAGULATION

Coagulation involves a finely maintained balance between the formation and destruction of clot. Alterations in this balance can cause disarray in the coagulation pathways. Several conditions can result, including disseminated intravascular coagulation. Although this disorder is most often associated with acute promyelocytic leukemia, its overall prevalence in cancer patients is approximately 10%. Any patient with cancer may be at risk for disseminated intravascular coagulation, particularly patients who have sepsis, trauma, or transfusion reactions.

Pathophysiology

Intuitively, the pathophysiology underlying disseminated intravascular coagulation appears to be an improbable reversal of the body's regulatory systems: bleeding occurring in response to a massive release of clotting factors. In reality, both formation of thrombus and hemorrhage are occurring simultaneously. The coagulation pathways determine the release of intrinsic clotting factors (factors VIII, IX, XI, and XII) as well as extrinsic factors (factor VII, thromboplastin) to produce prothrombin, thrombin, fibrinogen, and, ultimately, platelet aggregation and formation of a clot.

Stimulation of the coagulation pathways by the underlying tumor or infection results in increased formation and deposition of fibrin clots. The precise mechanism whereby this occurs is unknown. As quickly as coagulation factors are generated, they are also consumed, so coagulation is ineffective. At the same time, however, fibrinolysis is triggered, which breaks down the thrombi formed. By-products (e.g., fibrin degradation products) of this process are not totally cleared from the system. Thus, while clotting factors are accumulating, they are also being disseminated, and they inhibit further formation of platelets. As a result, minor localized bleeding can progress to severe hemorrhaging as disseminated intravascular coagulation continues.

Signs and Symptoms

Patients with acute promyelocytic leukemia should always be considered at risk for disseminated intravascular coagulation, but any cancer patient who has bleeding or thrombi should also be assessed for this condition. In addition to frank bleeding, patients may have bruising, petechiae, hematuria, guaiac-positive stool or emesis, hemoptysis, or other evidence of poor coagulation or blood loss. Laboratory tests indicate blood loss or a dysfunction in coagulation. Platelet count, hemoglobin level, hematocrit, and fibrinogen level are decreased, whereas prothrombin time, partial prothrombin time, thrombin time, and level of fibrin-split products are increased. As disseminated intravascular coagulation becomes more severe, patients may have signs and symptoms indicative of critical blood loss, including tachycardia, dyspnea, changes in level of consciousness, renal failure, and signs of shock.

Interventions

The basic goal in treating disseminated intravascular coagulation is to correct the underlying condition (e.g., chemotherapy for cancer, antibiotics for sepsis). A secondary goal is to address the accompanying signs and symptoms, by giving transfusions of red blood cells and fluid to replace blood loss and transfusions of platelets, fresh frozen plasma, or cryoprecipitate to restore missing or malfunctioning coagulation factors. Plasmapheresis may be done to deplete the circulation of coagulation factors and compounds that stimulate coagulation.

Administration of heparin to interfere with clot formation is a controversial intervention, except in patients with acute promyelocytic leukemia. The rationale for use of heparin is that disrupting the coagulation pathways, which are no longer effectively regulated, will ultimately restore balance to the system. Because the main side effect of heparin is bleeding, its use is contraindicated in patients who have intracranial bleeding or open wounds and immediately after surgery. Monitoring of heparin administration should include measuring the partial thromboplastin time; it should be kept at a level 1.5–2.0 times the normal value. Another drug that may be given with the heparin is ε-aminocaproic acid, which interferes with the breakdown of clots. Because the principal side effect of this drug is clotting, its use in conjunction with heparin may balance coagulation. The effectiveness of pharmacologic interventions may depend on concomitant use of medications, such as antihistamines or digitalis, that can interact with the heparin, so increased doses of heparin may be required.

The signs and symptoms of disseminated intravascular coagulation may be subtle at first or may be common side effects associated with cancer therapy. Therefore, nurses' judgment may be critical in evaluating physical indications and in reporting laboratory data that might usually be considered routine. Minor bleeding, anemia, and thrombocytopenia are prevalent among cancer patients; abnormal formation of thrombus may also be common with certain tumors (e.g., bone cancer, primary brain tumors, and lung cancer). Key roles for nurses are (1) recognition of patients at highest risk for disseminated intravascular coagulation and of patients who have early signs and symptoms of the disorder and (2) careful provision of interventions that address the primary deficits caused by disseminated intravascular coagulation (e.g., loss of blood and fluid).

STUDY QUESTIONS

Chapter 9

Questions 68–76

68. Superior vena cava syndrome is most often associated with which type of tumor?

    a. Breast
    b. Lung
    c. Bone
    d. Blood

69. The classic signs and symptoms of superior vena cava syndrome are:

    a. Bleeding, bone pain, abnormally high serum levels of creatinine
    b. Hyporeflexia, confusion, hypokalemia
    c. Seizures, lethargy, electrocardiographic changes
    d. Facial edema, engorgement of neck veins, confusion

70. Accumulation of fluid in the pericardial cavity can cause which of the following?

    a. Compromised cardiac output
    b. Pleural effusion
    c. Increased metastatic spread of tumor cells
    d. Bleeding

71. What is one possibly effective intervention for cardiac tamponade?

    a. Thoracentesis
    b. Formation of pericardial window
    c. Bronchoscopy
    d. Intravenous fluid therapy

72. The underlying pathophysiology of hypercalcemia of cancer may include:

    a. Bone pain
    b. Ileus
    c. Abnormally high serum levels of albumin
    d. Activation of osteoclasts

73. Nursing interventions in severe hypercalcemia of cancer should focus on:

    a. Reducing milk and milk products in the diet
    b. Increasing weight-bearing exercise
    c. Administering pharmacologic agents that reduce calcium
    d. Giving estrogen therapy

74. Signs and symptoms of compression of the spinal cord include:

    a. Shortness of breath, sternal pain, constipation
    b. Headache, tachycardia, dysrhythmia
    c. Change in motor function, deep back pain, incontinence
    d. Bone pain, hemorrhage, enlargement of thoracic veins

75. What tumor is most often associated with disseminated intravascular coagulation?

    a. Acute promyelocytic leukemia
    b. Chronic myelogenous leukemia
    c. Hepatoma
    d. Breast cancer

76. Signs and symptoms of disseminated intravascular coagulation may include:

   a. Increased levels of fibrinogen, thrombosis, pallor

   b. Decreased prothrombin time, increased urine output, neutropenia

   c. Decreased levels of hemoglobin, increased prothrombin time, petechiae

   d. Renal failure, increased hematocrit, constipation

CHAPTER 10

PSYCHOSOCIAL DIMENSIONS IN CANCER CARE

CHAPTER OBJECTIVE

After completing this chapter, the reader will be able to discuss the individual and family psychosocial dimensions that should be addressed when caring for cancer patients, recognize the importance of cultural differences among patients with cancer, specify the causes of sexual dysfunction associated with cancer and suggest appropriate nursing interventions, indicate issues of survivorship important to cancer patients and their families, and discuss concepts of care for elderly patients with cancer.

LEARNING OBJECTIVES

After studying this chapter, the reader will be able to

1. Specify the three major individual responses to a new diagnosis of cancer or recurrent disease.

2. Indicate nursing interventions for the three major individual responses to a new diagnosis of cancer or recurrent disease.

3. Specify a model of assessment of the family of a patient with cancer.

4. Indicate how acknowledging cultural differences among patients with cancer can improve quality care.

5. Recognize the importance of sexuality in cancer patients' lives.

6. Specify the side effects of chemotherapy that may interfere with a patient's sexual feelings and responses.

7. Recognize the definition of the term survivorship.

8. Indicate issues of survivorship that can effect cancer patients both psychosocially and practically.

9. Specify two myths about elderly patients and cancer.

10. Indicate the importance of cancer screening in the elderly.

INTRODUCTION

Recognition of a mind-body connection is a relatively new phenomenon. Although this connection had been suspected for some time, actual proof came only as recently as the late 19th century. We now know that some illnesses can improve or worsen as a result of a person's "state of mind." Current research has only scratched the surface of this connection, and the full impact of the link has not been explored. Recognition of the psychosocial component of illness is important, not only because of the intertwining of the mind and the body but also because of the outward manifestations this interrelationship can cause. In addition, many psychosocial factors and resulting behaviors are critical to the prevention and early detection of cancer. Recognizing these factors can help in designing educational materials and in targeting a particular group for prevention or detection (Cooper, 1984; Lederberg & Massie, 1993; Lickiss, 1980; McGee, 1993).

Because of the mind-body connection, addressing the psychosocial dimension of the cancer experience without considering the physical dimension is as inappropriate as addressing the physical without considering the psychosocial (Cooper, 1984; Lederberg & Massie, 1993; Lickiss, 1980; Maguire, 1985; McGee, 1993; Pasacretta & Massie, 1990). However, for the purposes of this chapter, the psychosocial aspects are reviewed without fully acknowledging the physical component.

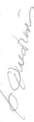

RESPONSES TO CANCER

Intuitively, it makes sense that patients become distressed when they learn that they have cancer or that their cancer has recurred. Although one might think that experiencing distress is a universal phenomenon among all cancer patients, it is not. In one study (Farber, Weinerman, & Kuypers, 1984), the prevalence of distress as a response to a diagnosis of cancer ranged from rare to 90%. Each patient has his or her own history and life

experiences, and these experiences shape the psychosocial dimensions of the patient's responses. This fact should be kept in mind during any assessment: The patient's feelings and perceptions should always be at the center of the assessment.

A diagnosis of diabetes, hypertension, or even cardiac disease does not evoke the same fear as a diagnosis of cancer. What is the reason for this difference? Possible explanations include the way cancer can appear without warning, the difficulty in diagnosing the disease, patients' loss of control over their own bodies, the possibility of no cure, the hopelessness associated with cancer, and the possibility of treatment without predictable response. In addition, patients with cancer are often stigmatized; somehow they are "unclean." Jobs may be lost, discrimination may take place, insurance may be canceled, and readjustment to the workplace or school after diagnosis or treatment may be a difficult challenge.

The results of a thorough psychosocial assessment can help the health care team anticipate problems and smooth a patient's adjustment. Often cancer is a chronic disease, involving complex and extended treatments and requiring frequent visits to the physician's office, the clinic, or the hospital, with no guarantee of response. Because of this, the psychosocial needs of cancer patients do not start and stop with the diagnosis of new or recurrent disease. Assessing a cancer patient's psychosocial health should be an ongoing process.

Patients' Responses

Each patient's response to cancer can be divided into two areas: (1) how the patient responds to distress; that is, whom does he or she seek support from, and (2) the actual responses the patient feels. Some generalities can be made about how a person might cope with the diagnosis of cancer. Most cancer patients have experienced other stressful events, and usually they attempt to cope with the diagnosis by using mechanisms that were successful before. Patients who cannot cope with the distress induced by the diagnosis are likely to seek help from significant others first and then from professionals (McGee, 1993). When help is sought from health care professionals, a thorough assessment can be done, and interventions can be started if necessary. Rarely, patients may have an underlying personality disorder or a history of psychiatric problems. These patients may not have any successful coping skills, and they may decompensate when given the diagnosis (Farber et al., 1984; Lederberg & Massie, 1993; Valente, Saunders, & Cohen, 1994).

Likely responses of patients include anxiety, depression, and hopelessness.

Anxiety. Anxiety can be defined as a vague uneasy feeling, the source of which often is unknown or nonspecific to the person who is experiencing it. Anxiety is a common reaction to the diagnosis of cancer. It is often a recurring response that can be elicited by many stimuli, both internal and external. The degree of anxiety can vary. Mild anxiety and moderate anxiety are defined as an increased level of arousal associated with expectation of a threat (unfocused) to the self or to significant relationships. The differences between mild and moderate anxiety can be seen in the manifesting characteristics. Patients with mild anxiety verbalize feelings of increased arousal and concern, feel restless, and may ask many questions. Patients with moderate anxiety express a feeling of unfocused apprehension and nervousness or concern. They may also express expectations of danger; they may pace; they may have tremors. Their voices may tremble and change in pitch during speech. They may have a narrowing focus of attention, tachycardia, diaphoresis, tachypnea, and sleep and eating disturbances. Mild and moderate anxiety can be very useful. These levels of anxiety can motivate patients to make decisions.

Severe anxiety (panic) shares the same definition as mild and moderate anxiety. However, patients with severe anxiety express a feeling of being unfocused and of having severe dread, apprehension, concern, or nervousness. They may be inappropriately verbal or may not verbalize at all. They may be either extremely agitated or immobile. Physical signs include tachycardia, tachypnea, diaphoresis, increased muscle tension, dilated pupils, and pallor. Patients experiencing this type of anxiety may be in the "fight or flight" mode and can be difficult to communicate with or control. Patients with severe anxiety may be nonfunctional. This level of anxiety is not an effective response, and referral to a psychiatrist or psychologist should be considered (Farber et al., 1984; Lederberg & Massie, 1993; Valente et al., 1994).

Nurses should know the range of anxiety possible and the manifestations of each level of anxiety. A response of anxiety can be viewed as fluid movement. Often patients move between the levels of anxiety, depending on their coping skills. If unable to cope, a patient experiencing mild or moderate anxiety could escalate to severe anxiety. On the other hand, patients experiencing severe (panic) anxiety may be able to de-escalate to mild or moderate anxiety.

Nurses should validate patients' feelings and let the patients know that anxiety is a normal response. Establishing a rapport that allows patients to acknowledge or deny that they feel anxious is also important. Such a rapport will also help patients prioritize the most disturbing responses they are feeling. If a patient wishes to reduce the level of anxiety he or she is experiencing, the nurse can help. The patient can be taught successful coping techniques, such as how to determine what the threat is, how to modify responses by using biofeedback or visualization, and how to channel the responses constructively. In some instances, especially when a patient is experiencing sustained severe anxiety, medication may be necessary.

Depression. Depression is an appropriate response to loss, either an anticipated or a current loss. The loss can be loss of a person (including oneself), or it can be loss of self-esteem, loss of control, or loss of a normal life. Recognizing depression can be difficult. Depression is often intricately woven into a patient's disease process, and it may be complicated to determine what is actually being caused by the disease itself and the treatment the patient is undergoing (Lederberg & Massie, 1993; McGee, 1993; Valente et al., 1994). A distinction should be made, if possible, so that proper treatment can be started. In addition, nurses should be aware that some persons are predisposed to depression. A new diagnosis of cancer may contribute to a patient's depressive nature, or patients may be depressed before any diagnostic workup is done. Distinguishing between these three entities—depression due to disease or treatment versus depression due to predisposition versus depression already present at the time of diagnosis—is important, because treatment of each type can be completely different (Farber et al., 1984; Lederberg & Massie, 1993; Maguire, 1985; Valente et al., 1994).

Depression is a common and normal reaction to the diagnosis of cancer or recurrent illness. According to estimates, up to 25% of hospitalized cancer patients and 20% of adults with cancer have signs and symptoms of depression during the course of their disease (Derogatis, Morrow, Fetting, et al., 1983; Farber et al., 1984; Massie & Holland, 1984; Valente et al., 1994). Patients frequently avoid mentioning depressive signs and symptoms unless asked, and some researchers think that clinically significant depression is underdiagnosed and undertreated (Farber et al., 1984). In one study (Hardman, Maguire, & Crowther, 1989), physicians and nurses recognized clinically significant depression only half of the time. Patients' behavior may be labeled as lazy, attention seeking, manipulative, or noncompliant. Because of the low energy these patients have, they may be unable to perform their activities of daily living or participate in treatment decisions. Behavioral indications of depression include sadness; poor concentration; discouragement; impaired cognitive functioning; perceptual, emotional, and somatic alterations such as anorexia or insomnia; and suicidal thoughts or acts. Depression is also a response that patients can move in and out of over time (Farber et al., 1984; Hardman et al., 1989).

A study (Maguire, 1985) of clinicians' ability to detect psychiatric problems in cancer patients found that oncology nurses and physicians were reluctant to talk in depth to patients with cancer, feeling that such discussions could be harmful or lead to subjects, such as death, that were uncomfortable for the patients. Overall, clinicians lacked confidence in their psychosocial skills or in their ability to answer difficult questions. If this is the case, then the nurse's role is to recognize the signs and symptoms of depression and notify the primary caregiver or make a referral to the psychiatric liaison team.

Depression can also be a side effect of some commonly used medications. These include analgesics, antiinflammatory agents, antihistamines, antihypertensives, antimicrobials (amphotericin), antiparkinsonian agents, hormones (steroids in particular), immunosuppressive agents, tranquilizers, stimulants, antineoplastics (vincristine, vinblastine, procarbazine, L-asparaginase, and interferon), anticonvulsants, and sedatives (Lehne, Moore, Hamilton, & Crosby, 1994). Nurses may be the first to notice the depressive side effects of a medication. If a patient experiences these side effects, and the medication cannot be discontinued, administration of antidepressant medication may be indicated. Other precipitating factors of depression include neurologic, metabolic, nutritional, and endocrine changes, such as abnormal concentrations of sodium, potassium, and calcium; anemia; vitamin deficiency; and adrenal insufficiency.

Patients at high risk for depression include those with a history of depression, alcoholism, advanced stages of cancer, poorly controlled pain, history of substance abuse, physical abuse or self-injury, concurrent illnesses, inadequate social supports, impaired body image, or changed work and family roles. Untreated depression can lower life expectancy and compliance with treatment. Patients experiencing depression also have decreased immune function.

Nurses should refer any patient with a history of depression to another member of the health care team, preferably a psychiatrist or psychologist, for assessment and treatment. Helping patients talk about their feelings of hopelessness, despair, failure, guilt, loss, and anger is useful. Patients should be reassured that these feelings are a normal reaction and that it is okay to discuss the feelings. Nurses can establish a relationship of trust with patients through active listening, use of open-ended questions, and a nonjudgmental attitude. During this period, patients become more vulnerable emotionally. If a nurse cannot deal with these emotions, an immediate referral should be made to someone who can. Because patients are so vulnerable in this situation, it is imperative that their nurses have no agenda. The nurse's role is to help patients describe their feelings. It is important not to put words into a patient's mouth, to let the patient discuss what he or she needs to discuss and not what the nurse thinks the patient should discuss. It is the nurse's responsibility to disseminate information during this time and to correct any misconceptions or misinformation the patient may have. Patients often feel better after discussing things openly and honestly in a safe environment, and often they reappraise their situation (Valente et al., 1994).

Hopelessness. Hopelessness is a subjective state in which a person sees limited or no alternative or personal choices available and cannot mobilize energy on his or her own behalf. This feeling waxes and wanes and may be difficult to detect. Outward manifestations of hopelessness include passivity. Patients may be withdrawn, have a decreased response to stimuli, lack initiative, turn away when someone speaks to them, lose weight because of decreased appetite, and sleep for long times. Nurses can help during this time by fostering supportive relationships. Possible nursing interventions include the following (Valente et al., 1994):

- Encourage the patient's significant others to continue interacting with the patient even though the patient does not appear to wish such interaction.

- Enhance the patient's personal power by giving him or her some control. Let the patient decide when some treatments or activities are to be done.

- Help create a future perspective; talk about future goals.

- Review changes in health status. If treatment is going well, remind the patient that it is.

- Confirm accurate perceptions and correct misconceptions. Correct any misinformation the patient has.

- Include the patient in planning care and in setting goals and schedules.

- Review coping strategies that the patient has used during other stressful times, and encourage the patient to use those strategies for this situation.

Families' Responses

The diagnosis of cancer is given to the patient, but it affects the patient's whole family. Consequently, assessment of a cancer patient's psychosocial needs should include some assessment of the patient's family. Relationships with family members help shape a patient's psychosocial profile (Clark & Gwin, 1993).

One analogy of the effect a diagnosis of cancer has on a family likens the family to a wind chime. Each individual chime is a family member. The wind is the diagnosis of cancer. As the family member who has the cancer is buffeted and recoils from the diagnosis, each of the other family members reacts to the shock wave, sometimes causing another shock wave, which again affects the patient (Wright & Leahey, 1994). In addition, just as the patient's responses to the diagnosis of cancer are influenced by previous life events, so are those of the patient's family.

Many models of family assessment are available. Perhaps the best known is the Calgary Family Assessment Model (Wright & Leahey, 1994; Table 10-1). In this framework, the family is divided into three major categories: structural, developmental, and functional. These are in turn divided into many subcategories, which are divided into subsubcategories. With this model of assessment, the nurse can decide which areas are relevant and need exploring with each family. Not all categories will be used for all families. This flexibility allows the nurse to focus on the areas he or she thinks are important and to ignore other subcategories. The assessment is designed to be completed over time, and not at the first family meeting. It can also be used to assess nontraditional families.

Generally, what family members want most is information. At the beginning, they usually want medical information about the diagnosis and treatment. As the patient's status improves, they may become more concerned with how to obtain insurance and information on job discrimination. If the patient's status deteriorates, information on how to deal with day-to-day demands, home care, and hospice care may be requested. Some information can be disseminated through group sessions, particularly if the information is general enough

Table 10-1
Calgary Family Assessment Model

Category	Subcategory	Subsubcategory
Structural	Internal	Family composition
		Gender
		Rank order
		Subsystem
		Boundary
	External	Extended family
		Larger systems
	Context	Ethnicity
		Race
		Social class
		Religion
	Environment	
Developmental	Stages	
	Tasks	
	Attachments	
Function	Instrumental	Activities of daily living
	Expressive	Emotional, verbal, nonverbal, and circular communication
		Problem solving
		Roles
		Influence
		Beliefs
		Alliances or coalitions

and required by many different family members. Some exchange of information may require individual discussion. In addition, use of audiovisual aids and written material is often helpful. Just as each patient is an individual and needs to have information tailored to meet his or her needs, so it is for the family unit. Not all families require the same information or the same style of delivery of information. Tailoring the information to meet the needs of the family unit is just as important as meeting the needs of an individual patient (Clark & Gwin, 1993).

The Calgary Family Assessment Model incorporates assessment of four different mechanisms of communica-

tion within the family. It is important to have an idea of how family members communicate with one another and with nonmembers. In particular, communication within the family unit and between the family unit and the health care system needs to be open and clear. It is not uncommon during a time of stress for a family's existing communication styles to become strained. A patient may be attempting to deal with all the new information he or she has received and not be capable of meeting the family's needs for communication. The patient may be experiencing anxiety, depression, or hopelessness and be unable to interact with family members, who in turn feel hurt and unable to help a loved one.

Nurses can help in this situation by recognizing areas of strained communication, communication styles that may have been successful before but are no longer working, and possible causes of problems in communications. Suggestions on how to improve communication, including concrete examples, can be helpful. It is not reasonable to expect to totally change a family's way of communicating. It is reasonable to offer new ways of communicating during this period of stress. The goal should be to keep the lines of communication as open as possible, intervening as appropriate. Interventions can include acting as a liaison between a patient and the patient's family, running interference for a patient who cannot communicate with his or her family members but wants certain information provided to them. Other interventions include coaching the patient to communicate, role playing, and referral of family members to other members of the health care team if necessary. Nurses should keep in mind that each member of the family is an individual and may experience all the feelings described in the beginning of this chapter. This in turn can hamper communication. Being able to detect these responses in family members or asking the patient how family members are doing helps nurses recognize ones who need intervention.

Family coping skills are similar to individual coping skills and vary from family to family. Supportive needs differ greatly according to sex, socioeconomic status, and age. Assessing all these factors provides an accurate evaluation. In addition, assessing the family for dysfunction can result in referral for counseling (Clark & Gwin, 1993; Wright & Leahey, 1994).

Once the psychosocial assessment has been completed, the family should also be assessed for practical support issues. For example, does child care need to be addressed so that the patient can keep appointments? Does the family require financial counseling or home management? What about transportation? These issues frequently get overlooked, but they contribute to the stress experienced by the family unit. Offering practical support may be all that the family needs to feel less stress and more normal. During this time, the patient is usually the focus of attention; the family tends to be an afterthought. A complete assessment is one that includes both the patient and the patient's family.

CULTURAL BELIEFS

The United States is indeed a melting pot, and today approximately 25% of its population are people of color, many of whom were not born in this country. This is an important fact for nurses to keep in mind when caring for a non–English-speaking person or one whose culture is different from theirs. Western medicine is exactly that, western, and unless a patient is from North America or Europe, his or her beliefs about medicine and the position that health care professionals hold probably will be much different from the nurse's beliefs.

For example, in some areas of Russia, two sets of charts are kept, one for the patient to see that minimizes the patient's health problems and one for the medical staff that has the real information in it. In these areas, patients are not told the truth about their condition. When someone from one of these areas comes to a clinic in the United States, and health caregivers want to share the truth with him or her, the situation can be difficult. The patient and his or her family members may resist knowing the truth.

In Asian societies, physicians are paternalistic and frequently make decisions for patients. Also, Eastern beliefs of how the body works differ from Western beliefs. These differences must be respected and honored as much as possible. Patients and their families may also have certain beliefs about illness in general and about how to treat an illness. Many persons believe that cancer can be a punishment for past transgressions.

Other differences include cultural and religious beliefs about death and dying. An incident that occurred in the intensive care unit of a major university hospital illustrates these differences (C. Viele, personal communication, 1994). A young Asian man with cancer did not respond to treatment and was eventually transferred to the intensive care unit. When it became apparent that no further intervention would help him, the focus of the health care team turned to palliative measures. Recognizing that the family was new to this country, and that their religious beliefs were not Christian, the primary nurse asked the family about their beliefs regarding death and dying. She found out that persons who died required several things on the journey in the afterlife. They needed to be dressed appropriately for the journey, and they required money (silver coins) to pay the spirits. The silver coins needed to be placed in the dying person's mouth at the moment of death so that he or she could take them on the journey. The nurses in the intensive care unit honored these beliefs. They bathed the patient and dressed him in a suit and tie and, at the moment of death, placed in his mouth the coins supplied by his family. Because these steps were taken, the family members were assured that the son would have a safe journey in the afterlife. Because the nurse took the time to ask about specific beliefs and rituals necessary to complete the process of death, the family only mourned the death of the son; they did not need to be concerned about his soul.

In other cultures and religions, the body is left in place for a period so the soul can return to it before leaving for the afterlife. It may also be unlucky for a patient to die in the family's house. This may mean that the family takes care of the patient at home until the time of death is near. Then the patient is admitted to the hospital or a free-standing hospice.

Some beliefs may be difficult to honor, for example, allowing a body to be left in a room for 8 hr. Others may require only simple acts on the part of the medical and nursing staff. Caregivers will not know what is required unless they ask.

SEXUAL DYSFUNCTION

Humans are sexual beings and need to be able to express the sexual component of their personalities. For many reasons, a patient with cancer may have sexual dysfunction. The tendency, however, is to ignore the sexual parts of patients, to treat patients as if they were asexual. When this is done, no one needs to deal with sexual dysfunction, except the patient and his or her significant other.

Nurses who are uncomfortable discussing sexual problems should, at the least, warn patients about any treatment-related side effects that may interfere with sexual functioning. For example, mucositis is not confined to the mouth; any mucous membrane can be affected, including those of the vagina. This can make sexual intercourse painful. If a woman is not warned, she may think something is abnormal (Lehne et al., 1994). If a nurse is comfortable discussing sexual issues and has a rapport with a patient, then more informative discussions can take place.

Educating patients about sexual issues is important. Patients should be warned that they may experience a decrease in their libido. Side effects of their treatment can interfere with their sexual feelings. Their treatment may leave them feeling nauseated, they may vomit, and often they will feel fatigued. Dispelling misinformation is a vital role nurses can play. For example, some persons may think that cancer is contagious and thus will not want to be intimate with a cancer patient. Treatment can leave patients with an altered body image because of removal of a body part, the tattoos necessary for radiation therapy, or changes in color caused by treatment. Discussing the possibilities with patients before treatment takes place is recommended, so they have time to process the information and ask questions. Offering options to help them continue feeling sexually attractive can be useful. For example, referral to the American Cancer Society's Look Better Feel Good program can help. Giving patients practical information can be helpful. That information can be as simple as informing them where to go to buy a wig or describing different sexual positions (Valente et al., 1994).

Fertility issues also should be discussed as appropriate. Chemotherapy, surgery, and radiation therapy can cause sterility. Sperm banking is a reasonably easy and cheap procedure that should be offered to young men who will be receiving treatment that may leave them sterile. This option should be offered even if the chance of sterilization is small. For women, the option is more labor intensive and expensive. Women's eggs can be harvested through a laparoscopic procedure and stored. The total cost is somewhere around $20,000, compared with approximately $250 for sperm banking.

SURVIVORSHIP

Once a patient has completed treatment, the waiting and watching begin. Patients often experience much anxiety during this time; fear of the unknown is a frequently voiced feeling. A patient is considered cured when he or she remains disease-free for a certain number of years; the exact number depends on the type of tumor. However, cure and survivorship are not necessarily synonymous. The exact moment a patient becomes a survivor is unknown. Some consider that the moment occurs at the time of diagnosis. Patients may live for long periods of time with stable disease, and if asked if they were survivors, they would most likely answer yes. Other patients call themselves survivors after their treatment is complete, before even their first checkup.

Survivorship can be defined as the state of being a survivor, one who *survives,* which means to remain alive and continue to function and manage despite some adverse circumstance or hardship. Survivorship, then, is in the eye of the beholder. Studies (Lederberg & Massie, 1993; Leigh, Boyle, Loescher, & Hoffman, 1993) of long-term survivors of cancer have shown what these patients struggle with on a regular basis. Often, they fear relapse and death and are preoccupied with minor physical problems. When new aches and pains occur, they cannot help but wonder if it is the cancer returning. They may also feel guilty, because they survived while others did not. Feelings of guilt are particularly common in the inpatient setting, where patients may get to know one another for longer periods.

For patients who cannot move past the diagnosis of cancer and its treatment, the future may always remain uncertain. These patients may fear planning for the future, because they are afraid that the cancer will come back. They may need help adjusting to life after cancer and its treatment. They may experience a persistent sense of vulnerability, similar to that felt by someone whose house has been burglarized. The sense of security that was present before the robbery or the cancer is forever gone. Patients may be left with physical reminders of their cancer and its treatment. In addition to the psychologic effects of survivorship, patients may also experience some practical problems, including discrimination by employers or insurance companies or feeling as if they have lost job mobility.

The nurse's role with cancer survivors is to facilitate the transition from being sick to being able to function in society. This does not mean that the nurse is responsible for the transition, but that he or she becomes more of a case manager. Referring patients to the necessary agencies so that the transition can occur can be beneficial. Patients may require occupational or physical therapy or referral to a social worker, legal aid society, or mental health worker. Nurses should be aware of and know how to contact the resources in their communities. One useful resource is the National Coalition of Cancer Survivors. This nonprofit organization offers support groups and counseling and advice about discrimination and financial concerns. It also lobbies Washington on behalf of cancer survivors.

CANCER AND THE ELDERLY

Cancer is a disease of the elderly, and the population of the United States is aging. More than 55% of all cancers occur in persons more than 65 years old, and the incidence increases with age. By the year 2010, the U.S. population will include approximately 39 million persons over the age of 65. Estimates project that by the year 2050, 23% of the population, or nearly 69 million persons, will be older than 65. It is safe to say then that the average nurse will be caring for a fair number of elderly patients who either have cancer or are at risk for cancer.

Cancer in the elderly may be underdiagnosed. Some clinicians may think, If a patient is old anyway, why put him or her through an extensive workup? Or once the cancer is diagnosed, treatment may not be offered, for the same reason. Because of the potential for discrimination, the Oncology Nursing Society wrote a position paper on cancer and the elderly in 1992 (Boyle, Engelking, Blesch, Dodge, Sarna, & Weinrich, 1992). This paper includes the following position statements:

1. It is imperative that oncology nurses recognize personal biases toward aging and the elderly that may interfere with the delivery of quality nursing care.

2. It is imperative that oncology nurses advocate cancer prevention and early detection activities for older adults.

3. It is imperative that oncology nurses acknowledge the dynamic and complex interrelationships between cancer and aging that affect cancer nursing care.

4. It is imperative that oncology nurses intervene to prevent or minimize the unique age-specific sequelae of cancer and its management.

5. It is imperative that oncology nurses integrate comprehensive gerontologic assessment into the nursing care of older adults.

6. It is imperative that oncology nurses assess the availability and capability of the support networks of elderly patients and their significant others.

7. It is imperative that oncology nurses increase communication with colleagues about older adults with cancer to enhance problem solving in a variety of settings and at different points along the cancer continuum.

8. It is imperative that oncology nurses consider age-related factors that affect learning and performance of self-care activities related to the cancer experience.

9. It is imperative that oncology nurses maximize their advocacy role in ethical decision making relative to quality of life of elderly people with cancer.

10. It is imperative that oncology nurses recognize the effects of health care policy on the nursing care of older adults who have or who are at risk for cancer.

The authors of the position paper defined old as 65 years or older. They then qualified this age range, designating the years of 65–74 as young-old, 75–84 as middle-old, and more than 85 as old-old. As one can see, the definition of elderly is ambiguous and somewhat arbitrary. In clinical practice, patients are assessed not only according to age but also by using the Karnofsky Performance Scale (Table 10-2; Karnofsky, Abelmann, Caver, et al., 1948). With this scale, patients are assigned a number that correlates with their ability to be out of bed and carry out their activities of daily living. A patient might be described as a young 70-year-old or an old 60-year-old, or someone might say that a patient appears younger or older than the patient's stated age. Descriptions other than those based on the Karnofsky Performance Scale can be subjective, and age alone should not be the deciding factor in decisions about who should have a thorough workup or receive treatment for cancer.

A radiation oncologist at a university hospital tells the story (D. Larson, personal communication, 1993) of an 85-year-old man who had stage II prostatic cancer and required radiation therapy. After a thorough assessment, the oncologist deemed the patient fit to undergo radiation therapy. The oncologist was chastised by his colleagues, who argued that the patient was too old and would die of natural causes before prostatic cancer would cause any problems. The oncologist goes on to report that the patient completed the course of therapy and now sends him a Christmas card every year. The patient is now 100 years old. This example illustrates how age should not be the only factor when assessing a patient's ability to undergo treatment for cancer. As shown by this anecdote, a patient's performance status is a better indicator of the patient's stamina and reserve than chronologic age.

Table 10-2
Karnofsky Performance Scale

Score (%)	Status
100	Normal, no complaints, no evidence of disease
90	Able to carry on normal activity, minor signs or symptoms of disease
80	Normal activity with effort, some signs or symptoms of disease
70	Cares for self, unable to carry on normal activity or to do active work
60	Occasionally requires assistance, but able to care for most needs
50	Requires considerable assistance and frequent medical care
40	Disabled, requires special care and assistance
30	Severely disabled, hospitalization indicated, although death not imminent
20	Very sick, hospitalization necessary, active supportive treatment necessary
10	Moribund, fatal processes progressing rapidly
0	Dead

BIBLIOGRAPHY

Boyle, D., Engelking, C., Blesch, K., Dodge, J., Sarna, L., & Weinrich, S. (1992). ONS position paper on cancer and aging. *Oncology Nursing Forum, 19*(6):913–933.

Cassileth, B., Lusk, E., & Walsh, W. (1986). Anxiety levels in patients with malignant disease. *Hospice, 2*:57–69.

Clark, J. (1993). Psychosocial responses of the patient. In S. Groenwald, M. Frogge, M. Goodman, & C. Yarbro (Eds.), *Cancer nursing: Principles and practice* (pp. 449–467). Boston: Jones and Bartlett.

Clark, J., & Gwin, R. (1993). Psychosocial responses of the family. In S. Groenwald, M. Frogge, M. Goodman, & C. Yarbro (Eds.), *Cancer nursing: Principles and practice* (pp. 468–483). Boston: Jones and Bartlett.

Cooper, C. (Ed.). (1984). The social psychological precursors to cancer. In *Psychosocial stress and cancer* (pp. 21–33). New York: Wiley.

Derogatis, L., Morrow, G., Fetting, J., et al. (1983). The prevalence of psychiatric disorders among cancer patients. *JAMA, 249*:751–757.

Farber, J., Weinerman, B., & Kuypers, J. (1984). Psychosocial distress in oncology outpatients. *Journal of Psychosocial Oncology, 2*:109–118.

Hardman, A., Maguire, P., & Crowther, D. (1989). The recognition of psychiatric morbidity on a medical oncology ward. *Journal of Psychosomatic Research, 33*(2):235–239.

Karnofsky, D., Abelmann, W., Caver, L., et al. (1948). The use of nitrogen mustards in the palliative treatment of carcinoma. *Cancer, 1*:634–656.

Lederberg, M., & Massie, M. (1993). Psychosocial and ethical issues in the care of cancer patients. In V. DeVita, S. Hellman, & S. Rosenberg (Eds.), *Cancer: Principles and practice of oncology* (pp. 2448–2463). Philadelphia: Lippincott.

Lehne, R., Moore, L., Hamilton, D., & Crosby, L. (1994). *Pharmacology for nursing care* (2nd ed.). Philadelphia: Saunders.

Leigh, S., Boyle, D., Loescher, L., & Hoffman, B. (1993). Psychosocial issues of long-term survival from adult cancer. In S. Groenwald, M. Frogge, M. Goodman, & C. Yarbro (Eds.), *Cancer nursing: Principles and practice* (pp. 484–498). Boston: Jones and Bartlett.

Lickiss, J. (1980). The growing edge: Psychosocial aspects of cancer. *Medical Journal of Australia, 1*:297–302.

Maguire, P. (1985). Improving the detection of psychiatric problems in cancer patients. *Social Science and Medicine, 20*:819–823.

Massie, M., & Holland, J. (1984). Diagnosis and treatment of depression in cancer patients. *Journal of Clinical Psychiatry, 45*:25–29.

McGee, R. (1993). Overview: Psychosocial aspects of cancer. In S. Groenwald, M. Frogge, M. Goodman, & C. Yarbro (Eds.), *Cancer nursing: Principles and practice* (pp. 437–448). Boston: Jones and Bartlett.

Pasacretta, J., & Massie, M. (1990). Nurses' report of psychiatric complication in patients with cancer. *Oncology Nursing Forum, 17*(3):347–353.

Valente, S., Saunders, J., & Cohen, M. (1994). Evaluating depression among patients with cancer. *Cancer Practice, 2*(1):65–71.

Wright, L., & Leahey, M. (1994). *Nurses and families: A guide to family assessment and intervention* (2nd ed.). Philadelphia: F. A. Davis.

CHAPTER 11

BASIC FACTS ABOUT MAJOR CANCERS

CHAPTER OBJECTIVES

After completing this chapter, the reader will be able to the discuss the epidemiology and etiology of the major cancers diagnosed in the United States today and suggest treatment options and specific nursing considerations for patients with these tumors.

LEARNING OBJECTIVES

After studying this chapter, the reader will be able to

1. Specify the two most frequently diagnosed malignant tumors in the United States.

2. Recognize appropriate measures for preventing lung cancer.

3. Indicate the mechanism by which tobacco smoke is thought to cause lung cancer.

4. Indicate three types of cancer associated with use of tobacco.

5. Specify risk factors for various types of cancer.

6. Recognize the components of screening for various types of cancer.

INTRODUCTION

The impact of cancer on the health care system of United States is staggering. The American Cancer Society (ACS) estimates that more than 1.2 million new cases of cancer will be diagnosed in 1995 (Wingo, Tong, & Bolden, 1995). The number of cases in men will be slightly higher than the number in women, and despite detection and treatment, almost half of all patients with newly diagnosed cancer will die of their disease. Cancer researchers are continually looking for better tests to detect tumors earlier, better treatment to control the disease once it has occurred, and ways to prevent cancer all together. Meanwhile, nurses should be familiar with the major cancers that affect the U.S. population.

CANCER OF THE LUNG

Cancer of the lung is the most frequently diagnosed cancer in men and the second most frequently diagnosed cancer in women. It is the second most common cancer in the United States, after prostatic cancer. In 1986, a milestone was reached: At that time, women achieved equality in the realm of cancer mortality, when deaths in women due to lung cancer exceeded deaths due to breast cancer (Bunn, 1992).

Epidemiology. Many epidemiologic studies have established a causal relationship between smoking cigarettes and the development of lung cancer. Up to 85% of all lung cancers could be prevented if cigarette smoking were eliminated (Bunn, 1992; McNaull, 1987). The risk of lung cancer appears to depend on the number of cigarettes smoked. The age at which a person starts smoking and the type of cigarettes smoked also influence the development of lung cancer. In addition, exposure to passive or secondhand smoke increases the risk. The risk is greater for someone who began smoking at age 15 than it is for someone who began smoking at age 25 (Elpern, 1993; Oleske, 1987; *Report of the Surgeon General,* 1986).

Occupational risks are also associated with the development of lung cancer. Persons exposed to asbestos, radon (a naturally occurring inert chemical present in soil and rocks), polycyclic aromatic hydrocarbons, bis ether, chromium, nickel, and inorganic arsenic have an increased incidence of lung cancer (Fraumeni, 1975). Industrial cities have the highest incidence of lung cancer and the highest number of deaths due to this cancer, suggesting that other environmental factors may have an effect.

Etiology. Many etiologic factors influence the development of lung cancer. Lung tumors seem to occur after exposure to substances that promote tissue irritation and inflammation. Generally, these substances are inhaled, either purposefully, as in the case of cigarette smoke, or along with ambient air (Fraumeni, 1975; Schmidt & Shell, 1994).

Despite the causal relationship between cigarette smoke and lung cancer, it is unclear exactly which chemical or chemicals within the smoke are the causative agent or agents. Cigarette smoke contains approximately 3,600 different chemicals, many of which are classified as carcinogens or mutagens (Schmidt & Shell, 1994). Most likely, these chemicals interact with both environmental and genetic factors to promote or cause cancer of the lung. The histologic type of the cancer that develops is also influenced by smoking. Squamous cell cancer and small-cell cancer occur almost exclusively in smokers; the relationship between smoking and carcinomas that arise in the bronchus is less clear cut. Estimates are that 12% of the annual number of deaths due to lung cancer can be attributed to smoking.

Long-term exposure to industrial carcinogens is also associated with an increased risk for lung cancer. Smoking and exposure to these carcinogens have a synergistic effect. The risk for lung cancer is 50 times greater for an asbestos worker who smokes than it is for a smoker who is not exposed to asbestos (Hammond, Selikoff, & Seidman, 1979).

Some research suggests the existence of an inverse relationship between vitamin A and lung cancer. Studies have consistently shown that patients with lung cancer consume a smaller quantity of foods rich in vitamin A or have lower blood levels of retinol or β-carotene than matched controls do (Willett, 1990). It is not clear whether dietary manipulation can influence lung cancer.

Finally, genetic makeup may play a role in the development of lung cancer, especially in younger men and women. Genes are thought to contribute to risk; however, no abnormality has been defined (Sellers, 1990).

Classification. Lung cancers are classified according to the World Health Organization's classification system. The four main categories of malignant tumors are squamous cell carcinoma (epidermoid), small-cell carcinomas (oat cell, intermediate cell, and combined oat cell), adenocarcinoma (acinar, papillary, bronchoalveolar, and mucus-secreting), and large-cell carcinomas (giant cell and clear cell) (Ginsberg, Dris, & Armstrong, 1993).

More and more, evidence indicates that all lung cancers evolve from a stem cell capable of differentiating into all the cells in the respiratory system (Ginsberg et al., 1993). This would explain why a single biopsy specimen often has two or more histologic patterns.

Adenocarcinoma accounts for 40% of all lung cancers in North America. The increase in the annual incidence of this type of tumor may be due to better radiologic detection techniques and the ability to better classify the tumor microscopically. Adenocarcinomas tend to be located on the periphery of the lung and originate from the epithelium or bronchial mucosal glands. They may be manifested as a solitary nodule, multifocal disease, or a rapidly progressing tumor (Ginsberg et al., 1993).

Squamous cell carcinoma often occurs in the proximal parts of the bronchi. The tumor cells tend to exfoliate, so cytologic examination of a sputum sample can be used to make the diagnosis. Squamous cell carcinoma is the second most commonly diagnosed type of lung cancer. Because of its location in the bronchus, the tumor can cause obstruction as it expands locally and intrudes into the bronchial lumen. Squamous cell carcinoma tends to be slow growing, taking up to 4 years to develop from carcinoma in situ to a clinically apparent tumor (Ginsberg et al., 1993).

Large-cell carcinoma is the least common of all lung cancers, accounting for approximately 15% of tumors. The incidence of this tumor type is decreasing, probably because of better histologic classification techniques (Ginsberg et al., 1993).

Small-cell carcinomas are biologically and clinically different from the other types of lung cancer. Hence, a broad division is made between non–small-cell lung cancer (i.e., adenocarcinoma, squamous cell carcinoma, and large-cell carcinoma) and small-cell lung cancer. Small-cell carcinomas account for approximately 18% of all lung cancers and are the most rapidly increasing cell type among lung cancers, especially in women. Epithelial in origin, small-cell carcinomas tend to metastasize both locally and distantly early in the disease. Often, this type of lung cancer arises in the central part of the endobronchus (Inde, Pass, & Glatstein, 1993).

Detection and Diagnosis. Lung cancer may be detected serendipitously when a patient has a chest radiograph obtained during a physical examination for employment or insurance coverage. More often, however, patients with lung cancer have respiratory complaints. These complaints are directly related to the location of the tumor. For example, a patient with small-cell lung cancer in the central part of the bronchus may have cough,

dyspnea, wheezing, hemoptysis, or chest pain or may have signs and symptoms of pneumonia due to obstruction. Patients with an adenocarcinoma, which generally occurs in the peripheral lung fields, may have signs and symptoms of pneumonia, atelectasis, or abscess formation (Sellers, 1990). If the tumor is large, the surrounding structures may be involved, including the pleura, bones, and nerves. In these instances, a patient's first complaint may be rib or shoulder pain or signs and symptoms of a plexopathy. If distant metastases are present, the signs and symptoms may reflect changes in the involved organ.

Routine screening chest radiographs have not been cost-effective in the detection of lung cancer. Diagnosis requires cytologic examination of sputum or histologic examination of a biopsy specimen. If the lesion is peripheral enough, computed tomography–guided fine-needle aspiration may be possible. A centrally located lesion may be accessible through a bronchoscopic procedure, and a biopsy specimen could be obtained by using that procedure. Mediastinoscopy, a more invasive procedure, may be used to obtain a biopsy specimen if the mediastinal lymph nodes are thought to be involved.

Staging. Lung cancers are staged according the TNM system, where T indicates the size of the tumor, N is the status of lymph node involvement, and M is the presence or absence of metastases. Obviously, small tumors, no tumor cells in the lymph nodes, and no evidence of metastases are prognostically better than large tumors, involvement of the lymph nodes, and distant metastases (Elpern, 1993; Ginsberg et al., 1993; Schmidt & Shell, 1994).

Small-cell lung carcinomas are further divided into limited and extensive disease, indicating disease contained within the thorax and distant metastases, respectively. Limited-stage small-cell lung cancer has a better prognosis than extensive-stage disease (Elpern, 1993; Inde et al., 1993; Schmidt & Shell, 1994).

Treatment. Surgery is appropriate treatment for patients with early stages of non–small-cell lung cancer and is the best chance for cure. This group accounts for approximately 25% of all patients with lung cancer. In some patients with later stages of disease, surgery may improve survival, when cure is not possible. Patients with squamous cell cancer have the best survival rates, perhaps because this tumor is detected during the early stages of disease, does not often metastasize, and grows more slowly than other types of tumors. Even with curative surgery, more than 70% of patients have relapses that involve distant metastases. This finding illustrates the inability to detect microscopic disease, which makes accurate staging of lung cancer difficult (Elpern, 1993; Ginsberg et al., 1993; Schmidt & Shell, 1994).

Radiation therapy for non–small-cell lung cancer consists of delivering approximately 60 Gy to the tumor bed over 6–7 weeks without interruption. This may eradicate the cancer but not affect overall survival (Elpern, 1993; Ginsberg et al., 1993; Schmidt & Shell, 1994). Radiation therapy may be indicated as curative treatment in patients whose tumors are inoperable and who have a good performance status. It is also indicated in patients with operable tumors for whom surgery is an increased risk because of age or illness. Preoperative radiation therapy can be used to sterilize a tumor and make an inoperable tumor operable. In this situation, survival is not improved and may be worse than when surgery alone is used for treatment. Postoperative radiation therapy is used to reduce local recurrence of tumor in patients with tumor involvement of mediastinal lymph nodes. Although local recurrence is reduced, survival may not be improved (Elpern, 1993; Ginsberg et al., 1993; Schmidt & Shell, 1994).

Chemotherapy may be used as adjuvant treatment with either radiation therapy or surgery. Non–small-cell lung cancers generally respond poorly to chemotherapy, and, at best, chemotherapy has limited benefits (Elpern, 1993; Ginsberg et al., 1993; Schmidt & Shell, 1994).

Small-cell lung cancer is considered a systemic disease regardless of the findings at diagnosis. Therefore, reliance on local treatment alone (e.g., surgery) for this type of lung cancer is ineffective. Combined techniques are generally used for treatment. If the tumor is small enough to be resected, a surgical procedure is done first and then chemotherapy is used. If the disease is in an advanced stage, chemotherapy can be used first and then radiation therapy to achieve local control. The prognosis for patients with untreated small-cell lung

cancer is poor (9–12 weeks survival). Treatment improves the survival rate, and although cure may not be possible, "buying" the patient some time may be. Among all patients with small-cell lung cancer, a small but consistent group survive long term, some of whom have been cured (Elpern, 1993; Inde et al., 1993; Schmidt & Shell, 1994).

Nursing Considerations. Perhaps nursing's greatest impact on lung cancer is not the care provided to the patient undergoing treatment but the influence nurses have on primary prevention. Smoking has been implicated in up to 40% of all deaths due to cancer and in one-sixth of deaths due to all causes. Decreasing the number of new smokers and helping current smokers quit would dramatically change these statistics. Morbidity and mortality associated with secondhand smoke would also be affected. Working with the ACS, promoting the national Great American Smoke-Out, disseminating information about support groups and smoking-cessation clinics and groups, and providing encouragement to neighbors and friends are all within nurses' spheres of influence.

Nurses also have a role, both professionally and personally, in the early detection of lung cancer. Assessing every patient's risk for lung cancer, educating patients about the signs and symptoms of lung cancer, and providing information on access to health care are all important tasks.

Finally, when caring for patients undergoing treatment, keeping them informed on side effects of treatment and involving them in their own care will help decrease anxiety and increase compliance. Nurses should encourage patients to stop smoking, even when lung cancer is diagnosed. If lung cancer is diagnosed at an early stage and curative therapy is planned, then stopping smoking can reduce the risk of a second lung cancer and of other chronic illnesses such as heart disease. If the disease is in an advanced stage when it is detected, and cure is unlikely, stopping smoking can improve respiratory status and eliminate the risk of exposing family members to secondhand smoke.

BREAST CANCER

According to estimates, cancer of the breast will be diagnosed in approximately 182,000 women and in 1,400 men in 1995. It is the most frequently diagnosed cancer in women, and it will account for 46,000 deaths among women and 240 deaths among men (Shimkin, 1963; Wingo et al., 1995).

Epidemiology. Approximately 70% of all breast cancers are diagnosed in women more than 50 years old. The annual incidence increases with age, and the lifetime risk that breast cancer will develop has been increasing also. In 1963, a woman's lifetime risk was 1 in 18. Today, the lifetime risk is 1 in 9 (ACS, 1993). Rates of breast cancer have increased steadily since 1980 (Boring, Squires, & Tong, 1992). Whether this is due to better screening, an aging population, or the result of more breast cancer is unknown. Although the incidence has increased, the mortality rate has remained unchanged despite earlier detection and new treatments. This is true for all populations. However, among minority populations, the mortality rate has increased. For example, the annual incidence of breast cancer has increased more for African-Americans than for whites, and the mortality rate remains high as well. In addition, breast cancer is diagnosed at a later stage of disease in African-American women than in white women, and African-Americans are 13% less likely than their white counterparts to be alive 5 years after the diagnosis. These findings may be a reflection of decreased access to care for African-Americans because of lower socio-economic status or a lack of information or education (ACS, 1991; Boring, 1992).

Most breast cancers are slow-growing tumors. However, an aggressive form of the disease exists, and, unfortunately, women with this form of the disease do poorly (ACS, 1986; Baquette, Horm, Gibbs, et al., 1991; Freeman, 1989).

Etiology. No single factor has been implicated in the development of breast cancer. Instead, many factors seem to contribute to a woman's cumulative risk. Interpreting and applying these risk factors in clinical practice should be done cautiously. One study (Seidman, Stellman, & Mushinski, 1982) showed that 75% of the breast cancers diagnosed were in women with no identifiable risk factor. So even though these trends exist, they do not account for all breast cancer; the element of chance is still present.

The biggest known risk factor is sex. The simple fact of being female increases a person's risk of breast cancer. A woman's risk that breast cancer will develop is 100 times greater than that of a man (Scanlon, 1991). Age is also considered a risk factor. The incidence of breast cancer is higher in older women than in young women. Cancers of the reproductive system, such as endometrial, ovarian, and breast cancer, increase the risk of subsequent breast cancer. Second primary malignant tumors develop in the contralateral breast in approximately 15% of women who have breast cancer (Callahan, Cropp, Merlo, Liscia, Cappa, & Lidereau, 1992; Garber, 1991; Hale, Lee, & Newman, 1990).

Family history of breast cancer, particularly in a first-degree relative (e.g., mother, sister), multiplies a woman' risk to two to three times the risk of the general population. The risk is even greater if two first-degree relatives have had breast cancer. Both maternal and paternal history are applicable. Genetics alone can account for the development of breast cancer in a few families. Generally, in these women, breast cancer develops at an early age, cancer occurs in both breasts, and often other types of cancers occur also. Although detection of a gene that allows some types of breast cancer to develop is scientifically important and may help determine which family members warrant close follow-up, the clinical significance is not yet apparent. Perhaps when gene therapy becomes more of a reality, this information will be useful (Callahan et al., 1992; Garber, 1991).

Hormones and menstrual history have long been implicated as risk factors. Women who have early onset of menarche (less than 12 years old), have late onset of menopause (more than 55 years old), are nulliparous, or have their first child after age 35 are all at increased risk. Exposure of breast tissue to estrogen seems to be the common thread. The greater the number of years of continuous exposure to endogenous estrogen, the greater is the incidence of breast cancer. The inverse of this is also true; that is, risk is reduced in women who have undergone menopause, either naturally or surgically, before age 45 and have received no hormone replacement therapy (Kelsey & Gammon, 1991).

Obesity has been associated with an increased risk. This is thought to be due to the ability of adipose tissue to produce estrone and estradiol from their precursors, which results in an increase in circulating levels of estrogen (Callahan et al., 1992; Garber, 1991). The relationship between diet and breast cancer has been the subject of many research studies, and as yet the definitive study has not been done. Some research reports that dietary fat plays a role in the development of breast cancer; other studies do not support this finding. The effect of drinking alcohol has also been studied, and again the findings are inconclusive (Mettlin, 1992).

Classification. Breast cancer is a heterogeneous group of several different histologic types. Infiltrating ductal cancer accounts for approximately 75% of all breast cancer and affects women in their early 50s. It may be well differentiated and slow growing or undifferentiated and aggressive. Ten-year survival rates for patients with this type of breast cancer are 50–60%. Invasive lobular cancer occurs in the same age group as infiltrating ductal cancer and accounts for 5–10% of all breast cancers. It is not uncommon for invasive lobular carcinoma to affect both breasts at the same time. Prognosis is similar to that of patients with infiltrating ductal carcinoma.

Tubular carcinoma is relatively uncommon; it accounts for only 2% of all breast cancers. This type of tumor affects women who are more than 55 years old. Because tubular carcinoma is usually calcified, it is easily detected on mammograms at an early stage. Medullary carcinoma accounts for 5–7% of all breast cancers and occurs in women less than 50 years old. It may be present in both breasts at the time of diagnosis. Medullary carcinomas tend to be large and circumscribed (Crane, 1994; Goodman & Chapman, 1993; Harris, Morrow, & Bonadonna, 1993).

Mucinous or colloid carcinoma is an uncommon type of tumor that accounts for only 3% of breast cancers. Bi-

opsy specimens contain large pools of mucin interspersed with small islands of tumor cells.

Detection and Diagnosis. Current ACS recommendations for the early detection of breast cancer include a baseline mammogram between the ages of 35 and 40 years, biannual mammograms from ages 40 to 50, and yearly mammograms thereafter. In addition, each woman should examine her breasts monthly. Studies suggest that compared with women who have not been formally trained, women who have had formalized instruction in breast self-examination and who practice it regularly can detect breast abnormalities more often and when the abnormalities are smaller (Goodman & Chapman, 1993).

If breast cancer is suspected, a biopsy is done to obtain tissue for diagnosis. If the lump is palpable, fine-needle aspiration may be used. If the abnormality is not palpable but is visible on mammograms, fine-needle aspiration may still be used; however, needle localization will be necessary to ensure that the biopsy specimen is obtained from the lesion. For this procedure, the area around the lesion is anesthetized, a double-lumen needle is inserted into the area detected on mammography, and more mammograms are obtained to guarantee accurate placement of the needle. If cytologic examination of a biopsy specimen obtained by fine-needle aspiration does not show any evidence of tumor cells, the possibility of breast cancer cannot be excluded. The patient should have an incisional biopsy for diagnosis. Fine-needle aspiration is the definitive biopsy only if cytologic examination shows tumor cells. If no tumor cells can be detected, another form of biopsy must be done.

Tumor cells in the biopsy specimen are examined microscopically for many different cellular characteristics, including the presence of receptors for estrogen and progesterone. The presence of these receptors is important because it indicates whether the tumor is hormone dependent, which can help determine treatment (Crane, 1994; Goodman & Chapman, 1993; Harris et al., 1993).

Treatment. Once a diagnosis of breast cancer is made, treatment options are explored with the patient. Invasive breast cancer is a systemic disease, whether or not systemic involvement can be detected. This concept guides the options offered to the patient.

The first option, surgical removal of the tumor, is indicated in all but the most advanced stages of breast cancer. The type of procedure used to remove the lesion depends on the size and location of the tumor. Breast conservation surgery (lumpectomy) has the best cosmetic result when the tumor is small (4–5 cm in diameter), is located on the periphery of the breast, and has not spread to axillary lymph nodes. Additionally, the tumor-to-breast ratio influences the cosmetic result. In a modified radical mastectomy, the entire breast is removed, leaving the chest muscles intact. Women whose tumors exceed 5 cm are candidates for modified radical mastectomy. Dissection of axillary lymph nodes is usually done with a modified radical mastectomy.

Radiation therapy is used for local control. It is mandatory in patients who have breast conservation therapy and is useful, even after modified radical mastectomy, in patients who have large tumors. Radiation therapy can also be used palliatively, in the event that metastases are detected. It is especially useful in controlling pain caused by bony metastases, treating brain lesions, and controlling recurrent breast cancer in the chest wall.

Chemotherapy is indicated in several circumstances. First, it can be used as adjuvant treatment, that is, given as treatment even though no evidence of disease can be found. The rationale for this is usually based on historical data, which suggest that untreated tumors will recur. Second, it may be the first line of treatment in patients who have a large tumor or an advanced stage of disease. Sometimes chemotherapy is given before surgery (neoadjuvantly) in the hope that it will reduce the size of the tumor enough to make a surgical resection possible. If a patient has distant metastases, chemotherapy can also be useful, especially in patients who have not previously received chemotherapy. Many different agents are effective against breast cancer. The most common ones are doxorubicin (Adriamycin), cyclophosphamide (Cytoxan), methotrexate (Mexate), and 5-fluorouracil (5-FU, Fluracil). Recently, an agent used to treat ovarian cancer was approved for the treatment of advanced stages of breast cancer unresponsive to standard therapy. That agent is paclitaxel (Taxol). Research

studies are currently under way to determine the effectiveness of new chemotherapeutic agents. Bone marrow transplantation is also being investigated as a therapeutic option for women with breast cancer (Crane, 1994; Goodman & Chapman, 1993; Harris et al., 1993).

Patients with tumors that have receptors for estrogen may be given oral tamoxifen (Novaldex) at a dosage of 10 mg twice a day. This drug is particularly useful in postmenopausal women with breast cancer. Tamoxifen is an estrogen antagonist. It is thought to block the estrogen receptors of the tumor cells, thereby limiting the cells' exposure to estrogen and retarding tumor growth. It may also be given to premenopausal women undergoing chemotherapy.

Prognosis. Lymph node involvement has long been an indicator of overall prognosis in breast cancer. The more axillary lymph nodes that contain tumor cells, the poorer is the prognosis. However, in one large study, even women with no lymph node involvement still had a 25% recurrence rate at 5 years. The 5-year recurrence rates according to number of lymph nodes involved were 40% for 1–3 nodes, 49% for 4–6 nodes, 58% for 7–9 nodes, and 78% for 10 or more nodes.

Tumor size also has some predictive value for mortality. More than 99% of women with tumors less than 0.5 cm in diameter were alive 5 years after diagnosis. Chances of surviving 5 years were 80% if the tumor was 2–5 cm in diameter and 50–60% if it was more than 5 cm in diameter (Goodman & Chapman, 1993; Harris et al., 1993).

Nursing Considerations. Nurses' most important functions with regard to breast cancer are educating women and disseminating information about the disease. The benefits of teaching all women how to perform monthly breast self-examinations and reinforcing the need for regular mammograms cannot be overstated. Early detection is the key to cure.

Women who have had a modified radical mastectomy may wish to have breast reconstruction surgery. In some patients, the breast is reconstructed at the time of the mastectomy, by using adipose tissue from the abdomen. For other women, reconstruction is done after therapy is

HtN 40% oral/larynx 25

complete. Nurses perform a great service when they inform patients about these procedures. Women who have had reconstructive surgery should be reminded to include the reconstructed breast when they do breast self-examination.

Lymphedema can be a problem for women who have had axillary lymph nodes removed. Because the architecture of the lymphatic system is altered, drainage of lymph is not as efficient as before, and swelling of the arm on the side of the dissection can occur. This swelling can be painful, limit range of motion, and cause embarrassment. Treatment of lymphedema is difficult. Exercise and compression sleeves produce some results, but generally this complication is a chronic problem. Support groups are available for patients with this side effect, and a national lymphedema network offers support and services.

HEAD AND NECK
CANCER

Cancer of the head and neck can be a visible disabling disease. In Western society, the face is how a person presents himself or herself to the world. Persons with scars or acne often are obsessed about these blemishes when the abnormalities occur on the face. The impact of having cancer in the same area can be devastating (Parzuchowski, 1994).

Epidemiology. Cancer of the head and neck accounts for 5% of all tumors in humans. This type of cancer occurs mostly in men; the male-to-female ratio is 3:1. Age at onset is 40–70 years, and the annual incidence increases as age increases. The overall yearly incidence for the U.S. population is approximately 17 per 100,000 persons. This increases to 45 per 100,000 for persons 50–70 years old, 70 per 100,000 for those 71–80 years old, and 100 per 100,000 for those more than 80 years old (Bildstein, 1993; Parzuchowski, 1994; Schantz, Harrison, & Hong, 1993).

Most head and neck tumors (40%) occur in the oral cavity. Other sites, in order, are the larynx (25%), the orohypopharynx (15%), major salivary gland (7%), and all other locations (13%). Most patients (more than 60%) have locally advanced disease at the time of diagnosis.

Etiology. Constant exposure to carcinogens is the probable cause of head and neck cancer. Tobacco use is the primary risk factor, either through smoking or by using smokeless tobacco. Use of alcohol and tobacco appears to have a synergistic effect. The incidence of head and neck cancer associated with the use of alcohol and tobacco together exceeds the sum of the incidences associated with the use of either alone (Bildstein, 1993; Schantz et al., 1993).

Some research also suggests that persons exposed to wood, metal, leather, or textile dust have a higher incidence of cancer of the head and neck than persons not exposed to these materials. Cancer also may develop in areas of mechanical irritation within the mouth, particularly areas of irritation due to poorly fitting dentures. Infection with Epstein-Barr virus has long been associated with nasopharyngeal cancer, although the exact mechanism is unknown (Bildstein, 1993; Schantz et al., 1993).

Genetic predisposition is also suspected to be a factor. Researchers have detected a specific HLA profile in Cantonese patients with this type of cancer (Bildstein, 1993). Finally, nutritional deficiencies may play a role, particularly deficiencies in iron, vitamin A, and retinoids (Bildstein, 1993; Schantz et al., 1993).

Classification. Head and neck tumors are staged according to the TNM staging system. The system varies however, for each specific type of tumor.

95% HANal squamous cell epi

As mentioned previously, 95% of all head and neck tumors are squamous cell carcinomas that arise from the epithelium, either the mucosa or the submucosa. Invasion usually occurs through local extension along tissue planes or nerves. Bone invasion is a late manifestation of the disease and occurs through a preexisting anatomic opening. Perineural and lymphatic spread is the doorway to distant metastases. Local and regional lymph nodes are typically involved by the time the patient seeks medical attention. Prognosis depends on the number of lymph nodes involved, the degree of involvement of those nodes, and whether the tumor has spread to soft tissues. Prognosis is poor for patients with involvement of the lower neck; 5-year survival rates are decreased in these patients (Bildstein, 1993; Parzuchowski, 1994; Schantz et al., 1993).

In approximately 30% of patients with head or neck cancer, a second primary tumor develops within 3 years after diagnosis of the original tumor. Typically, the second tumor is a squamous cell cancer of the lung. Regular follow-up is essential (Bildstein, 1993; Schantz et al., 1993).

Detection and Diagnosis. Generally, patients with head or neck cancer notice either an enlarging lesion located with in the oral cavity or have a sore or ulcer that will not heal. Many cancers of the head and neck are detected by dentists during routine oral examinations. If the tumor is locally advanced, the patient may have dysphagia, odynophagia (pain on swallowing), obstruction of one side of the nose, lymphadenopathy in the cervical or supraclavicular region, or persistent hoarseness.

Diagnosis is based on the results of biopsy, usually an incisional biopsy. This can be done with either local anesthesia or, if the lesion is not readily accessible, general anesthesia.

Treatment. Treatment of head or neck cancer, regardless of the site, requires a multidisciplinary approach. Treatment may mean the loss of physiologic function of the affected area or gross disfigurement or both. The physical and emotional impact on the patient is best dealt with in a team approach.

For most early-stage tumors, surgery or radiation therapy is equally effective. However, most tumors are not early stage at the time of diagnosis. For these tumors, combined therapy is indicated. If extensive surgery is required, reconstruction offers hope of restoring a cosmetically appealing and functional face (Bildstein, 1993).

Chemotherapy may be used before surgery to reduce the size of the tumor and perhaps limit the amount of surgery necessary to remove it. Drug delivery to the tumor is better when chemotherapy is given before either surgery or radiation therapy, because the vessels of the tumor are intact (Bildstein, 1993; Schantz et al., 1993).

Radiation therapy offers many different treatment options. In addition to external-beam radiation, implants have been useful, and hyperthermia has also gained acceptance. In some institutions, intraoperative radiation therapy may be available (Bildstein, 1993; Parzuchowski, 1994; Schantz et al., 1993).

Combined therapy can mean concomitant radiation therapy and chemotherapy, surgery and radiation therapy, or surgery and chemotherapy. All are used to improve responses and prolong disease-free survival in the event that curative therapy is not available (Bildstein, 1993; Schantz et al., 1993).

Nursing Considerations. Primary intervention to prevent head and neck cancer is encouraging patients to stop smoking and to limit alcohol intake. Once a diagnosis has been made and treatment has begun, nursing considerations include educating the patient about the treatment and its side effects, managing the patient's airway, and monitoring the patient for signs and symptoms of adverse effects of therapy. In addition, depending on the extent of surgery, patients may need rehabilitation to relearn how to swallow or speak or both. The psychosocial issues in patients with head and neck cancer can be overwhelming. Referral to a social worker or other member of the health care team is appropriate if a nurse encounters a problem he or she cannot deal with.

GASTROINTESTINAL CANCERS

Gastrointestinal cancers are tumors that occur anywhere along the gastrointestinal tract, including the pancreas, gall bladder, stomach, and colon. This section reviews stomach and colon cancers only.

Stomach Cancer

Epidemiology. The annual incidence of stomach cancers is declining in some parts of the world and increasing in others. In the United States, it has been declining steadily since the 1930s, when stomach cancer was the leading cause of death.

Japan has the highest incidence of stomach cancer in the world, and this disease is a major cause of death for Japanese people. In the United States, only 22,800 new cases are expected to be diagnosed in 1995. More cases occur in men than in women, and ethnic minorities within the United States have a higher incidence (especially African-Americans, Japanese, and Chinese) than non-Hispanic whites. Incidence varies considerably among native Hawaiians, Native Americans of New Mexico, and Hispanic Americans (Alexander, Kelsen, & Tepper, 1993; Daniel, 1994; Frogge, 1993; Wingo et al., 1995).

Etiology. Among immigrants to the United States, risk for stomach cancer remains the same as that in their country of origin, suggesting that genetics may contribute to the development of this disease. Increased risk is also associated with eating pickled, highly salted food; nitrites; and processed foods and with drinking water from certain areas. One hypothesis is that since the advent of refrigeration and an increase in the amount of ascorbic acid consumed, formation of nitrates has decreased, resulting in a decreased incidence of stomach cancer (Alexander et al., 1993; Daniel, 1994; Frogge, 1993). ↑ amt of ascorbic acid consumed

Other risk factors include lower socioeconomic status, poor nutritional habits, vitamin A deficiency, family history of stomach cancer, pernicious anemia, achlorhydria, chronic gastritis, gastric polyps, and benign peptic ulcer disease. In addition, coal miners, nickel refiners, timber and rubber processors, and asbestos workers all have higher rates of stomach cancer than the general public does (Alexander et al., 1993; Daniel, 1994; Frogge, 1993).

Classification. More than 90% of stomach cancers are adenocarcinoma. Most often the tumor is located in the antrum. The second most common site is the lesser curvature of the stomach. Lesions in the greater curvature occur less often (Daniel, 1994; Frogge, 1993).

Detection and Diagnosis. Vague gastrointestinal complaints in patients with undiagnosed stomach cancer are common. As the disease progresses, patients may experience signs and symptoms of ulceration, hemorrhage, obstruction, and distant metastases. Tumors of the stomach metastasize by direct extension and infiltration into the surrounding mucosal surface, stomach wall, vasculature, and lymphatic system. Vascular embolism and local invasion of the lymphatic system lead to involvement of regional lymph nodes and distant metastases. As the tumor grows, direct extension into the liver, pancreas, and esophagus also occurs (Daniel, 1994; Frogge, 1993).

The pattern of spread depends on the size and location of the tumor. Because the signs and symptoms can be vague, several months may pass between their onset and the time the patient seeks medical intervention. Pain in the epigastric area, back, or retrosternal area is often ignored and rationalized as a pulled muscle. Sensations of early satiety, distension after meals, and a feeling of fullness or heaviness may prompt a visit to a physician. In the late stages of disease and as the cancer progresses, patients may experience weight loss, nausea, vomiting, fatigue, anemia, dysphagia, hematemesis, melena, and a change in bowel habits. These signs and symptoms almost always prompt medical consultation. Unfortunately, these are all signs and symptoms of advanced disease (Alexander et al., 1993; Daniel, 1994; Frogge, 1993).

Unless an epigastric or an abdominal mass is palpable, further testing is necessary to determine the cause of the patient's signs and symptoms. Examination of the upper part of the gastrointestinal tract (barium swallow), endoscopic sonography, and computed tomography can be used to delineate the abnormality and are helpful in determining the nature and extent of the disease. However, a definitive diagnosis requires examination of a biopsy specimen. Obtaining the specimen usually entails endoscopy or a surgical procedure.

Staging. Tumors involving the stomach are staged according the TNM system.

satiety

Treatment. Once the tumor is staged, a treatment plan can be designed. In approximately 50% of patients, stomach cancer is localized, and the focus is on curative treatment. *50% curative*

Surgery is the treatment of choice for patients who have localized disease and for whom a cure is possible. The surgical procedure is tailored to the size and location of the tumor but may be either a total or a subtotal gastrectomy. If cure is not possible, surgery may still be recommended for palliation of pain or obstruction.

Although stomach cancer tends to be radiosensitive, its location deep within the abdomen makes the morbidity associated with treatment intolerable for most patients. Radiation therapy is difficult in patients with this type of tumor. It does have a role in the treatment of locally advanced or recurrent disease, when the treatment field can be more focused and few other organs affected (Alexander, Kelsen, & Tepper, 1993; Daniel, 1994; Frogge, 1993).

Chemotherapy has been used in the treatment of stomach cancer with variable results. Many different combinations of agents have been tried, with responses ranging from 20% to 50%. However, the response rarely lasts, and the morbidity associated with chemotherapy may not be tolerable to the patient. No one regimen has proven effectiveness (Alexander et al., 1993; Daniel, 1994; Frogge, 1993).

Nursing Considerations. Nutrition is compromised in patients with stomach cancer, either because of the cancer itself or as a result of the treatment. Patients who have had total or subtotal gastrectomy must be reeducated about eating. They cannot tolerate three large meals a day. Small frequent feedings are better tolerated. Consultation with a dietitian may be necessary to instruct patients about maximizing nutrients and calories in the small feedings.

Colorectal Cancer

It is estimated that an infant born today in the United States has a 5% lifetime chance of having either colon or rectal cancer. Obviously, colorectal cancer is a significant problem.

Epidemiology. Colorectal cancer accounts for 15% of all malignant tumors in both men and women. The incidence is increased in the northeastern part of the country and in urban areas. According to estimates, approximately 100,000 new cases of colon cancer and 38,200 cases of rectal cancer will be diagnosed in 1995. This type of cancer generally affects those more than 40 years old; the mean age at onset is 63 years for men and 62 years for women. At age 75, the incidence decreases. The incidence is about 50% lower in Native Americans than in whites, and certain religious groups have a lower risk. One hypothesis is that these religious groups have a lower risk because they forbid the use of meat, alcohol, and tobacco, resulting in less colorectal cancer. However, no studies have causally linked these substances to the development of cancer of the colon or rectum (Cohen, Minsky, & Friedman, 1993; Cohen, Minsky, & Schilsky, 1993; Daniel, 1994; Frogge, 1993; Wingo et al., 1995).

Etiology. Dietary causes of colorectal tumors have been extensively explored, and as yet no causal relationship has been established. Calcium, fat, protein, and fiber are suspected to contribute, in some way, to either the development of or protection against colorectal cancer. Bacteria, viruses, and parasites have also been suspected. One theory suggests that by-products or metabolites of bacteria, viruses, or parasites within the bowel initiate malignant changes. The impetus for this theory comes from the observation that patients who have had schistosomiasis tend to have a higher incidence of colorectal cancer (Cohen, Minsky, & Friedman, 1993; Cohen, Minsky, & Schilsky, 1993; Daniel, 1994; Frogge, 1993).

Researchers are also studying the effects of agents that may be chemoprotectants (substances that may actually prevent the development of colorectal cancer). So far, results have shown an inverse relationship between flavones and indoles contained within cruciferous vegetables and ascorbic acid and the development of colorectal cancer (Cohen, Minsky, & Schilsky, 1993; Frogge, 1993). *ascorbic acid / crucif veg*

One known factor associated with development of colorectal cancer is familial adenomatous polyposis. Patients with this disease are likely to have

schistomiasis ⊃ ↑ → colorectal CA

adenocarcinoma of the colon or rectum develop. Risk is increased if a patient has a primary relative who has or had colorectal cancer. Research suggests that cancer will develop in 60–100% of patients who have active bowel disease, either inflammatory bowel syndrome or ulcerative colitis, for 30 years. Patients who have had an appendectomy, cholecystectomy, or previous pelvic radiation and patients with Crohn's disease have an increased risk of colon cancer. Inactivity also increases risk, as does exposure to asbestos (Cohen, Minsky, & Friedman, 1993; Cohen, Minsky, & Schilsky, 1993; Daniel, 1994; Frogge, 1993).

Classification. Adenocarcinomas arising from the glandular epithelium account for 94% of colorectal tumors. Invasion occurs by direct extension into surrounding organs. However, lymphatic and hematogenous spread may occur, resulting in distant metastases (Cohen, Minsky, & Friedman, 1993; Cohen, Minsky, & Schilsky, 1993; Frogge, 1993).

Detection and Diagnosis. Patients with colorectal cancer are asymptomatic in the early stages of tumor development. They may notice minor changes in bowel habits or intermittent rectal bleeding. The latter is typically attributed to internal hemorrhoids. Cramping, aching pressure, pain that resembles that of cholecystitis in character and distribution, or appendicitis may occur. Patients may be constipated or obstipated. If the lesion occludes the lumen of the bowel, patients experience signs and symptoms of obstruction. If the tumor is located in the rectum, tenesmus, rectal pressure, or fullness may occur. The caliber of the stool may decrease, and patients may have a dull aching in the perineal or sacral area, radiating down the legs. Less commonly, weight loss or fever may occur.

In advanced cases of colorectal cancer, patients may have a palpable mass in the abdomen. Further testing is necessary to determine the cause of the mass. A barium enema usually shows a classic apple-core lesion within the large bowel. Half of all colorectal tumors are located within the distal 50 cm of the colon. Therefore, proctosigmoidoscopy (rigid or flexible) is better for characterizing the lesion, and a biopsy can be done at the same time. Blood for determination of carcinoembryonic antigen should be obtained before treatment (surgical or chemotherapeutic). Carcinoembryonic antigen belongs to a class of antigens normally found in fetuses. Originally, researchers noted that many patients with colon cancer had detectable serum levels of carcinoembryonic antigen and thought that this "marker" could be measured periodically to evaluate tumor response or recurrence. Unfortunately, it was later determined that this antigen is not specific for colon cancer. Other types of cancer also produce it, and some patients with colon cancer do not have detectable amounts of it in their blood.

Tests useful in detecting obstruction include radiographs of the abdomen and barium enema. Liver function tests should be done. Levels of liver enzymes will be increased if the liver is extensively involved with tumor. An excretory urogram is useful for evaluating the urinary tract. Computed tomography, magnetic resonance imaging, and endoluminal sonography are helpful in staging rectal cancer (Cohen, Minsky, & Friedman, 1993; Cohen, Minsky, & Schilsky, 1993; Daniel, 1994; Frogge, 1993).

Staging. The Duke staging system was originally developed in the 1930s and has been revised over the years. In 1987, the Duke system was converted to the TNM system of staging.

Treatment. Colorectal cancer is difficult to treat. Over the past 20 years, the mortality rate has not changed despite better screening and intervention.

Surgery is the treatment of choice. The extent of resection is determined by the size and location of the tumor and the extent of involvement of lymph nodes or vessels. Formation of a colostomy is often part of the surgical procedure.

Radiation therapy is used to control regional and local recurrence of tumor. It can be used preoperatively to decrease the size of the tumor, thereby decreasing the number of viable cells. Lymph nodes may be included in the treatment field to sterilize them. In this situation, surgery is done 2–3 weeks after completion of radiation therapy. It is unclear whether this combination of therapies has any benefit. Sometimes, radiation therapy is given both preoperatively and postoperatively; this is called "sandwich" therapy. The goals of preoperative radiation are the same as those stated earlier. The goal of postoperative therapy is to treat the tumor bed when pathologic examination confirms advanced-stage disease. This treatment option is experimental. Postoperative surgery is used routinely when the risk of local recurrence is increased, as indicated by a perforated bowel at surgery or the presence of tumor cells in the lymph nodes. Even though local recurrence of tumor may be controlled, distant metastases are still a problem.

Chemotherapy is used as adjunctive treatment when residual tumor is left at the time of surgery, the tumor is in an advanced stage, or metastatic disease is present. Chemotherapy is used as adjuvant treatment in patients who have limited disease, have undergone surgery, and have no evidence of residual tumor. In patients with limited-stage disease, adjuvant chemotherapy can increase survival. The two most commonly used regimens are a combination of 5-fluorouracil and leucovorin or a combination of 5-fluorouracil and levamisole (Cohen, Minsky, & Friedman, 1993; Cohen, Minsky, & Schilsky, 1993; Daniel, 1994; Frogge, 1993).

Nursing Considerations. Educating patients about the signs and symptoms of colorectal cancer can help them recognize these indications. Encouraging patients to seek medical attention when these signs and symptoms occur is another step in the direction of early detection. Screening with guaiac cards and sigmoidoscopies may or may not be useful. The U.S. Preventive Services Task Force (1989) deemed that evidence was insufficient to either promote or discourage screening. Their recommendation was that it may be prudent to screen patients 50 years or older who have known risk factors for colorectal cancer.

Once colorectal cancer has been diagnosed, nursing care focuses on the impact of the disease and treatment on the patient. Strategies for managing the side effects of treatment should be explored with patients to improve quality of life. Information on psychosocial issues such as body image and sexuality should be mixed with information on practical issues such as bowel training and use of public rest rooms. Nurses should be prepared to address these concerns or to refer patients to someone who can.

CANCER OF THE URINARY SYSTEM

Cancer of the urinary system includes tumors of the bladder and kidney.

Bladder Cancer

Epidemiology. Bladder cancer is the second most common genitourinary cancer. It accounts for up to 5% of all cancer. It is estimated that 50,500 cases will be diagnosed in 1995. The annual incidence is twice as high in white men as in African-American men. Among whites, the male-to-female ratio is 4:1. This disease affects older men, typically around the age of 50 years. In Egypt, bladder cancer has been associated with infections caused by *Schistosoma haematobium* (Davis, 1994; Fair, Fuks, & Scher, 1993; Kravitz & Grieg, 1993; Wingo et al., 1995).

Etiology. Smoking cigarettes may contribute to the development of bladder cancer in up to 50% of cases. Occupational exposure to aromatic amines also appears to increase the risk that this kind of cancer will develop. Weak links have also been established between development of bladder cancer and use of alcohol, saccharin, coffee, and phenacetin. In Egypt, ova of the parasite *S. haematobium* have been found on the bladder wall in patients who have bladder cancer (Davis, 1994; Fair et al., 1993; Kravitz & Grieg, 1993).

Classification. The bladder is lined with transitional epithelium (urothelium). Ninety to ninety-five percent of all tumors of the bladder arise from this epithelial layer and thus are transitional-cell cancers. Of the remaining tumors, 7% are squamous cell cancers, and 2% are adenocarcinomas. Bladder tumors are categorized by their pattern of growth (in situ vs. papillary vs. solid), depth of invasion, and differentiation. Metastases develop by direct extension into the surrounding structures (Davis, 1994; Kravitz & Grieg, 1993).

Detection and Diagnosis. Painless hematuria, gross or microscopic, is usually the first indication of a bladder cancer. Bladder irritability usually accompanies the hematuria. When it does, patients complain of dysuria, frequency, urgency, and burning. If the tumor is large or is located near the base of the bladder, urinary obstruction can occur. Hesitancy and decreased force and caliber of the urinary stream occur. Ureteral obstruction produces pain in the flank and hydronephrosis. Pain in the suprapubic region, back, or rectum may be a symptom of bone, lung, or liver metastases (Davis, 1994; Kravitz & Grieg, 1993).

Because bladder cancers grow into the lumen of the bladder, exfoliated tumor cells are present in the urine. Cytologic examination of urine specimens thus is an easy, cost-effective way of diagnosing bladder cancer. A full-void urine specimen obtained late in the morning or early in the afternoon is best. Bladder washings can also be used for cytologic examination. Another method of diagnosing bladder cancer is flow cytometry. This technique, which examines the DNA content of cells in the urine, is also useful in defining malignant characteristics. Cystoscopy is used for direct visualization and biopsy of bladder tumors (Davis, 1994; Fair et al., 1993; Kravitz & Grieg, 1993).

About 50% of patients with late-stage disease have elevated levels of carcinoembryonic antigen. Levels of this antigen are useful in determining response to treatment or recurrence of tumor. Additional tests include excretory urography, computed tomography, magnetic resonance imaging, and sonography.

Staging. Many staging systems exist for bladder cancer. The TNM system is the most recent addition. Bladder cancers are also graded to predict aggressiveness of the tumor (Davis, 1994; Fair et al., 1993; Kravitz & Grieg, 1993).

Treatment. Removal of the tumor is the treatment of choice in bladder cancer. This can be done through a transurethral resection, if the tumor is small enough, or by electrocautery, laser treatment, or cystectomy. Radi-

cal cystectomy with urinary diversion is required for invasive tumors. Radiation therapy is used after radical cystectomy as part of curative treatment (Davis, 1994; Fair et al., 1993; Kravitz & Grieg, 1993).

Chemotherapeutic agents, such as thiotepa (Thio-Tepa), mitomycin C (Mutamycin), doxorubicin (Adriamycin), and live bacille Calmette-Guérin (BCG), are often instilled into the vesicle of the bladder and left there for approximately 2 hr. This local application of a chemotherapeutic agent produces few systemic side effects and is efficacious (Davis, 1994; Fair et al., 1993; Kravitz & Grieg, 1993).

Chemo- in vesicle of bladder x2

White males with localized disease have an 88% chance of surviving 5 years. With disseminated disease, the chance decreases to 41%, and for all stages of disease, the overall 5-year survival rate is 79%. For African-American males, the numbers are much different. The 5-year survival rate for African-American males with localized disease is 80%. With disseminated disease, the rate decreases to 25%, and the overall 5-year survival rate for all stages is 59% (Davis, 1994; Fair et al., 1993; Kravitz & Grieg, 1993).

AA - Survival rate 59%

Nursing Considerations. Tobacco is implicated in the development of bladder cancer. Preventive measures include helping patients to stop smoking. (For more information, see the section on lung cancer.)

For patients receiving therapy for bladder cancer, nursing considerations include wound care and side effects of radiation therapy and intravesicular chemotherapy. If a surgical procedure has been done, patients may have altered body image. They may also be concerned about sexual issues. Preparing patients for these possibilities can help alleviate anxiety. Offering concrete information on sexual dysfunction and alternative options is also useful. Patients should be educated about bladder cancer and the need for regular follow-up.

Cancer of the Kidney

Epidemiology. Renal cell cancer accounts for 85% of all cancers of the kidney; the remaining 15% are made up of the cancers of the renal pelvis. These two types of tumors occur in men twice as often as they do in women. Age at onset is 40–50 years. According to estimates, approximately 28,800 new cases of kidney cancer will be diagnosed in 1995. The annual incidence of this disease is one-third higher in Hispanic American males and females than in whites (Davis, 1994; Kravitz & Grieg, 1993; Lineham, Shipley, & Parkinson, 1993; Wingo et al., 1995).

Etiology. Cigarette smoking has been associated with about 24% of kidney cancers in women and 30% in men. Persons who work with cadmium, asbestos, and lead have an increased risk for kidney cancer. Use of aspirin, acetaminophen, and phenacetin has been associated with an increase in risk. Obesity in women is associated with kidney cancer; however, it is unclear whether the obesity or the altered estrogen metabolism common in obese women is what increases the risk. Additionally, kidney cancer is more prevalent in patients on dialysis (Davis, 1994; Kravitz & Grieg, 1993; Lineham et al., 1993).

Classification. Renal cell cancer arises from the tubular epithelium and grows toward the medullary part of the kidney. Cancer of the renal pelvis is usually papillary and originates in the epithelial tissue within the pelvis. It tends to grow toward the ureteropelvic junction, invading the muscular coats of the submucosa. Lymphomatous and hematogenous spread are common and are the mechanisms for distant metastases. At the time of diagnosis, 30–50% of patients have metastases (Davis, 1994; Kravitz & Grieg, 1993; Lineham et al., 1993).

Detection and Diagnosis. Gross hematuria, dull aching pain, and a palpable abdominal mass are considered the classic triad of signs and symptoms for kidney cancer. However, this presentation is uncommon. Patients may be asymptomatic for a long time. Fever, weight loss, an increase in sedimentation rate, and anemia may be present at the time of diagnosis (Davis, 1994; Kravitz & Grieg, 1993).

A radiograph of the kidneys, ureters, and bladder and an excretory urogram are recommended studies if kidney cancer is suspected. Magnetic resonance imaging, renal angiography, nephrotomography, renal sonography, and computed tomography can help delineate the location and size of the tumor and involvement of surrounding organs. If cancer of the renal pelvis is suspected, urinary cytology may be useful in establishing a diagnosis (Davis, 1994; Kravitz & Grieg, 1993; Lineham et al., 1993).

Staging. Kidney cancers are staged according to the TNM system. The stages are similar to those used for bladder cancer.

Treatment. Surgical removal of the tumor is the treatment of choice for kidney cancer. Unfortunately, this is possible in only about 50% of patients at the time of diagnosis. Including dissection of lymph nodes as part of the surgical procedure is controversial, because the added information gained does not lead to better survival rates. Kidney cancers are generally radioresistant and chemoresistant (Davis, 1994; Kravitz & Grieg, 1993; Lineham et al., 1993).

In advanced stages of the disease, surgery may be appropriate as palliative treatment to relieve either pain or bleeding, and radiation therapy may be used palliatively to treat distant metastases. Hormonal manipulation has been tried, mostly because of good results in an animal model. Progestin or antiestrogens are most commonly used, including medroxyprogesterone acetate (Depo-Provera), megesterol acetate (Megace), testosterone, and tamoxifen (Novaldex). Responses have been equivocal, but morbidity associated with these agents is low (Davis, 1994; Kravitz & Grieg, 1993; Lineham et al., 1993).

Biological response modifiers such as α-interferon and interleukin-2 have been modestly effective in treatment of kidney cancer, but no statistical improvement in survival has been noted (Davis, 1994; Kravitz & Grieg, 1993; Lineham et al., 1993).

Median survival of patients with metastatic disease at the time of diagnosis of kidney cancer is 4 months. Only 10% of these patients survive 1 year. In early-stage renal cell cancer, 5-year survival rates are 60–100%. For late-stage disease, the rates are 0–20%. For cancer of the renal pelvis, the 5-year survival rates are 60–90% for patients with early-stage disease and 0–33% for those with late-stage disease (Kravitz & Grieg, 1993; Lineham et al., 1993).

Nursing Considerations. Smoking cessation can decrease the incidence of kidney cancer by approximately 25%. Offering to help patients through smoking-cessation classes, support groups, or medication can be useful.

Nursing care of patients with advanced stages of kidney cancer focuses on palliation. Giving transfusions to patients who are anemic, controlling pain, and keeping patients as comfortable as possible are key goals. Patients with early-stage disease should be closely monitored for evidence of tumor recurrence and encouraged to stick to their follow-up schedule.

CANCER OF THE REPRODUCTIVE SYSTEM

Cancers of the reproductive system include ovarian, cervical, and uterine cancer in females and prostatic and testicular cancer in males.

Ovarian Cancer

Epidemiology. Approximately 29% of all gynecologic tumors are ovarian. Although this type of cancer accounts for less than one-third of gynecologic cancers, it accounts for 59% of the deaths due to gynecologic tumors. According to estimates, 26,600 new cases of ovarian cancer will be diagnosed in 1995, and more than half of these cases will result in death. Ovarian cancer affects women in their late 50s; the annual incidence in the United States is 1 in 71 women. Five-year survival rates for all stages of the disease are about 35%. This is a disease of industrialized nations; it is rarely seen in developing countries (Clark, 1994; Walczak & Klemm, 1993; Wingo et al., 1995; Young, Perez, & Hoskins, 1993).

Etiology. The incidence of ovarian cancer is increased in women of high socioeconomic status and in women who have delayed child bearing until later in life. It appears that continuous ovulation produces chronic irritation of the ovarian epithelium, resulting in cancer. Women with a family history of ovarian cancer also have an increased risk. Use of oral contraceptives seems to have a protective effect (Clark, 1994; Walczak & Klemm, 1993; Young, et al., 1993).

Classification. Eighty to ninety percent of all ovarian tumors originate in the epithelium on the surface of the ovary. The tumors spread by direct extension into surrounding tissues and structures. In addition, in a seeding effect, exfoliated tumor cells spread to the peritoneal and abdominal cavity (Clark, 1994; Walczak & Klemm, 1993; Young et al., 1993).

Detection and Diagnosis. Early indications of ovarian cancer include vague gastrointestinal discomfort, dyspepsia, indigestion, flatulence, loss of appetite, eructations, pelvic pressure, and urinary frequency. As the tumor progresses, an abdominal mass becomes palpable and ascites develops.

No screening tools are available for diagnosis of ovarian cancer. The tumor may be detected during routine pelvic examinations by palpation of the uterine adnexa. Once ovarian cancer is suspected or detected, further testing is needed. Pelvic or abdominal sonography, computed tomography, magnetic resonance imaging, and chest radiography are important diagnostic procedures. If a diagnosis has already been made, these procedures are used to complete the staging workup. Blood tests should include an assay for the antigen CA-125. Serum levels of this tumor marker are increased in approximately 82% of women with advanced stages of ovarian cancer. As with carcinoembryonic antigen, levels of CA-125 can be serially followed to determine response to therapy or recurrence of tumor.

For diagnosis, a biopsy specimen is obtained by using a surgical procedure, specifically a laparotomy. Fine-needle aspiration or incisional biopsies are not appropriate for this type of tumor. It is thought that these types of biopsies may actually spread the tumor.

Staging. During the surgical biopsy, staging is done. This relies on a meticulous surgical debulking proce-

Early stage — surgery 90% curative (handwritten)

dure and a thorough examination of the peritoneal and abdominal cavities. Most women have at least stage III disease at the time of diagnosis; in 70–85% of women, the tumor is either stage III or stage IV (Clark, 1994; Walczak & Klemm, 1993; Young et al., 1993).

Treatment. In patients with early stages of ovarian cancer, surgery can be curative in up to 90%. Unfortunately, few patients have early-stage disease at the time of diagnosis. All other stages require chemotherapy. If the tumor persists or recurs after chemotherapy, salvage treatment offers little hope (Clark, 1994; Walczak & Klemm, 1993; Young et al., 1993). The chemotherapeutic agents are usually given intravenously. In some instances, they may be delivered directly into the peritoneal cavity by way of a surgically implanted access device. The efficacy of this method of administration is still being debated. The agents used most often to treat ovarian cancer are cisplatin (Platinol), carboplatin (Paraplatin), and cyclophosphamide (Cytoxan). Other agents that may be combined with these three include doxorubicin (Adriamycin), 5-fluorouracil (5-FU), methotrexate (Mexate), and hexamethylmelamine (HMBA).

Radiation therapy is most effective in early-stage disease. It is also used palliatively in advanced-stage ovarian cancer to relieve pain (Clark, 1994; Walczak & Klemm, 1993; Young et al., 1993).

Nursing Considerations. Nurses are in a position to educate women about the importance of routine pelvic examinations. A bimanual examination includes palpation of the ovaries and can be used to detect masses. An experienced practitioner can detect a mass of 2 cm or less, which can be an early sign of ovarian cancer (U.S. Preventive Services Task Force, 1989).

Once a diagnosis of ovarian cancer has been made, other issues become prominent. Psychosocial aspects of the extensive surgery used for treatment include altered body image, concerns of sexual attractiveness, and physical issues such as pain control and dressing changes. For patients undergoing chemotherapy, nurses should focus on assessment and management of signs and symptoms to improve quality of life.

Cervical Cancer

Epidemiology. Since the advent of routine Pap smears, the annual incidence of cervical cancer has decreased steadily. However, this cancer is still a problem, especially in elderly women. Twenty-four percent of new cases of cervical cancer occur in women more than 65 years old, and 40% of these women die of their disease. Estimates are that 15,800 new cases of cervical cancer will be diagnosed in 1995 and that 4,800 deaths will be attributable to this disease (Clark, 1994; Hoskins, Perez, & Young, 1993; Walczak & Klemm, 1993; Wingo et al., 1995).

Etiology. Many factors have been associated with an increased risk for cervical cancer. They include low socioeconomic status, smoking, sexual activity before the age of 17 years, number of sexual partners, being the daughter of a woman who was treated with diethylstilbestrol, and exposure to human papovaviruses. African-American and Hispanic American women have an increased risk. Wives of men with penile cancer have an increased risk of cervical cancer, as do women who marry men whose wives have died of cervical cancer (Clark, 1994; Hoskins et al., 1993; Walczak & Klemm, 1993). A decreased risk is associated with using a barrier method of birth control; high dietary levels of vitamin A, β-carotene, and vitamin C; low number of sex partners; and later age at first coitus (Clark, 1994; Hoskins et al., 1993; Walczak & Klemm, 1993.

↓ risk / high VitA / β Carotene / Vita C (handwritten)

Classification. The cervix is the neck of the uterus. It is divided into the endocervix and the exocervix. Although these two areas are contiguous, the cells that make up each area are different. The exocervix is composed of squamous epithelial cells, whereas the endocervix is made up of columnar epithelial cells. The location where these areas meet is called the squamocolumnar junction or the transition zone (T-zone). All cervical cancer occurs within the T-zone; 80–90% of the tumors detected in the T-zone are squamous cell in origin; the other 10–20% are adenocarcinoma. Before malignant transformation, cells in the T-zone show various degrees of dysplasia, which is referred to as either cervical intraepithelial neoplasia or squamous intraepithelial neoplasia. These premalignant lesions can be detected early and are evaluated for the degree of invasion into the cervix. Once a lesion has progressed beyond the basement membrane and invades cervical stroma, it becomes invasive cervical cancer. With the use of yearly Pap smears, most lesions are detected during the premalignant stages (Clark, 1994; Hoskins et al., 1993; Walczak & Klemm, 1993).

Detection and Diagnosis. Invasive cervical cancer is relatively asymptomatic. A watery vaginal discharge may be observed early in the disease, but this is usually ignored or attributed to a vaginal infection. As the disease progresses, painful intercourse, postcoital bleeding, intermenstrual bleeding, or heavy menstrual flow may occur. If the bleeding is heavy enough or persists for a long time, patients may have signs and symptoms of anemia, and the watery discharge eventually becomes foul smelling (Clark, 1994; Hoskins et al., 1993; Walczak & Klemm, 1993).

Later in the disease, pain in the pelvis, hypogastrium, flank, or leg may occur. If the cancer is not detected, the pelvic wall, ureters, lymph nodes, and sciatic nerve roots can be affected. Signs and symptoms of urinary or rectal invasion are indications of later stage, progressive disease (Clark, 1994; Hoskins et al., 1993; Walczak & Klemm, 1993).

Once a mass is detected, a biopsy must be done to make a diagnosis. Other studies should include computed tomography or magnetic resonance imaging of the pelvis and abdomen and blood tests to detect anemia.

Staging. Lesions of the cervix are staged according to the Bethesda staging system. In this system, the staging report includes an evaluation of the adequacy of the biopsy specimen and a descriptive diagnosis. This can include information on infections (fungal, bacterial, viral, protozoan) or reactive and reparative changes (inflammation and miscellaneous). Finally, cellular abnormalities are described. Depending on the degree of cellular abnormality, the lesion is classified as cervical intraepithelial neoplasia stage I, II, or III (Walczak & Klemm, 1993). Once invasive cervical cancer is diagnosed, the TNM system is used.

Treatment. Cervical intraepithelial neoplasia can regress, persist, or become invasive. Generally, when le-

sions are detected, treatment consists of electrocautery or cryosurgery, laser surgery, loop electrosurgical excision, cone biopsy, or, in the most advanced cases, hysterectomy.

Surgery is used for early-stage invasive disease. If the disease is diagnosed at a later stage, then radiation therapy to the lesion, with parametrial boosts, intracavitary radiation, or pelvic exenteration, is indicated.

Chemotherapy has not been effective as initial treatment of cervical cancer. It can be useful as second-line therapy if other treatments are unsuccessful. Unfortunately, by the time a woman has completed radiation and surgical therapy, the vascularization of the tumor bed has been severely altered, and delivery of chemotherapeutic agents to the area is questionable at best. Poor renal function and poor bone marrow reserve can further limit the use of chemotherapy. Responses of 10–40% have been reported, but no long-term benefit has been shown, and responses on the average last only 4–8 months.

Thirty-five percent of all women with cervical cancer have persistent disease or have recurrences, usually within 2 years of treatment. Most have local recurrence; only 25% have distant metastases (Clark, 1994; Hoskins et al., 1993; Walczak & Klemm, 1993).

Nursing Considerations. The most important responsibility of nurses with regard to cervical cancer is to strongly encourage women to have yearly Pap smears and to have follow-up examinations when the results are abnormal. Probably the second most important responsibility is to educate women about safe sex practices. It is suspected that cervical intraepithelial neoplasia is caused by human papillomavirus. Using a barrier method of birth control can decrease exposure to this virus as well as exposure to human immunodeficiency virus (U.S. Preventive Services Task Force, 1989).

When caught early, cervical intraepithelial neoplasia is easily eradicated. Morbidity and mortality associated with early lesions are less than those associated with invasive cervical cancer. Women may have concerns about sexual functioning and fertility. Treatment for cervical intraepithelial neoplasia rarely causes any physiologic sexual dysfunction. Difficulty with conception may be experienced after treatment, so women should be informed about this possibility. For patients with invasive disease, nursing care should focus on managing signs and symptoms and providing psychosocial support.

Uterine Cancer

Epidemiology. Uterine cancer, also called endometrial cancer, is currently the predominant gynecologic cancer; according to estimates, 32,800 new cases will be diagnosed in 1995. The good news is that little more than 20% of patients will die of their disease. Uterine cancer most often occurs in postmenopausal women in their 60s (Clark, 1994; Hoskins et al., 1993; Walczak & Klemm, 1993; Wingo et al., 1995).

Etiology. Obesity (being more than 20 lb [9 kg] overweight) has been linked to the development of uterine cancer. It is unclear if the important factor is the obesity or the effect obesity has on hormones. Nulliparity, late onset of menopause, diabetes, hypertension, infertility, irregular menses, failure of ovulation, history of breast or ovarian cancer, adenomatous hyperplasia, and prolonged use of exogenous estrogen replacement therapy increase a woman's risk for uterine cancer. Use of oral contraceptives, however, has a protective effect, and the effect lasts for up to 15 years after discontinuance of the hormone. Ironically, smoking also appears to have a protective effect (Clark, 1994; Hoskins et al., 1993; Walczak & Klemm, 1993).

Classification. Ninety percent of all uterine cancers are adenocarcinoma; 10% are clear-cell carcinoma. Uterine cancer can invade locally by spreading up the fallopian tubes, involving the ovaries and going into the peritoneal cavity. As a result, tumor cells can be present in pelvic and paraaortic lymph nodes even in early-stage disease. Hematogenous spread can also occur (Clark, 1994; Hoskins et al., 1993; Walczak & Klemm, 1993).

Detection and Diagnosis. In most women, uterine cancer is a localized disease at the time of diagnosis. The reason for this finding is probably the signs and symptoms caused by the cancer. The most frequent sign is postmenopausal vaginal bleeding. This usually prompts women to seek immediate medical attention, because

they recognize that such bleeding should not happen. Medical caregivers know that this sign is pathognomonic (characteristic) for uterine cancer, so a workup is done quickly. Twenty percent of all women with postmenopausal bleeding have uterine cancer. In the advanced stages of disease, pyometra; hematometra; or pain in the lumbosacral, hypogastric, and pelvic areas may occur (Clark, 1994; Hoskins et al., 1993; Walczak & Klemm, 1993).

Staging. Uterine cancer is staged according to the corpus cancer staging system, which is a surgical staging system. The degree of infiltration and spread of the tumor are assessed. Metastases are determined to be either local or distant. In addition, the histopathologic degree of differentiation is reported. This grading of the tumor gives the practitioner some idea about the aggressiveness of the disease (Clark, 1994; Hoskins et al., 1993; Walczak & Klemm, 1993).

Treatment. Surgery for treatment of uterine cancer includes total abdominal hysterectomy, bilateral salpingo-oophorectomy, thorough bimanual examination in the operating room, cytologic examination of cells obtained from the peritoneal cavity, inspection and palpation of all peritoneal surfaces, biopsy of any lesions that may be tumorous, sampling of pelvic and paraaortic lymph nodes, possible omentectomy, and resection of all visible tumors. After the surgical procedure is complete, patients usually have adjuvant radiation therapy, in an attempt to eliminate any microscopic areas of disease that might remain.

In advanced or recurrent disease, treatment is difficult. Involvement of the upper part of the vagina may be treated by surgical resection or radiation. Disease in other areas requires hormonal manipulation or chemotherapy (Clark, 1994; Hoskins et al., 1993; Walczak & Klemm, 1993).

Nursing Considerations. Nursing's focus in uterine cancer is early detection. Educating women about the need to seek prompt medical attention in the event of postmenopausal bleeding can save lives. Encouraging women on hormonal replacement therapy to have regular gynecologic checkups is also important. Patients with newly diagnosed disease may be concerned about body image, treatment side effects, sexuality, and pain. Nurses can offer psychologic support and practical information that may alleviate fears.

Prostatic Cancer

Epidemiology. Prostatic cancer is the most common cancer in males in the world and is the most frequently diagnosed cancer in the United States. According to estimates, 244,000 new cases will be diagnosed in 1995, and 40,400 patients will die of the disease. Prostatic cancer accounts for 23% of all cancers in men and 12% of all deaths. The incidence in African-American men has increased. This cancer rarely affects men less than 40 years old; the risk of developing it increases with age (Davis, 1994; Hanks, Myers, & Scardino, 1993; Kravitz & Grieg, 1993; Wingo et al., 1995).

Etiology. Endogenous hormones are the only clear factor implicated in prostatic cancer. Promoting and initiating factors include genetics; sexual history; exposure to viruses and other pathogens, industrial chemicals, and cadmium; and urbanization. Dietary fat alters hormone metabolism and may increase the risk that prostatic cancer will develop (Davis, 1994; Hanks et al., 1993; Kravitz & Grieg, 1993).

Classification. Almost all prostatic cancers are adenocarcinomas that arise from the posterior lobe of the prostate. They tend to be multifocal lesions, growing and spreading locally. Lymphatic and hematogenous spread of disease can occur also. At the time of diagnosis, one-third of patients have metastatic disease (Davis, 1994; Hanks et al., 1993; Kravitz & Grieg, 1993).

Detection and Diagnosis. Men are usually asymptomatic in the early stages of prostatic cancer. Often, an enlarged prostate is detected on routine rectal examination, prompting further investigation. Weight loss, back pain, prostatism, urinary frequency, nocturia, dysuria, hematuria, and decreased force and size of urinary stream may be indications of advancing disease. At the time of diagnosis, 56% of patients have localized disease, 20% have regional involvement, and 24% have distant metastases (Davis, 1994; Hanks et al., 1993; Kravitz & Grieg, 1993).

Diagnosis requires a biopsy. Complete staging consists of a thorough rectal examination, cytologic examination of urine and prostatic cells, computed tomography or magnetic resonance imaging, laboratory studies including an assay for prostate-specific antigen (PSA), bone scan, and excretory urography (optional).

Staging. Many different systems are used to stage prostatic cancer. The one used most often is the Whitmore-Jewett system, which stages disease A to D. More recently, the TNM system has been applied to prostatic cancer. With the Gleason scale, the cancer is both staged and graded. The tumor is examined histopathologically and given a grade of 2 to 10 on the basis of the glandular features; grade 10 tumors are the most aggressive (Davis, 1994; Hanks et al., 1993; Kravitz & Grieg, 1993).

Treatment. Treatment of prostatic cancer depends on the size of the tumor and the presence or absence of metastases. Surgery is the treatment of choice for early-stage disease. Radical peritoneal prostatectomy provides the best chance of cure. Because of the extent of this surgical procedure, sexual dysfunction may result. Patients should be fully informed of this possibility before surgery.

Use of radiation therapy as curative treatment has only recently been accepted. Diarrhea, proctitis, and urinary frequency may occur after radiation therapy. Some men will also be impotent; the prevalence of impotence increases with age. Internal radiation implants, specifically radioactive gold or iodine, deliver a dose of radiation to the tumor bed equivalent to that provided by external-beam radiation, and morbidity and the prevalence of impotence are reduced.

Endocrine manipulation is an effective treatment of advanced-stage prostatic cancer. Approximately 85% of prostatic tumors are androgen dependent, and decreasing circulating levels of androgen gives a response rate of 70–90%. The decrease can be accomplished by using either surgical or chemical castration. Surgical castration entails a bilateral orchiectomy; for chemical castration, patients are given medication that reduces the concentration of circulating androgens. Examples of these medications are diethylstilbestrol, goserlin acetate

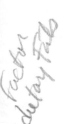

(Zoladex), and leuprolide acetate (Lupron). To suppress adrenal production of androgens, patients can take aminoglutethimide, ketoconazole, spironolactone, or glucocorticoids. Flutamide (Eulixin), an antiandrogen, is also useful in the treatment of prostatic cancer. Chemotherapy has a limited role in the treatment of prostatic cancer. It can help stabilize the disease, but generally the poor responses and the morbidity associated with the therapy limit its use.

Five-year survival rates for patients with early-stage disease are good. Eighty-eight percent of these patients will be alive at 5 years; however, only 57% will be alive at 10 years. Patients with intermediate-stage disease have survival rates of 73% at 5 years and 53% at 10 years. The 5-year survival rate for patients with more advanced disease is 62%, and only 28% will be alive at 10 years (Davis, 1994; Hanks et al., 1993; Kravitz & Grieg, 1993).

Nursing Considerations. Early detection and diagnosis are important for long-term survival in prostatic cancer. Most practitioners include a digital examination of the prostate as part of the routine physical examination of older men. However, the effectiveness of this examination as a screening test for prostatic cancer is a matter of dispute. Nevertheless, informing patients of recommended screenings and encouraging them to participate may lead to early detection (U.S. Preventive Services Task Force, 1989).

Bone metastasis can be a particular problem for men with prostatic cancer. Most patients have some bone involvement at some time during their disease. Aggressive management of this condition can improve a patient's quality of life dramatically. Medications such as nonsteroidal antiinflammatories provide good relief of bone pain. Spot irradiation of the site causing the pain is also effective. In addition, treatment with strontium 89, a bone-seeking radionuclide that emits a low-energy β-particle, may be helpful.

Patients with prostatic cancer who have undergone treatment may need urinary retraining as part of their rehabilitation. They may also be left impotent as a result of the treatment. Providing patients with a safe environment to discuss their feelings or concerns, information

about alternative methods of sexual gratification, and referrals to other health care team members for additional resources can be helpful.

Testicular Cancer

Epidemiology. Testicular cancer is a relatively rare tumor, accounting for about 1% of all tumors in men. Only 7,100 cases will likely be diagnosed in 1995, and only 370 deaths will be due to this cancer. Testicular cancer is a disease of younger men, 15–35 years old, and it occurs mostly in whites with higher socioeconomic status. The incidence in African-American men seems to be decreasing (Davis, 1994; Einhorn, Richie, & Shipley, 1993; Kravitz & Grieg, 1993; Wingo et al., 1995).

Etiology. Testicular cancer has consistently been associated with atrophic or undescended testes. No other risk factors have been detected (Davis, 1994; Einhorn et al., 1993; Kravitz & Grieg, 1993).

Classification. Testicular cancer can be divided into two broad categories: germ cell and stromal. Within the category of germ cell tumor, further distinction can be made between seminomatous and nonseminomatous cancers (embryonal cancer, teratocarcinoma, choriocarcinoma). Stromal tumors are either Leydig cell tumors or gonadal-stromal tumors. Because stromal tumors are so rare, only germ cell tumors are discussed here (Davis, 1994; Einhorn et al., 1993; Kravitz & Grieg, 1993).

Detection and Diagnosis. Most boys and men with testicular cancer first notice a painless enlargement of one testicle. Eventually, scrotal heaviness is felt; this can be followed by pain in the lumbar area of the back. Masses in the abdomen or supraclavicular area may be noticed. If the lungs are involved, a cough can develop, and eventually obstruction occurs. At some point, the person will seek medical attention (Davis, 1994; Einhorn et al., 1993; Kravitz & Grieg, 1993).

Once the mass is felt in the scrotum, testicular sonography is done to better define the lesion. Chest radiography and computed tomography of the chest and abdomen are also necessary for staging. Blood tests should also be done, including assays for lactate dehydrogenase and α-fetoprotein and measurement of serum levels of β-human chorionic gonadotropin. -Fetoprotein and β-human chorionic gonadotropin are substances that may be secreted by the tumor; serial measurements of serum levels of these can be used to monitor response to treatment. A radical inguinal orchiectomy is used to obtain biopsy specimens (Davis, 1994; Einhorn et al.,, 1993; Kravitz & Grieg, 1993).

Testicular cancers spread by direct extension, through the lymph nodes or through the blood (Davis, 1994; Einhorn et al., 1993; Kravitz & Grieg, 1993).

Staging. Testicular tumors are staged according to the TNM system.

Treatment. Surgical removal of the primary tumor is indicated regardless of whether distant metastases exist. Complete surgical staging requires a high radical inguinal orchiectomy, with a radical retroperitoneal lymph node dissection. In early-stage disease, surgery alone is curative for up to 75% of patients with nonseminomatous tumors (Davis, 1994; Einhorn et al., 1993; Kravitz & Grieg, 1993).

For patients with seminomas, either stage I or II, treatment is surgery followed by radiation therapy. This results in a cure rate of more than 90%. For patients with more advanced-stage seminomas or nonseminomatous tumors, treatment is surgery followed by chemotherapy.

Prognosis for patients with testicular cancer is excellent. Survival rates for patients with all stages of seminomas are 71–98%. The rates for patients with nonseminomatous cancers are 55–100%, depending on the stage of the tumor (Davis, 1994; Einhorn et al., 1993; Kravitz & Grieg, 1993).

Nursing Considerations. Early detection of testicular cancer depends on testicular self-examination. Patients should be educated as to what is normal and what should be reported to their medical provider. In most males, one testicle is slightly larger than the other. Assuring patients that this size difference is normal will alleviate fear. However, if one testicle is markedly enlarged, medical attention should be sought (U.S. Preventive Services Task Force, 1989).

Because all patients with testicular cancer undergo unilateral orchiectomy, they may be concerned about fertility and sexual performance. Patients should be assured that the remaining testicle will provide enough testosterone to maintain masculinity. The few patients who have bilateral orchiectomy require testosterone after treatment. The hormone can be given as intramuscular injections every other week, or the patient can wear a testosterone patch that dispenses a steady dose of testosterone. The patch is worn on the scrotum.

Even though most patients still have one testicle, they may have a decreased sperm count. The additive effect of treatment may make patients infertile. Because of this, sperm banking should be discussed before any therapy is started.

CANCERS OF THE BRAIN AND CENTRAL NERVOUS SYSTEM

The brain is contained within a closed system. When tumors occur within this system, morbidity and mortality are high. According to estimates, approximately 17,200 new cases of central nervous system tumors will be diagnosed in 1995, and nearly 75% of all patients with these tumors will die of their disease. Tumors of the central nervous system occur slightly more often in men than in women (Levin, Gutin, & Leibel, 1993; Murphy, 1994; Wegmann, 1993; Wingo et al., 1995).

Epidemiology. Fifty percent of the tumors occurring within the brain and central nervous system are malignant. These tumors account for 1.5% of all malignant neoplasms. Occurrence of the tumors has a bimodal distribution. The first peak is from birth to 6 years. The second peak begins after age 45 and steadily increases. Although no racial differences in incidence exist, the 5-

year survival rates are 32% for blacks and 24% for whites (Levin et al., 1993; Murphy, 1994; Wegmann, 1993).

Etiology. No specific causes or risk factors have been detected as promoters of central nervous system tumors. Viral agents and chemical carcinogens have induced these types of tumors in animal models. Extrapolation from animal models to humans suggests the following factors may be important: vinyl chloride, petrochemicals, inks, solvents, acrylonitrile, lubricating oils, and radiation (especially in children who received prophylactic brain radiation as part of their treatment of acute lymphocytic leukemia) (Levin et al., 1993; Murphy, 1994; Wegmann, 1993). Recent concern has also focused on low-frequency electromagnetic fields, such as those created by cellular telephones.

Classification. Tumors within the central nervous system can be either primary tumors or metastases. This section addresses only the primary tumors arising from either the brain or the spinal cord. Intracerebral tumors can arise from neuroepithelial cells, neurons, and the cells of the blood vessels and connective tissues within the brain.

Glioblastomas account for 60% of primary brain tumors in adults, astrocytomas for 10%, and oligodendrogliomas for less than 5%. Extracerebral tumors include those that originate in the meninges, the acoustic nerve, and the pituitary and pineal glands. Schwannomas and meningiomas involve the spinal cord (Levin et al., 1993; Murphy, 1994; Wegmann, 1993).

Detection and Diagnosis. Clinical features of primary tumors of the central nervous system depend on the size and location of the lesion. For tumors affecting the brain, the effects can be classified as general, secondary, and focal. General effects include all the signs and symptoms of increased intracranial pressure. When a tumor grows within the closed space of the skull, the brain has three mechanisms to compensate for increasing mass: decreased production of cerebrospinal fluid, increased absorption of cerebrospinal fluid, and decreased blood flow to the brain. These compensatory mechanisms are effective for a short time, but eventually the growth of the tumor exceeds the brain's ability to com-

pensate, and signs and symptoms of increased intracranial pressure occur. These include changes in mental status, decreased level of consciousness, confusion, short-term memory loss, personality changes, headache, vomiting, and papilledema. If the signs and symptoms are not recognized and treated, nerve cell damage occurs and, ultimately, death (Levin et al., 1993; Murphy, 1994; Wegmann, 1993).

Secondary effects are the result of actual displacement or shifts of brain structures. In the worse case, complete herniation may occur. If a supratentorial herniation occurs, a change in the level of consciousness may be noticed as well as ocular, motor, and respiratory signs and symptoms. In the event of an infratentorial herniation, loss of consciousness may be the first indicator; later, respiratory and cardiac changes occur (Levin et al., 1993; Murphy, 1994; Wegmann, 1993). The focal effects of a brain tumor depend on the location of the tumor within the brain.

Seizure activity is present in 20–50% of all patients with brain tumors and occurs most often when the tumor affects the parietal or temporal lobe. Sometimes, patients with brain tumors are brought to a health care provider by their family members, who find the patients acting strangely. Occasionally, patients seek medical care themselves because of similar complaints. All too often, the first sign of a brain tumor is a seizure, so many of these patients are seen in emergency departments. Once a lesion has been detected by either computed tomography or magnetic resonance imaging, a biopsy is done. Only 50% of all masses appearing in the brain are malignant, so other causes of a lesion must be eliminated.

Cerebral angiograms or nuclear medicine studies may be done to evaluate the blood vessels surrounding the tumor. A lumbar puncture should only be done after increased intracranial pressure has been ruled out. A lumbar puncture can be useful. Opening pressure can be accurately measured and cerebrospinal fluid obtained for pathologic examination and for tests to determine the presence of white blood cells and to measure protein and glucose levels. Generally, the number of white blood cells and levels of protein and glucose are increased in patients who have a malignant tumor (Levin et al., 1993; Murphy, 1994; Wegmann, 1993).

Definitive diagnosis requires a biopsy. This is important because the brain is a frequent site of distant metastases. Tissue can be obtained either through an open biopsy, in which the brain is exposed, or through stereotaxic biopsy performed through burr holes.

Staging. The TNM system with one modification is used for staging central nervous tumors. Because no lymph nodes are present within the brain, the *N* information is not reported. Tumors are graded as well as staged. The degree of cellular differentiation provides some indication of how aggressive the tumor is and can be used to predict prognosis.

Treatment. Surgery is the only chance of cure for patients with low-grade brain tumors. All other categories of brain tumors are incurable. Some tumors of the central nervous system are radiosensitive (medulloblastomas and high-grade astrocytomas) and may respond to external-beam radiation or radioactive implants. In addition, hyperthermia may be used during surgery to kill tumor cells. The gamma knife offers yet another treatment option.

Chemotherapy is used in combination with radiation therapy or surgery for treatment of gliomas and medulloblastomas; success has been limited. Response rates are 20–40%, probably because of the blood-brain barrier. The most effective drugs are carmustine and lomustine. Responses are of short duration, and usually the tumor recurs (Levin et al., 1993; Murphy, 1994; Wegmann, 1993).

Nursing Considerations. Safety is the number one concern for patients with tumors of the central nervous system. Patients with these tumors may be confused, disoriented, and unable to care for themselves. Ensuring that they have safe surroundings and adequate care is important. Achieving this goal may require placing the patient in either a skilled nursing facility or a hospice. In addition, keeping patients and, perhaps more importantly, their family members informed of tests and treatment side effects is always useful.

LYMPHOMA

Lymphomas are a group of heterogeneous diseases first identified by Thomas Hodgkin in 1832. Essentially, lymphomas are divided into two categories: Hodgkin's disease and non-Hodgkin's lymphoma.

Non-Hodgkin's Lymphoma

Epidemiology. Estimates indicate that approximately 50,900 new cases of lymphoma will be diagnosed in 1995. Fifteen percent will be classified as Hodgkin's disease and 85% as non-Hodgkin's lymphoma. Close to half of the patients with lymphoma of any type die of their disease. Non-Hodgkin's lymphoma occurs more often in men than in women and more often in whites than in blacks. Occurrence of this cancer has a bimodal distribution: The first peak begins in preadolescence and continues into the teens. The second peak starts in the 40s and increases steadily with age (Longo, DeVita, Jaffe, et al., 1993; McFadden, 1993; Moore, 1994; Wingo et al., 1995).

Etiology. The etiology of non-Hodgkin's lymphoma is unknown. What is known is that this cancer is linked in some way to the immune system. Non-Hodgkin's lymphoma is more likely to occur in patients who are immunocompromised. The immunosuppression can be primary, acquired, or iatrogenic (Longo et al., 1993; McFadden, 1993; Moore, 1994).

Viruses have been long suspected in the development of non-Hodgkin's lymphoma. However, with the exception of Epstein-Barr virus, which is causally related to African Burkitt's lymphoma, and human T-lymphotropic virus (type 1), which has been implicated in T-cell lymphoma in adults, no causal relationship has been established (Longo et al., 1993; McFadden, 1993; Moore, 1994).

Finally, exposure to certain drugs may increase the risk of developing non-Hodgkin's lymphoma. Second malignant tumors occur in patients treated with chemotherapy for leukemia and Hodgkin's disease, and diphenylhydantoin has been associated with an increased risk (Longo et al., 1993; McFadden, 1993; Moore, 1994).

Detection and Diagnosis. Patients with non-Hodgkin's lymphoma generally have a rapidly enlarging mass, usually in the oral cavity or cervical or axillary area. Rarely, an inguinal tumor occurs, although involvement of the scrotum occurs in about 7% of patients with lymphoma. Patients may also have certain constitutional signs and symptoms, including fever, weight loss, and night sweats. Patients with constitutional signs and symptoms are thought to have more advanced stages of disease than those without these findings. If the enlarging mass is abdominal, the patient may have gastrointestinal signs and symptoms and pain (Longo et al., 1993; McFadden, 1993; Moore, 1994).

Fine-needle aspiration may be used to diagnose non-Hodgkin's lymphoma, but usually a larger tissue sample is needed to better classify the lesion. In addition, chest radiography; computed tomography of the chest, abdomen, and pelvis; laboratory work including measurement of serum levels of lactic dehydrogenase, which can be an indicator of tumor burden, and tests for human immunodeficiency virus; and bilateral bone marrow biopsies are done. Lumbar puncture may be done also (Longo et al., 1993; McFadden, 1993; Moore, 1994).

Staging. Once all testing is completed, and the biopsy specimen has been thoroughly examined, the tumor is staged. Stage of disease in non-Hodgkin's lymphoma is assigned according to the Ann Arbor staging system. In this system, the location of the tumor and the number of lymph node chains involved are the main factors. The body is divided in half at the diaphragm. Involvement of one side of the diaphragm, either above or below, is stage I or II. Involvement on both sides of the diaphragm is stage III, and any extralymphatic involvement is considered stage IV (Longo et al., 1993; McFadden, 1993; Moore, 1994).

Non-Hodgkin's lymphomas are also graded. The tumors are classified as low, intermediate, or high grade, depending on the histologic cell type. Low-grade lymphomas are indolent and slow growing, intermediate-grade tumors progress somewhat faster,

and high-grade lymphomas tend to be aggressive and fast growing.

Treatment. Treatment of non-Hodgkin's lymphoma is depends on tumor histology, stage of disease, and the physiologic status of the patient. Although surgery is used to obtain the biopsy specimen, it has no other role in the treatment of this tumor. Radiation therapy alone may be curative for patients with early-stage, low-grade tumors. A growing body of evidence suggests that patients with late-stage, low-grade tumors may benefit from aggressive chemotherapy or bone marrow transplantation (Longo et al., 1993; McFadden, 1993; Moore, 1994).

Chemotherapy is the mainstay of treatment of all other types of non-Hodgkin's lymphoma. The exact regimen is less important than the drugs used in the regimen. Cyclophosphamide (Cytoxan) is the single most effective agent against non-Hodgkin's lymphoma, and any regimen that contains cyclophosphamide is considered effective (Longo et al., 1993; McFadden, 1993; Moore, 1994). Radiation therapy may be used for palliation in recurrent disease or to consolidate an area of persistent disease after chemotherapy.

Age at onset is clearly an important factor in prognosis, as is performance status. Patients with large tumor burdens or high levels of lactic dehydrogenase are more likely to do poorly than those with smaller tumors and lower levels of the enzyme. Most patients have complete or partial responses to treatment; however, only 20–50% will be cured (Longo et al., 1993; McFadden, 1993; Moore, 1994).

Nursing Considerations. Nursing care of patients with newly diagnosed non-Hodgkin's lymphoma includes educating them about the disease and treatment options. When treatment begins, aggressive assessment and management of signs and symptoms help improve patients' quality of life.

Hodgkin's Disease

Epidemiology. According to estimates, 7,800 cases of Hodgkin's disease will be diagnosed in 1995, and 1,400 patients will die because of this tumor. Although it accounts for less than 1% of all cancers, Hodgkin's disease is the most common cancer of young adults. The incidence peaks in the teens and twenties and then gradually declines until age 45, when a second gradual increase occurs, which peaks in the 50s to 60s. Men have this cancer slightly more often than women do and have a poorer prognosis (DeVita, Hellman, & Jaffe, 1993; McFadden, 1993; Moore, 1994; Wingo et al., 1995).

Etiology. The cause of Hodgkin's disease is unknown. No one etiologic factor has been determined; however, research suggests that immune status and exposure to viruses may contribute to the development of this cancer. The virus most frequently associated with Hodgkin's disease is Epstein-Barr virus, and this cancer may be the rare result of infection with this virus. No causal relationship has been established. The risk of Hodgkin's disease is increased in siblings of patients who have or had this cancer and in woodworkers (DeVita et al., 1993; McFadden, 1993; Moore, 1994).

Detection and Diagnosis. A rapidly enlarging mass may be the only indication of Hodgkin's disease. The mass is usually nontender and discrete and may feel rubbery. If lymphadenopathy occurs in the mediastinum, patients may have a cough, shortness of breath, dyspnea on exertion, chest pain, or signs and symptoms of superior vena cava syndrome. Occasionally, Hodgkin's disease is discovered with routine chest radiography. Abdominal involvement produces gastrointestinal complaints and pain. Patients may also have constitutional signs and symptoms, including weight loss, fevers, and night sweats. Prognosis is poorer for patients with constitutional signs and symptoms than for patients who do not have them. In addition, patients may have generalized pruritus, and consumption of alcohol may cause pain in the lymph nodes. Reasons for the pain are unclear (McFadden, 1993).

Diagnosis of Hodgkin's disease requires pathologic examination of a biopsy specimen. The presence of Reed-Sternberg cells within the biopsy tissue is the diagnostic hallmark. Fine-needle aspiration may be the first step in determining whether an enlarged mass is malignant, but the amount of tissue obtained by this procedure is not sufficient for diagnosis of Hodgkin's disease. A com-

plete staging workup includes a thorough history and physical; computed tomography of the chest, abdomen, and pelvis; blood tests; and bilateral bone marrow biopsies. Exploratory laparotomy was once an integral part of the staging workup for this cancer, to accurately assess the extent of disease. However, since the advent of computed tomography, which is a less invasive method of assessing the abdomen, laparotomies are performed less often (DeVita et al., 1993; McFadden, 1993; Moore, 1994).

Staging. Hodgkin's disease is staged according to the Ann Arbor staging system. In addition, histopathologic classification is done; the results can be used to predict prognosis. The four histopathologic classifications are lymphocyte predominance, nodular sclerosing, mixed cellularity, and lymphocyte depleted. Each distinct subtype has well-defined characteristics and manifests certain features of natural history. In the past, differences were also noted in survival between patients with different subtypes, but with recent therapeutic advances, those differences have disappeared (DeVita et al., 1993; McFadden, 1993).

Treatment. In Hodgkin's disease, the goal of treatment is cure. This is crucial, because in most patients, the tumor is curable if the optimal regimen is used.

Early-stage disease is treated with radiation therapy to the affected area and to other lymph node chains. An alternative approach includes irradiating the affected area and then using combination chemotherapy. Later stages of the disease are usually treated with combination chemotherapy, although radiation therapy may be added, especially if abdominal involvement is extensive.

Survival depends on the stage of disease, the size of the tumor, the presence of constitutional signs and symptoms, and use of curative therapy. Seventy to eighty percent of patients with early-stage Hodgkin's disease survive 10 years after the diagnosis. Ten-year survival rates for those with later stage disease who are treated with either radiation therapy or chemotherapy are 40-75%.

Patients who have a relapse after treatment with radiation therapy alone can be treated with combination chemotherapy. For patients treated with chemotherapy who have a relapse, the time between therapy and relapse must be determined. If the patient was in remission for 12 months or more, chances are good that retreatment will produce long-term survival, but probably not a cure. If the remission was less than 12 months, the prognosis is worse; most likely, the remission will not last (DeVita et al., 1993; McFadden, 1993; Moore, 1994). Bone marrow transplantation may be a treatment option for patients with recurrent disease who are responsive to chemotherapy. Approximately 30–50% of these patients have complete remission; however, 75% of those who respond to treatment have a relapse within 5 years (Kessinger & Armitage, 1994).

Nursing Considerations. Nurses' most important tasks when caring for patients receiving therapy for Hodgkin's disease are to educate and offer support. Most patients experience complications of their curative therapy for years after completion of treatment (e.g., thyroid dysfunction due to mantle radiation). Warning patients about these complications and offering means of coping are useful interventions. The major long-term complication is other malignant tumors. Gonadal dysfunction and sterility are also common long-term effects. Sperm banking should be discussed with men undergoing treatment. For women, the technology of storing eggs exists, but the cost is in the tens of thousands of dollars and is out of reach for all but the most wealthy. In women, primary ovarian failure is usually the cause of gonadal dysfunction. This affects close to 50% of women, and 20–30% have permanent amenorrhea.

LEUKEMIA

Leukemia is defined as a group of neoplasms characterized by malignant proliferation of myeloblasts or lymphoblasts that replace normal bone marrow elements and infiltrate normal tissues. The acute leukemias are characterized by the proliferation of immature blood cells with a short natural history; the chronic leukemias, by an excessive accumulation of apparently more ma-

ture cells that are dysfunctional, with a longer progressive course (Meili, 1994; Wingo et al., 1995; Wujik, 1993).

Epidemiology. According to estimates, in 1995, leukemias will account for 25,700 cases of cancer. Half will be chronic and half acute. Three-quarters of these patients will die of their disease. Men have leukemia more often than women do, and race and age do not appear to influence occurrence. The types of leukemia diagnosed most often in adults are acute myelogenous leukemia and chronic lymphocytic leukemia (Deisseroth, Andreeff, Champlin, et al., 1993; Keating, Estey, Kantarjian, 1993; Wujik, 1993).

Etiology. The etiology of most leukemias is still uncertain; however, many factors have been associated with an increased risk. These include exposure to radiation, chemicals, drugs, and viruses and genetic factors (Deisseroth et al., 1993; Keating et al., 1993; Wujik, 1993). Results of the explosion of the atomic bomb in the 1940s and the nuclear accident at Chernobyl show that persons exposed to ionizing radiation have an increased risk for leukemia, especially acute myelogenous leukemia.

Certain chemicals have been associated with the development of leukemia. This phenomenon was first detected in Turkish cobblers in the early 1900s. Further epidemiologic research has shown that persons who work with explosives, distillers, dye users, painters, and shoemakers have an increased incidence of leukemia. Additionally, cancer patients treated with alkylating agents have an increased risk of developing a second tumor, usually acute myelogenous leukemia.

Some families seem to be at particularly high risk for leukemia; the risk may be up to four to seven times higher than in other families. Certain genetic disorders also are associated with an increased risk of leukemia. These include Down syndrome, Bloom syndrome, Fanconi's anemia, Klinefelter's syndrome, and Ellis–van Creveld syndrome. The exact role of genetic factors remains a mystery (Deisseroth et al., 1993; Keating et al., 1993; Wujik, 1993).

The role of viruses in the development of leukemia is also unclear. T-cell leukemia in adults in Japan and the Caribbean is associated with human T-cell leukemia virus type 1, and human T-cell leukemia virus type 2 has been associated with a rare form of hairy cell leukemia. Other than these isolated diseases, other viruses have not been implicated (Keating et al., 1993).

Classification. Leukemia can be divided into two broad categories: acute and chronic. These categories are further differentiated according to the cell line involved. Acute myelogenous, acute lymphoblastic, chronic myelogenous, and chronic lymphocytic leukemias are the major subtypes. The subtypes are based on the cell type that predominates and the location of arrested cellular maturation (Keating et al., 1993; Meili, 1994; Wujik, 1993).

Detection and Diagnosis. Signs and symptoms of acute myelogenous or lymphoblastic leukemia have a short duration. Generally, these types of leukemia grow rapidly within the bone marrow, and typical complaints are due to the crowding out of normal cells within the marrow. Signs and symptoms may include fatigue (caused by anemia), fever and infection (the result of granulocytopenia), bleeding (thrombocytopenia), and bone and joint pain (proliferation of the leukemic cells within the marrow) (Deisseroth et al., 1993; Meili, 1994; Wujik, 1993).

Patients with either subtype of chronic leukemia may be asymptomatic or may have malaise, loss of appetite, weight loss, low-grade fever, and night sweats. These signs and symptoms are due to the presence of dysfunctional cells and the accumulation of these cells in various organs (spleen, liver). Onset of signs and symptoms is gradual. Fever is a rare in chronic myelogenous leukemia until the terminal phase of the disease (Meili, 1994; Wujik, 1993).

Findings on smears of peripheral blood are the first indication that a patient may have leukemia. However, diagnosis of acute leukemia requires bone marrow aspiration and biopsy. Pathologic examination of biopsy specimens shows leukemic cells within the architecture of the marrow. Specific staining and chromosomal evaluation are also done. In approximately 50% of patients with acute leukemia, a lumbar puncture is necessary to determine whether the central nervous system is involved. No further testing is necessary in these patients (Keating et al., 1993).

Patients with chronic leukemia usually have leukocytosis; the white cell counts are 20,000 to more than 100,000 cells/mm^3. This may be the first indication that something is wrong. In cases of chronic leukemia, a diagnosis can be made by examining a stained smear of peripheral blood. Chromosomal testing shows a specific abnormality in 90% of patients with chronic myelogenous leukemia (Philadelphia chromosome). Approximately 50% of patients with chronic lymphocytic leukemia also have hypogammaglobulinemia (Deisseroth et al., 1993).

Treatment. The mainstay of treatment of acute leukemia is chemotherapy. If a complete response is achieved, the chemotherapy may be followed by bone marrow transplantation. Age is a factor in bone marrow transplantation. Generally patients more than 60 years old are not good candidates for transplantation (Deisseroth et al, 1993; Keating et al., 1993; Meili, 1994; Wujik, 1993).

Chronic leukemia is also treated with chemotherapy at some point. Chronic myelogenous leukemia can be cured by destroying the Philadelphia chromosome. This requires high-dose chemotherapy and allogeneic bone marrow transplantation. In patients for whom this regimen is not an option, an alternative is the use of α-interferon, which can produce long-term remission (Deisseroth et al., 1993; Meili, 1994; Wujik, 1993). Chronic lymphocytic leukemia does not require treatment until signs or symptoms occur, either cytopenias or organomegaly. In these patients, the benefits of treatment do not outweigh the associated morbidity. Treatment options include chemotherapy, corticosteroids, radiation therapy, or a combination of these. The goal is palliation, because cure is not possible (Deisseroth et al., 1993; Meili, 1994; Wujik, 1993).

Average survival time of patients with acute leukemia who do not have treatment is 3 months after diagnosis. Treatment can improve that. Median survival of patients with acute lymphocytic leukemia who respond to therapy is 16 months. For patients with acute myelogenous leukemia, median duration of first remission is 6–25 months. These patients survive an average of 30 months. Thirty percent of patients with acute myelogenous leukemia are disease-free 5 years after treatment (Deisseroth et al., 1993; Keating et al., 1993; Meili, 1994; Wujik, 1993).

Survival of patients with chronic myelogenous leukemia has not changed since the 1920s. Average survival time after diagnosis is 2.5–3.5 years. Curative therapy for these patients is allogeneic bone marrow transplantation. Less than 50% of these patients are actually cured. For patients with chronic lymphocytic leukemia, median survival time varies from less than 4 years to more than 6 years. The degree of infiltration of the tumor into organs influences survival. Patients with less organ involvement can survive up to 10 years (Deisseroth et al., 1993).

Nursing Considerations. Nursing care of patients with leukemia is directed at treating the anemia, thrombocytopenia, and granulocytopenia. Most therapy is intense, and many patients need continuing support to complete their treatment.

MELANOMA

Melanoma is among the most refractory of tumors in humans. Its annual incidence is increasing faster than that of any other malignant tumor except lung cancer in women. The difference, however, is that in lung cancer, the reason for the increase is clear: More women are smoking. In melanoma, the reason is less clear (Balch, Houghton, & Peters, 1993; Ketchum & Loescher, 1993; Otto, 1994).

Epidemiology. According to estimates, 34,100 new cases of melanoma will be diagnosed in 1995. The tumor occurs slightly more often in men than in women (18,700 vs. 15,400 cases, respectively). The estimated number of deaths that will be attributed to melanoma in 1995 is 7,200; nearly twice as many men as women will

die (Balch et al., 1993; Ketchum & Loescher, 1993; Otto, 1994; Wingo et al., 1995).

In the United States, the age-adjusted yearly incidence is 12–30 cases per 100,000 persons. In 1935, melanoma developed in only 1 in 1500 persons. In 1980, that figure changed dramatically to 1 in 250, and by 1987, it had changed even more, to 1 in 135. If this trend continues, by the year 2000, melanoma will develop in 1 in 90 persons. The increases in annual incidence may be due to exposure to sunlight during recreation, increased exposure to ultraviolet light, or earlier detection (Balch et al., 1993; Ketchum & Loescher, 1993; Otto, 1994).

Melanoma is a disease mainly of whites who have a fair complexion and a tendency to sunburn rather than tan. Skin coloring plays a role in the development of this tumor. Having red hair increases a person's risk for melanoma by 300%; having blond hair increases it by 60%. Patients with more than 20 nevi and patients with a history of melanoma have a threefold increase in risk. An uncommon, but defined, risk group is patients with a family history of melanoma (Balch et al., 1993; Ketchum & Loescher, 1993; Otto, 1994).

The "latitude" effect is a phenomenon associated with melanoma. The nearer a location is to the equator, the higher are the incidence of this tumor and the number of deaths due to it.

Although melanoma affects men and women almost equally, the distribution of lesions differs between the sexes. Men typically have lesions on the trunk, neck, and face. Women usually have tumors on the extremities (Balch et al., 1993; Ketchum & Loescher, 1993; Otto, 1994).

Etiology. Although the cause of melanoma is unknown, the cell of origin is the melanocyte, and more than 90% of all melanomas originate in the skin. A small percentage originate in the eye, and in approximately 4% of patients with melanoma, no primary tumor is found (Balch et al., 1993; Ketchum & Loescher, 1993; Otto, 1994).

Detection and Diagnosis. Patients with melanoma have "moles" that have changed in some way. In some cases, a friend or family member may notice a suspicious-looking mole in an area not visible to the patient. The mnemonic for the classic features of a malignant melanoma is ABCD:

A = asymmetry. Most lesions are asymmetric.

B = borders. Most melanomas have irregular borders.

C = color. Lesions vary from deep purple or black to brown. Some are variegated.

D = diameter. The diameter of most lesions is greater than the diameter of an eraser on a pencil (6 mm).

If melanoma is suspected, a complete history and a physical examination are indicated, including liver function tests and chest radiograph. The biopsy of choice is an excisional one with narrow margins. Once the biopsy specimen has been examined and the tumor staged, a determination is made about the need for further excision. Elective dissection of regional lymph nodes may be done also. It is thought that melanoma metastasizes in a sequential manner, involving the regional lymph nodes first. An examination of these lymph nodes provides a complete picture of tumor involvement (Balch et al., 1993; Ketchum & Loescher, 1993; Otto, 1994).

Staging. Melanoma is staged according to the TNM system. In melanoma, the *T* (tumor size) is measured in millimeters, not centimeters. *N* still indicates the involvement of lymph nodes, and *M* reflects the presence or absence of metastases. In addition, melanomas are microstaged, which determines the level of invasion into the skin. This is an important prognostic indicator and correlates with the Clark stage (Balch et al., 1993; Ketchum & Loescher, 1993; Otto, 1994).

Treatment. Surgery is the only curative therapy available for melanoma. Therefore, early detection is a must in patients at risk.

Melanoma is relatively resistant to chemotherapy. The most effective chemotherapeutic agent is dacarbazine (DTIC), which produces a response in about 20% of patients. However, the response usually does not last, and tumor recurrence is common. Radiation therapy is not helpful, because the tumor is radioresistant. Biotherapy

and hormonal manipulations have been tried, with limited success.

For patients with lesions less than 0.76 mm thick, the 5-year survival rate is almost 98%; for patients with localized disease and tumors thicker than 0.76 mm, the rate is 90%. If regional lymph nodes are involved, the 5-year survival rate decreases to 50%, and if distant metastases are present, it drops to 14% (Balch et al., 1993; Ketchum & Loescher, 1993; Otto, 1994).

Nursing Considerations. Detecting patients at risk for melanoma and educating them about the disease are important. For patients with nevi, establishing a relationship with a health care provider who will examine the patients' skin on a regular basis can mean the difference between early detection and disseminated disease. In addition, providing information on skin care, such as using sun-blocking agents on all exposed parts of the body when outside and wearing hats with wide brims to protect the face, can help the next generation avoid this tumor.

HIV-RELATED TUMORS

Patients infected with human immunodeficiency virus (HIV) have an increased propensity for certain types of malignant tumors. These tumors are often called "opportunistic" cancers, ones that typically develop in persons who are immunocompromised. The Centers for Disease Control and Prevention designates four specific malignant tumors as defining or indicator conditions for acquired immune deficiency syndrome (AIDS): Kaposi's sarcoma, non-Hodgkin's lymphoma, primary lymphoma of the central nervous system, and invasive squamous cell cancer of the cervix (Moran, 1993).

Kaposi's Sarcoma

Epidemiology. Nearly 95% of all Kaposi's sarcomas occur in homosexual or bisexual men. The reason for this is unknown, although acquiring HIV through the sexual route seems to be linked with the development of Kaposi's sarcoma. The prevalence of this tumor is higher among women who acquire HIV through sex than it is among women who acquire the virus through use of injectable drugs. This finding suggests that perhaps another sexually transmitted agent promotes the development of Kaposi's sarcoma (Brogden, 1994; Karp, Groopman, & Broder, 1993; Moran, 1993).

Etiology. Before the widespread occurrence of Kaposi's sarcoma in patients with AIDS, three classifications of the tumor existed. The first was the classic form of the disease, described by Kaposi in 1872. This form of the disease tended to be an indolent, slow-growing tumor that affected men of Jewish or Mediterranean descent in the sixth to eighth decade of life. In 1970, Kaposi's sarcoma was described in Africa, unrelated to HIV infection, as an aggressive disease involving mucocutaneous surfaces, the viscera, and lymph nodes. This form affected patients of all ages, from infants to the elderly, and occurred equally in women and men. The third form of the disease was also reported In 1970. Clinicians found that Kaposi's sarcoma developed in patients who were purposefully immunosuppressed to prevent organ rejection. In about half of these patients, the tumor resolved spontaneously when the immunosuppressive drug was discontinued. The 1980s saw the addition of a new category of Kaposi's sarcoma, the form detected in homosexual men exposed to HIV. Interestingly, HIV-related Kaposi's sarcoma does not seem to correlate with degree of immunosuppression. The tumor is just as likely to develop in patients with CD4 counts of 1000 cells/mm^3 as in those with CD4 counts less than 200 cells/mm^3 (Brogden, 1994; Karp et al., 1993; Moran, 1993).

Detection and Diagnosis. Patients with Kaposi's sarcoma often have bruises that do not resolve. If biopsy of the lesions shows Kaposi's sarcoma, no further workup is indicated unless the patient has other signs or symptoms. Seventy percent of patients with mucocutaneous Kaposi's sarcoma may have visceral involvement at the time of diagnosis. This involvement is only important if it causes signs and symptoms (Brogden, 1994; Karp et al., 1993; Moran, 1993).

Staging. The AIDS Clinical Treatment Group has established a system for staging Kaposi's sarcoma. It consists of evaluating the number of tumors, the status of the immune system, and the presence of other signs and symptoms. Once all data are collected, patients can be divided into good and poor prognostic categories (Moran, 1993).

Treatment. Kaposi's sarcoma is multifocal, so surgical removal of the lesions is impractical. Radiation therapy with a superficial electron beam is useful in treating lesions that are unsightly, cause pain, or involve the oropharyngeal area. This treatment causes few systemic side effects (Brogden, 1994; Karp et al., 1993; Moran, 1993).

Chemotherapy is used to treat indolent, localized, aggressive, or disseminated disease. It consists of small doses of drugs given intralesionally or regular doses given systemically. Agents such as vincristine (Oncovin), vinblastine (Velban), and bleomycin (Blenoxan) are used alone or combined with doxorubicin (Adriamycin) to treat more disseminated disease. Other procedures that have some efficacy in the treatment of Kaposi's sarcoma include use of liquid nitrogen and photodynamic light therapy.

The treatment goal of therapy for Kaposi's sarcoma is palliation. In patients with HIV disease, this tumor is not curable. Prognosis usually has more to do with the status of the patient's immune system than with the presence of Kaposi's sarcoma (Brogden, 1994; Karp et al., 1993; Moran, 1993).

Nursing Considerations. Often, the most important nursing consideration in patients with HIV-related Kaposi's sarcoma is support and education about their HIV disease. For some patients, Kaposi's sarcoma may be the first AIDS-indicator disease, heralding the progression from simply being HIV positive to having AIDS. For others, it may be one other disease that must be treated. Recognizing where the patient is on the relative health-illness continuum helps determine the appropriate nursing intervention.

Patients with Kaposi's sarcoma often have lesions on the face. These lesions can become grossly disfiguring, and patients may become isolated, not wanting to leave their home because of the disfigurement. Referring the patient to a local cosmetologist or to a camouflage clinic, if one is available, can be useful. Lesions can be masked by certain types of makeup. This may be all a patient needs to regain confidence and resume activities of daily living.

HIV-Related Non-Hodgkin's Lymphoma

For information on the epidemiology, etiology, detection, diagnosis, and staging of HIV-related non-Hodgkin's lymphoma, see the earlier section on non-Hodgkin's lymphoma in general. The only distinguishing characteristics of HIV-related non-Hodgkin's lymphoma are that this disease tends to be manifested at an advanced stage in an extralymphatic manner and that the tumors uniformly have either intermediate or high-grade characteristics. HIV-related non-Hodgkin's lymphoma also tends to be a late manifestation of HIV disease. Typically, the CD4 count is less than 200 cells/mm^3 before non-Hodgkin's lymphoma occurs. Exceptions to this happen, and the tumor has developed in patients with higher CD4 counts (Brogden, 1994; Karp et al., 1993; Moran, 1993).

Treatment. Treatment options for patients with HIV-related non-Hodgkin's lymphoma are limited to chemotherapy. Dosages are reduced because of the infection with HIV and poor bone marrow reserve. In addition, patients are given prophylactic treatment against opportunistic infections, particularly *Pneumocystis carinii* pneumonia. In patients who have residual disease after treatment with chemotherapy, radiation therapy may be used to control the disease.

Most patients with HIV-related non-Hodgkin's lymphoma respond to treatment, and complete responses occur in close to 50% of those treated. The problem is that the responses do not last, and most patients either die of their lymphoma or of HIV infection. A few patients have had responses that have lasted years (Brogden, 1994; Karp et al., 1993; Moran, 1993).

Nursing Considerations. Patients undergoing treatment for HIV-related non-Hodgkin's lymphoma may experience exaggerated side effects due to the treatment. Aggressive management of signs and symptoms is indicated, and patients should be examined by a physician if even minor side effects occur.

Primary Lymphoma of the Central Nervous System

Epidemiology. Primary lymphoma of the central nervous system is essentially non-Hodgkin's lymphoma that develops in the brain. Before HIV disease became so widespread, this tumor was most common in elderly, immunocompromised patients and occurred slightly more often in women than in men. Currently, the age at onset is 40–50 years, and the tumor occurs more often in men than in women. Primary lymphoma of the central nervous system is a late manifestation of immune dysfunction. In most patients, the CD4 count is less than 75 cells/mm^3 (Brogden, 1994; Karp et al., 1993; Moran, 1993).

Etiology. The cause of primary lymphoma of the central nervous system is closely linked with immunosuppression. The tumor typically occurs when the immune system is severely depressed and the CD4 count is 75 cells/mm^3 or less. In almost all patients with this lymphoma, the Epstein-Barr virus genome can be detected within the tumor. The significance of this finding is not known. It may be an incidental finding or an indication of a causal relationship (Brogden, 1994; Karp et al., 1993; Moran, 1993).

Detection and Diagnosis. No one knows how long the signs and symptoms of primary lymphoma of the central nervous system exist before they are reported. The onset is usually so insidious that it may be many months before the tumor is diagnosed, and often the patient's family or significant other reports the changes. All the signs and symptoms are the result of either the location of the tumor within the brain or the enlargement of the tumor.

Primary lymphoma of the central nervous system in patients with HIV disease is a diagnosis of exclusion. Because of the morbidity associated with biopsy of the brain in these patients, any brain mass detected is treated as if it were an indication of toxoplasmosis. The treatment continues for 7–10 days. If improvement occurs, the mass was probably toxoplasmosis, and the treatment continues. If no improvement occurs, the mass is presumed to be a lymphoma, and other treatment is undertaken (Brogden, 1994; Karp et al., 1993; Moran, 1993).

Treatment. No good treatment for primary lymphoma of the central nervous system exists. Usually the patient is too ill and the tumor is too deep for surgical removal. The blood-brain barrier prevents adequate doses of chemotherapeutic agents from reaching the tumor, and radiation therapy is only mildly effective.

A brief "honeymoon" period may occur in which all signs and symptoms decrease and the patient "wakes up." This is the result of decreased cerebral edema. Duration of response can be up to 8 weeks. Median survival time is 3–4 months (Brogden, 1994; Karp et al., 1993; Moran, 1993).

Nursing Considerations. Once palliative treatment of any signs or symptoms the patient may be experiencing has been completed, focus should turn to the patient's family or significant other. Primary lymphoma of the central nervous system is a disease that occurs at the end of the continuum of HIV disease, and the patient's family or significant other will most likely need support during this time.

Invasive Squamous Cell Cancer of the Cervix

Etiology. Women dually infected with HIV and human papillomavirus 16,18 have a higher incidence of both cervical intraepithelial neoplasia and invasive squamous cell carcinoma of the cervix. The increased risk usually begins when the CD4 count is 200 cells/mm^3 or less (Maimen, Fruchter, Guy, et al., 1993; Mandelblatt, Fahs, Garibaldi, et al., 1992).

For specifics on clinical features and diagnosis of this tumor, see the section on cervical cancer. Other risk factors associated with invasive squamous cell carcinoma of the cervix in noninfected woman do not apply to women with HIV infection.

Treatment. Treatment of invasive squamous cell carcinoma of the cervix in women with HIV disease is not standardized. Because they are infected with HIV, have poor marrow reserve, and may have concomitant oppor-

tunistic infections, the treatment of choice is unclear. Most clinicians follow the guidelines for treating cervical intraepithelial neoplasia in women without HIV disease. For invasive squamous cell carcinoma of the cervix, the benefits of chemotherapy may not outweigh the associated morbidity (Maimen et al., 1993; Mandelblatt et al., 1992).

Nursing Considerations. Many women with HIV disease care for children who are also infected with HIV. If a woman's chance of survival is diminished because she has HIV disease, legal issues arise, and she may need to make arrangements for the children. Nurses can play an important role in supporting women through this difficult time.

SARCOMAS OF THE BONE AND SOFT TISSUES

Sarcomas differ from carcinomas in their cells of origin. Sarcomas are derived from connective tissue, formed by the proliferation of mesodermal cells.

Epidemiology. Sarcomas tend to be uncommon tumors. According to estimates, 2,070 new cases of sarcoma will be diagnosed in 1995, and 1,280 deaths will be due to these tumors. Sarcomas occur equally in both sexes, and no racial differences have been detected. The age of onset has a bimodal distribution. The first peak occurs at the ages of 15–19 years; the second peak occurs after age 65 (Chang, 1994; Malawer, Link, & Donaldson, 1993; Piasecki, 1993; Wingo et al., 1995; Yang, Rosenberg, Blatstein, et al., 1993).

Etiology. Because sarcomas of the bone and soft tissues are such uncommon tumors, little is known about their etiology. Prevention and detection are difficult because of the tissues involved. Persons exposed to high doses of radiation, usually as a result of treatment for cancer, have a higher annual incidence of bone and soft tissue sarcomas. Vinyl chloride gas, arsenic, and dioxin (agent orange) also appear to be associated with an increased incidence. Sarcomas develop more often in patients who are immunocompromised, especially those purposefully immunosuppressed to prevent organ rejection and those infected with HIV, than in persons who are immunocompetent.

Bone sarcomas may develop in patients who have a preexisting bone condition, such as Paget's disease, or skeletal maldevelopment and specific types of skeletal pattern growth. Lymphangiosarcoma is common in patients with prolonged lymphedema, and neurofibrosarcomas develop in almost 10% of patients who have neurofibromatosis (Chang, 1994; Malawer et al., 1993; Piasecki, 1993).

Soft-tissue sarcomas may occur after prolonged exposure to herbicides and other chemicals. Alkylating chemotherapeutic agents also appear to increase the incidence of sarcomas. These include melphalan, procarbazine, chlorambucil, and the nitrosoureas (Chang, 1994; Malawer et al., 1993; Piasecki, 1993).

A familial tendency may exist. Cases of osteosarcoma, Ewing's sarcoma, and chondrosarcoma in siblings have been reported (Chang, 1994; Malawer et al., 1993; Piasecki, 1993).

Classification. Bone sarcomas arise from the primitive mesoderm or ectoderm and can be divided into three main groups. The first group consists of the sarcomas that originate from collagen-producing cells: osteogenic sarcoma, chondrogenic sarcoma, and fibrogenic sarcoma. The second group consists of the sarcomas derived from the bone marrow reticulum: Ewing's sarcoma and reticulum cell sarcoma. Blood vessels of the bone account for the third group: angiosarcoma and epithelioid sarcoma that has no known cell of origin (Chang, 1994; Malawer et al., 1993; Piasecki, 1993).

Soft-tissue sarcomas generally invade the surrounding tissue along the anatomic planes. As the tumors enlarge, they compress the tissues and form a pseudocapsule. Examples of these tumors include rhabdomyosarcoma, synovial sarcoma, and liposarcoma. Some soft-tissue sarcomas such as alveolar soft-part sarcomas and epithelioid sarcomas have no known cell of origin (Chang, 1994; Malawer et al., 1993; Piasecki, 1993).

Detection and Diagnosis. Pain or the detection of a mass is what usually prompts someone with a sarcoma to seek medical attention. Other causes of the signs and symptoms must be excluded, including trauma, hematoma, and myositis ossificans. The onset of signs and symptoms is usually gradual. The pain is often worse at night, and the tumors do not cause pain until they impinge on vital structures or nerves. Indications of distant metastases may be present. Patients may have chest pain, hemoptysis, cough, fever, chills, weight loss, or malaise (Chang, 1994; Malawer et al., 1993; Piasecki, 1993).

A complete staging workup is done if sarcoma is suspected. Computed tomography, magnetic resonance imaging, and routine radiography may show the abnormality. A bone scan may also be helpful in delineating the tumor. If a soft-tissue sarcoma is suspected, sonography can be useful in determining the dimension of the mass and the involvement of other structures (Chang, 1994; Malawer et al., 1993; Piasecki, 1993).

An incisional or fine-needle biopsy is used to establish the diagnosis. The biopsy is routinely done before staging.

Staging. Sarcomas are classified according to their cell of origin and are staged by using the TNM staging system. Additional information included in this staging system is whether the lesion is intracompartmental or extracompartmental. This is reported as A or B, respectively. Sarcomas are also graded, to help predict their degree of aggressiveness (Chang, 1994; Malawer et al., 1993; Piasecki, 1993; Yang et al., 1993).

Treatment. Twenty years of research supports the fact that no procedure short of ablation can control or eradicate aggressive forms of osteosarcoma, fibrosarcoma, or chondrosarcoma. A typical surgical procedure is amputation of the affected limb and the joint above the lesion. In 1984, the National Institutes of Health convened a meeting of physicians noted for their care of sarcoma patients. At that meeting, information was presented that supported the use of limb-sparing surgery, citing no difference in disease-free survival among those who had undergone the new procedure and those treated the conventional way. Contraindications for the new procedure include likely difficulty in obtaining an adequate surgical margin free of tumor cells, involvement of neurovascular bundle by tumor, and patient's age less than 10 years (Chang, 1994; Malawer et al., 1993; Piasecki, 1993). Limb-sparing therapy works best on those sarcomas that tend to metastasize later in the disease (Chang, 1994; Malawer et al., 1993; Piasecki, 1993).

Radiation therapy is not very useful in treating primary bone sarcomas, because most are radioresistant. In contrast, soft-tissue sarcomas tend to be radiosensitive. Chemotherapy is used preoperatively to treat micrometastases and decrease tumor size, increasing the likelihood of a limb-sparing procedure. It is used postoperatively when metastases are suspected.

Soft-tissue sarcomas are also difficult to treat. Surgical removal of the mass often results in local recurrence of the tumor. Radiation to the surgical site offers local control, but the prognosis is still poor (Chang, 1994; Malawer et al., 1993; Piasecki, 1993). Even when the tumor can be controlled locally, distant metastases remain a problem. Although theoretically systemic chemotherapy could prevent distant metastases, no good chemotherapeutic agents exist for this group of diseases. Prognosis varies according to the type, size, and location of the tumor and the presence of metastases.

Nursing Considerations. Nursing considerations for care of patients with bone and soft-tissue sarcomas focus on the psychologic impact of amputation and rehabilitation. For patients undergoing chemotherapy or radiation therapy, the goal is management of signs and symptoms.

BIBLIOGRAPHY

Alexander, H., Kelsen, D. P., & Tepper, J. E. (1993). Cancer of the stomach. In V. DeVita, S. Hellman, & S. Rosenberg (Eds.), *Cancer: Principles and practice of oncology* (4th ed., pp. 818–848). Philadelphia: Lippincott.

American Cancer Society. (1986). *Special report on cancer in the economically disadvantaged.* New York: Author.

American Cancer Society. (1991). *Cancer facts and figures 1991.* Atlanta: Author.

American Cancer Society. (1993). *Cancer facts and figures 1993.* Atlanta: Author.

Balch, C. M., Houghton, A. N., & Peters, L. J. (1993). Cutaneous melanoma. In V. DeVita, S. Hellman, & S. Rosenberg (Eds.), *Cancer: Principles and practice of oncology* (4th ed., pp. 1612–1661). Philadelphia: Lippincott.

Baquette, C. R., Horm, J. W., Gibbs, T., et al. (1991). Socioeconomic factors and cancer incidence among blacks and whites. *Journal of the National Cancer Institute, 83,* 551–556.

Bildstein, C. Y. (1993). Head and neck cancer. In S. Groenwald, M. Frogge, M. Goodman, & C. Yarbro (Eds.), *Cancer nursing: Principles and practice* (3rd ed., pp. 1114–1148). Boston: Jones and Bartlett.

Boring, C. C. (1992). Cancer statistics for African-Americans. *CA—A Cancer Journal for Clinicians, 42*(1), 7–17.

Boring, C. C., Squires, T. S., & Tong, T. (1992). Cancer statistics 1992. *CA—A Cancer Journal for Clinicians, 42*(1), 19–38.

Brogden, C. (1994). HIV and related cancers. In S. Otto (Ed.), *Oncology nursing* (2nd ed., pp. 261–277). St. Louis: Mosby.

Bunn, P. (1992). *Lung cancer: Current understanding of the biology, diagnosis, staging and treatment.* Princeton, NJ: Bristol-Myers.

Callahan, R., Cropp, C. S., Merlo, G. R., Liscia, D. S., Cappa, A. P., & Lidereau, R. (1992). Somatic mutations and human breast cancer. *Cancer, 69,* 1582–1586.

Chang, S. (1994). Bone cancers and soft tissue sarcomas. In S. Otto (Ed.), *Oncology nursing* (2nd ed., pp. 59–73). St. Louis: Mosby.

Clark, J. C. (1994). Gynecological cancer. In S. Otto (Ed.), *Oncology nursing* (2nd ed., pp. 190–220). St. Louis: Mosby.

Cohen, A. M., Minsky, B. D., & Friedman, M. A. (1993). Rectal cancer. In V. DeVita, S. Hellman, & S. Rosenberg (Eds.), *Cancer: Principles and practice of oncology* (4th ed., pp. 978–1005). Philadelphia: Lippincott.

Cohen, A. M., Minsky, B. D., & Schilsky, R. L. (1993). Colon cancer. In V. DeVita, S. Hellman, & S. Rosenberg (Eds.), *Cancer: Principles and practice of oncology* (4th ed., pp. 929–977). Philadelphia: Lippincott.

Crane, R. (1994). Breast cancer. In S. Otto (Ed.), *Oncology nursing* (2nd ed., pp. 90–129). St. Louis: Mosby.

Daniel, B. T. (1994). Gastrointestinal cancers. In S. Otto (Ed.), *Oncology nursing* (2nd ed., pp. 145–167). St. Louis: Mosby.

Davis, M. (1994). Genitourinary cancer. In S. Otto (Ed.), *Oncology nursing* (2nd ed., pp. 168–189). St. Louis: Mosby.

Deisseroth, A. B., Andreeff, M., Champlin, R., et al. (1993). Chronic leukemias. In V. DeVita, S. Hellman, & S. Rosenberg (Eds.), *Cancer: Principles and practice of oncology* (4th ed., pp. 1965–1984). Philadelphia: Lippincott.

DeVita, V. T., Hellman, S., & Jaffe, E. S. (1993). Hodgkin's disease. In V. DeVita, S. Hellman, & S. Rosenberg (Eds.), *Cancer: Principles and practice of oncology* (4th ed., pp. 1819–1858). Philadelphia: Lippincott.

Einhorn, L. H., Richie, J. P., & Shipley, W. U. (1993). Cancer of the testis. In V. DeVita, S. Hellman, & S. Rosenberg (Eds.), *Cancer: Principles and practice of oncology* (4th ed., pp. 1126–1152). Philadelphia: Lippincott.

Elpern, H. E. (1993). Lung cancer. In S. Groenwald, M. Frogge, M. Goodman, & C. Yarbro (Eds.), *Cancer nursing: Principles and practice* (3rd ed., pp. 1174–1199). Boston: Jones and Bartlett.

Fair, W. R., Fuks, Z. Y., & Scher, H. I. (1993). Cancer of the bladder. In V. DeVita, S. Hellman, & S. Rosenberg (Eds.), *Cancer: Principles and practice of oncology* (4th ed., pp. 1052–1072). Philadelphia: Lippincott.

Fraumeni, J. F. (1975). Carcinogenesis: An epidemiological appraisal. *Journal of the National Cancer Institute, 55,* 1039–1046.

Freeman, H. P. (1989). Cancer in the socioeconomically disadvantaged. *CA—A Cancer Journal for Clinicians, 39,* 266.

Frogge, M. H. (1993). Gastrointestinal cancer: Esophagus, stomach, liver and pancreas. In S. Groenwald, M. Frogge, M. Goodman, & C. Yarbro (Eds.), *Cancer nursing: Principles and practice* (3rd ed., pp. 1004–1043). Boston: Jones and Bartlett.

Garber, J. E. (1991). Familial aspects of breast cancer. In J. R. Harris (Ed.), *Breast disease* (2nd ed.). Philadelphia: Lippincott.

Ginsberg, R. J., Dris, M. G., & Armstrong, J. G. (1993). Non-small cell lung cancer. In V. DeVita, S. Hellman, & S. Rosenberg (Eds.), *Cancer: Principles and practice of oncology* (pp. 673–723). Philadelphia: Lippincott.

Goodman, M., Chapman, D. (1993). Breast cancer. In S. Groenwald, M. Frogge, M. Goodman, & C. Yarbro (Eds.), *Cancer nursing: Principles and practice* (3rd ed., pp. 903–958). Boston: Jones and Bartlett.

Hale, J. M., Lee, M. K., & Newman, B. (1990). Linkage of early-onset familial breast cancer to chromosome 17q21. *Science, 256,* 1684–1689.

Hammond, E. C., Selikoff, I. J., & Seidman, H. (1979). Asbestos exposure, cigarette smoking and death rates. *Annals of the New York Academy of Science, 330,* 473–490.

Hanks, G. E., Myers, C. E., & Scardino, P. T. (1993). Cancer of the prostate. In V. DeVita, S. Hellman, & S. Rosenberg (Eds.), *Cancer: Principles and practice of oncology* (4th ed., pp. 1073–1113). Philadelphia: Lippincott.

Harris, J. R., Morrow, M., & Bonadonna, G. (1993). Cancer of the breast. In V. DeVita, S. Hellman, & S. Rosenberg (Eds.), *Cancer: Principles and practice of oncology* (4th ed., pp. 1264–1332). Philadelphia: Lippincott.

Hoskins, W. J., Perez, C. A., & Young, R. C. (1993). Gynecological tumors. In V. DeVita, S. Hellman, & S. Rosenberg (Eds.), *Cancer: Principles and practice of oncology* (4th ed., pp. 11152–1225). Philadelphia: Lippincott.

Inde, D. C., Pass, H. I., & Glatstein, E. J. (1993). Small cell lung cancer. In V. DeVita, S. Hellman, & S. Rosenberg (Eds.), *Cancer: Principles and practice of oncology* (pp. 723–758). Philadelphia: Lippincott.

Karp, J. E., Groopman, J. E., & Broder, S. (1993). Cancer in AIDS. In V. DeVita, S. Hellman, & S. Rosenberg (Eds.), *Cancer: Principles and practice of oncology* (4th ed., pp. 2093–2110). Philadelphia: Lippincott.

Keating, M. J., Estey, E., & Kantarjian, H. (1993). Acute leukemia. In V. DeVita, S. Hellman, & S. Rosenberg (Eds.), *Cancer: Principles and practice of oncology* (4th ed., pp. 1938–1964). Philadelphia: Lippincott.

Kelsey, J. L., & Gammon, M. D. (1991). The epidemiology of breast cancer. *CA—A Cancer Journal for Clinicians, 41,* 146.

Kessinger, A., & Armitage J. O. (1994). Blood stem cell transplants in lymphomas. In R. Gale, C. Juttner, & P. Henon (Eds.), *Blood stem cell transplants* (pp. 128–135). New York: Cambridge University Press.

Ketchum, M., & Loescher, L. J. (1993). Skin cancers. In S. Groenwald, M. Frogge, M. Goodman, & C. Yarbro (Eds.), *Cancer nursing: Principles and practice* (3rd ed., pp. 1238–1257). Boston: Jones and Bartlett.

Kravitz, D., & Grieg, B. (1993). Urologic and male genital malignancies. In S. Groenwald, M. Frogge, M. Goodman, & C. Yarbro (Eds.), *Cancer nursing: Principles and practice* (3rd ed., pp. 1258–1315). Boston: Jones and Bartlett.

Levin, V. A., Gutin, P. H., & Leibel, S. (1993). Neoplasms of the central nervous system. In V. DeVita, S. Hellman, & S. Rosenberg (Eds.), *Cancer: Principles and practice of oncology* (4th ed., pp. 1679–1739). Philadelphia: Lippincott.

Lineham, W. M., Shipley, W. U., & Parkinson, D. R. (1993). Cancer of the kidney and ureter. In V. DeVita, S. Hellman, & S. Rosenberg (Eds.), *Cancer: Principles and practice of oncology* (4th ed., pp. 1023–1051). Philadelphia: Lippincott.

Longo, D. L., DeVita, V. T., Jaffe, E. S., et al. (1993). Lymphocytic lymphoma. In V. DeVita, S. Hellman, & S. Rosenberg (Eds.), *Cancer: Principles and practice of oncology* (4th ed., pp. 1859–1927). Philadelphia: Lippincott.

Maimen, M., Fruchter, R. G., Guy, L., et al. (1993). Human immunodeficiency virus infection and invasive cervical carcinoma. *Cancer, 71*(2), 402–406.

Malawer, M. M., Link, M. P., & Donaldson, S. S. (1993). Sarcomas of the bone. In V. DeVita, S. Hellman, & S. Rosenberg (Eds.), *Cancer: Principles and practice of oncology* (4th ed., pp. 1509–1566). Philadelphia: Lippincott.

Mandelblatt, J. S., Fahs, M., Garibaldi, K., et al. (1992). Association between HIV infection and cervical neoplasia: Implications for clinical care of women at risk for both conditions. *AIDS, 6*(2), 173–178.

McFadden, M. E. (1993). Malignant lymphomas. In S. Groenwald, M. Frogge, M. Goodman, & C. Yarbro (Eds.), *Cancer nursing: Principles and practice* (3rd ed., pp. 1200–1229). Boston: Jones and Bartlett.

McNaull, F. (1987). Lung cancer: What are the odds? *American Journal of Nursing, 87,* 1428–1432.

Meili, L. (1994). Leukemia. In S. Otto (Ed.), *Oncology nursing* (2nd ed., pp. 278–301). St. Louis: Mosby.

Mettlin, C. (1992). Breast cancer risk factors. *Cancer, 69*(Suppl.), 1904–1911.

Moran, T. A. (1993). AIDS-related malignancies. In S. Groenwald, M. Frogge, M. Goodman, & C. Yarbro (Eds.), *Cancer nursing: Principles and practice* (3rd ed., pp. 861–877). Boston: Jones and Bartlett.

Moore, J. G. (1994). Malignant lymphomas. In S. Otto (Ed.), *Oncology nursing* (2nd ed., pp. 340–355). St. Louis: Mosby.

Murphy, J. E. (1994). Cancer of the brain and central nervous system. In S. Otto (Ed.), *Oncology nursing* (2nd ed., pp. 74–89). St. Louis: Mosby.

Oleske, D. M. (1987). Epidemiology of lung cancer. *Seminars in Oncology Nursing, 3,* 165–173.

Otto, S. E. (1994). Skin cancers. In S. Otto (Ed.), *Oncology nursing* (2nd ed., pp. 361–375). St. Louis: Mosby.

Parzuchowski, J. (1994). Head and neck cancer. In S. Otto (Ed.), *Oncology nursing* (2nd ed., pp. 221–260). St. Louis: Mosby.

Piasecki, P. A. (1993). Bone and soft tissue sarcomas. In S. Groenwald, M. Frogge, M. Goodman, & C. Yarbro (Eds.), *Cancer nursing: Principles and practice* (3rd ed., pp. 877–902). Boston: Jones and Bartlett.

Report of the Surgeon General: The health consequences of involuntary smoking. (1986). Washington, DC: Dept. of Health and Human Services.

Scanlon, E. F. (1991). Breast cancer. In A. L. Holleb, D. J. Fink, & G. P. Murphy (Eds.), *ACS textbook of clinical oncology.* Atlanta: American Cancer Society.

Schantz, S. P., Harrison, L. B., & Hong, W. K. (1993). Tumors of the nasal cavity and paranasal sinuses, nasopharynx, oral cavity and oropharynx. In V. DeVita, S. Hellman, & S. Rosenberg (Eds.), *Cancer: Principles and practice of oncology* (4th ed., pp. 574–630). Philadelphia: Lippincott.

Schmidt, S. P., & Shell J. A. (1994). Lung cancer. In S. Otto (Ed.), *Oncology nursing* (2nd ed., pp. 302–339). St. Louis: Mosby.

Seidman, H., Stellman, S. D., & Mushinski, M. H. (1982). A different perspective on breast cancer risk factors: Some implications of the nonattributable risk. *CA—A Cancer Journal for Clinicians, 32,* 301–312.

Sellers, T. A. (1990). Evidence for Mendelian inheritance in the pathogenesis of lung cancer. *Journal of the National Cancer Institute, 82,* 1272–1275.

Shimkin, J. D. (1963). Cancer of the breast. *Journal of the American Medical Association, 183,* 358–361.

U.S. Preventive Services Task Force. (1989). *Guide to clinical preventive services: An assessment of the effectiveness of 169 interventions.* Baltimore: Williams & Wilkins.

Walczak, J. R., & Klemm, P. R. (1993). Gynecological cancers. In S. Groenwald, M. Frogge, M. Goodman, & C. Yarbro (Eds.), *Cancer nursing: Principles and practice* (3rd ed., pp. 1065–1113). Boston: Jones and Bartlett.

Wegmann, J. A. (1993). Central nervous system cancers. In S. Groenwald, M. Frogge, M. Goodman, & C. Yarbro (Eds.), *Cancer nursing: Principles and practice* (3rd ed., pp. 959–984). Boston: Jones and Bartlett.

Willett, W. C. (1990). Vitamin A and lung cancer. *Nutritional Reviews, 48,* 201–211.

Wingo, P. A., Tong, T., & Bolden, S. (1995). Cancer statistics 1995. *CA—A Cancer Journal for Clinicians, 45*(1), 8–30.

Wujik, D. (1993). Leukemia. In S. Groenwald, M. Frogge, M. Goodman, & C. Yarbro (Eds.), *Cancer nursing: Principles and practice* (3rd ed., pp. 1149–1174). Boston: Jones and Bartlett.

Yang, J. C., Rosenberg, S. A., Blatstein, E. J., et al. (1993). Sarcomas of the soft tissues. In V. DeVita, S. Hellman, & S. Rosenberg (Eds.), *Cancer: Principles and practice of oncology* (4th ed., pp. 1436–1488). Philadelphia: Lippincott.

Young, R. C., Perez, C. A., & Hoskins, W. J. (1993). Cancer of the ovary. In V. DeVita, S. Hellman, & S. Rosenberg (Eds.), *Cancer: Principles and practice of oncology* (4th ed., pp. 1226–1263). Philadelphia: Lippincott.

STUDY QUESTIONS

Chapter 11

Quesitons 77–81

77. Which of the following is a risk factor for melanoma?

   a. Having blond or red hair and a fair complexion
   b. Residing in Canada
   c. Eating large amounts of red meat
   d. Smoking tobacco

78. Risk factors for HIV-related Kaposi's sarcoma include:

   a. Using injectable drugs
   b. Being gay or bisexual
   c. Smoking tobacco
   d. Being a vegetarian

79. Increased risk for ovarian cancer is associated with:

   a. Obesity
   b. Alcohol consumption
   c. Higher socioeconomic class
   d. Use of oral contraceptives

80. Which of the following has been implicated in the development of prostatic cancer?

   a. Celibacy
   b. Endogenous hormones
   c. Wearing restrictive clothing
   d. Living in a undeveloped country

81. An increased risk for cancer of the stomach is associated with which of the following?

   a. Eating fresh fruits and vegetables
   b. Eating highly salted or pickled foods
   c. Drinking large amounts of alcohol
   d. Trauma

CHAPTER 12

PATIENTS WITH ADVANCED STAGES OF CANCER

CHAPTER OBJECTIVE

After completing this chapter, the reader will be able to discuss the important aspects of palliative care and advance directives for patients with advanced stages of cancer, describe various models of hospice care and the importance of management of signs and symptoms in patients who are terminally ill, and indicate the importance of bereavement counseling for families of cancer patients after the patients' death.

LEARNING OBJECTIVES

After studying this chapter, the reader will be able to

1. Specify characteristics of patients who have advanced stages of cancer.

2. Recognize the types of treatment included in palliative care.

3. Indicate the characteristics of advance directives.

4. Specify features of hospice care.

5. Recognize signs and symptoms that commonly occur in patients who are terminally ill.

6. Recognize the purpose of bereavement counseling for families of terminally ill patients who have died.

INTRODUCTION

According to statistics, in 1994, approximately 1.2 million new cases of cancer were diagnosed, and 538,000 persons died of cancer (Boring, Squires, Tong, & Montgomery, 1994). However, no estimates are available of the number of patients who have advanced stages of cancer at the time of diagnosis or who eventually will have advanced stages of cancer even after aggressive treatment.

Just what constitutes the advanced stages of cancer? One might say that these stages begin when the tumor has metastasized, when the chance of cure, remission, or long-term survival is small even with aggressive treatment. However, this characterization does not include tumors that generally do not metastasize (e.g., certain brain tumors) but are just as recalcitrant to treatment as metastatic cancer is. These nonmetastatic tumors tend to progress locally, causing damage as they either invade surrounding organs or expand in a confined space. In addition, some tumors are simply resistant to chemotherapy or radiation therapy. If they are not detected when they are small enough to be removed surgically or if they are unresponsive to treatment, it is just a matter of time before they progress to an advanced state. During this time, when there is no response to aggressive treatment, whether chemotherapy or radiation, the transition is made to palliative care.

PALLIATIVE CARE

Palliative care is care that a patient receives when the emphasis of treatment has shifted from prolonging life through cure or remission to alleviating suffering through management of signs and symptoms. Acknowledging that the time a patient has left is finite, caregivers make a conscious effort to make the patient's death as painless, symptom-free, and peaceful as possible.

At this time, nurses assume a pivotal part in assessment and management of the patient's condition. Before care shifts from aggressive treatment to palliation, the patient should be informed about the change and about the reason for the change, that remission or cure is no longer possible. Often, patients, knowing their bodies and feeling that the cancer is growing or has recurred, have expected the information. They may even feel relief that this knowledge is "out in the open" and can be discussed freely. Often patients have already thought about how much further intervention they wish, and if they are assertive enough, they convey this information to their primary caregiver.

The primary caregiver may be a physician, a nurse practitioner, or a physician's assistant. Patients who are not comfortable telling the caregiver about their feelings often feel comfortable sharing their feelings with their nurse. The nurse may then act as intermediary in several ways. For example, he or she may act as a liaison between the patient and the primary caregiver, sharing the patient's preferences and needs, or act as a coach or facilitator, encouraging patients to speak for themselves and providing the necessary support for them to do so. In either case, the nurse is the one who is with the patient no matter where the patient is, in the hospital, at home, or in a hospice.

The change from aggressive treatment, with the goal of curing, inducing remission, or providing disease-free survival, to palliative care should not mean that the patient is abandoned. It also should not mean that the patient stops coming to the clinic or private office. Less care is not what palliation is about. Patients may be receiving therapy to help relieve some signs or symptoms. Often patients continue to receive either chemotherapy or radiation therapy to help control pain caused by a progressing tumor. More care is often necessary when the patient begins to become sicker and has more signs and symptoms. The focus of palliation may expand to include the patient's family or significant others (Martinez & Wagner, 1994; Mills, 1992).

ADVANCE DIRECTIVES

Beginning in December of 1991, the federal Patient Self-Determination Act mandated that hospitals, clinics, health care agencies, and hospices provide written information to patients at the time of admission about two areas of concern: (1) patients' right to accept or refuse treatment and (2) ways in which patients can execute advance directives. The purpose of the Patient Self-Determination Act is to ensure that a patient's desires and wishes about health care are carried out even if the patient becomes mentally incapacitated.

Patients who are aware that their treatment has become ineffective or who have been told that "things are not going well" may have initiated an advance directive. Advance directives are legal documents that give another person the authority to make decisions about the patient's health care in the event the patient cannot make those decisions (Wadill, 1991). Advance directives may include a document called a durable power of attorney for health care. Living wills are also thought of as advance directives; however, in some states, these wills are not legally binding. The unfortunate consequence is that even though a patient has spelled out exactly how much medical intervention he or she wishes, once the patient cannot speak for himself or herself, the primary health care provider is not legally bound to abide by the patient's wishes.

A durable power of attorney for health care is a legally binding document, and primary health care providers must comply with its provisions. The person appointed to act on behalf of the patient can be anyone the patient wishes. Some advocate picking a close friend to be the appointed agent, because they think it would be too difficult or cause too much guilt for a spouse or significant other to withhold treatment even if withholding treatment is what the patient wants. Patients must make their wishes about life support and continued treatment known to the appointed person.

Advance directives are used only if a patient cannot speak for himself or herself (Wadill, 1991). They are not meant to be used by patients as a way to abdicate the responsibility for making decisions about health care, and they can be revoked by the patient at any time. The nurse's role in the execution of advance directives is to provide patients with any information necessary so that an informed decision can be made. When a patient executes a durable power of attorney for health care, he or she is asked to check a box on the form that indicates his or her wishes about being resuscitated or being given feedings or intravenous hydration. In addition, a space is provided for the patient to address any other health care issues of concern to him or her.

Nurses who provide information to patients deciding on a durable power of attorney for health care should be aware of the survival statistics for cardiopulmonary resuscitation. In an acute care setting, approximately 11% of patients with cancer who undergo cardiopulmonary resuscitation survive; unfortunately, their quality of life is poor (Bedell, Pelle, Maher, et al., 1986; Vitelli, Cooper, Rogatko, et al., 1991; VonGunten, 1991). The likelihood of surviving resuscitation is 0% for patients with metastatic disease and 2.3% for those who do not have

metastatic disease but are bedridden (Bedell et al., 1986; Vitelli et al., 1991). It is unlikely that a patient with an advanced stage of cancer would survive cardiopulmonary resuscitation. This is important information for patients with advanced stages of cancer. Ultimately, the patient must decide on the aggressiveness of therapy. It is essential that the patient and the entire health care team have an opportunity to discuss all aspects of care and alternative treatment before the patient becomes unable to make decisions about health care (Vitelli et al., 1991; VonGunten, 1991).

HOSPICE CARE

Hospice care was developed to meet one simple objective: to facilitate a comfortable and natural death. For patients who are terminally ill, this concept can be comforting. With the advent of acquired immune deficiency syndrome, death has stopped being a taboo topic. More and more feature films and television programs depict stories about persons who are terminally ill. Society continues to emphasize youth and wellness, but the face of death has started to appear. As a result of this shift, death is being talked about more openly. The population of the United States is aging, and many patients have thought about their death and have definite feelings of how they would like to die. Hospice care is a way to help them achieve their goal.

Unfortunately, in today's society, a "natural death" requires planning. Because of medical technology and advances, the tendency is to do "more" in an attempt to save a patient, rather than to withhold treatment and allow the patient to die peacefully and with dignity. This trend, however, is being challenged. Voters in Oregon have approved a right-to-die initiative, and individuals like Dr. Kevorkian have brought physician-assisted suicide to the forefront of society's consciousness.

Many different models of hospice care are available. These include community-based programs in which a multidisciplinary team focuses on providing care in the home. The goal of this type of hospice program is to provide comfort; autonomy; and physical, emotional, and spiritual support to the patient and the patient's family. The program has no associated facility other than an office. One disadvantage of this type of hospice care is that patients must be hospitalized to receive respite care when the family needs a break from caring for the patient at home. This type of hospice care requires a good deal of organization and mobilization of family, friends, and volunteers. Not all patients will be able to mobilize the number of friends or family members required to make this type of program work.

Hospices can also be hospital based. The program may be either an inpatient or a hospital-based home care program. Such a program provides for inpatient stays if and when respite care is required. The difference between this program and the community-based program is the allocation of non–acute care beds for respite care. This type of program also takes a multidisciplinary approach to care, and the primary goal is still to provide patients autonomy; comfort; and physical, emotional, and spiritual support. A hospital-based hospice team adds a different dimension to hospice care. Patients who are terminally ill may be referred to the hospice team while the patients are still hospitalized. A patient gets to meet the team members before he or she is discharged from the hospital, making a smooth transition between hospital and home possible. Members of the hospice team may be the same primary health care providers who cared for the patient while the patient was undergoing aggressive treatment. A hospice team can also be instrumental in providing palliative care. They can make daily rounds and recommend steps to improve control of signs and symptoms and the patient's quality of life.

The final model of hospice care is the free-standing hospice. This is usually a free-standing facility associated with a home care agency. Patients who cannot be maintained at home have the option of being admitted to the hospice facility for terminal care. Hospice care is not interrupted, because the same team members facilitate transition from home to the hospice facility. This model of care also has the advantage of avoiding miscommunication. Everyone admitted to the hospice facility is there for one reason: to die a natural and peaceful death. Unlike in a hospital setting, where care during off hours may be provided by a physician who is not familiar with a patient's situation and who may order aggressive therapy in response to reported signs and symptoms, in the hospice setting, patients receive comfort care only.

Advantages of hospice care include 24-hr availability of staff personnel; aggressive control of signs and symptoms; improved communication between patient, family, and interdisciplinary team; and use of volunteers as members of the care team. In addition, the hospice program also provides bereavement counseling for patients' family members after death has occurred. Each hospice program drafts its own eligibility criteria for admission of patients to the program. Some of the general criteria include the following:

- The patient has less than 6 months to live.

- The patient has a primary caregiver willing to assume responsibility for the patient's care.

- If the patient is to be cared for at home, he or she must live within the geographic constraints of the hospice program.

- The patient has agreed to have palliative care only and must understand that curative treatment is not an option.

Some hospice programs also require that patients have a written "do not resuscitate" order before they are admitted to the program.

It is important to recognize that there is not one "right" way to die and that a natural, peaceful death is defined by the person who is dying. There seems to be an idealistic belief that dying at home is the right way to die and that all efforts should focus on achieving this goal. In some instances, dying at home is not what the family or patient wants, and it is not an achievable outcome for patients with few family members and friends. Dying at home takes a great deal of commitment from all involved, and if family members or friends cannot help a patient achieve this goal, they should not feel that they have failed. Rather the goal of peacefulness and dignity should be valued. Cultural differences also should be respected and mutually agreeable goals worked toward.

Payment for a hospice program often is covered by insurance. If it is not, negotiations with the insurance company can sometimes be useful. In 1983, funding became available to certified hospice programs for Medicare-eligible patients. Medicaid is trying to formulate a similar type of hospice package.

MANAGEMENT OF SIGNS AND SYMPTOMS IN DYING PATIENTS

One of the most important tasks of any nurse who cares for cancer patients who are dying is to assess the patients and aggressively manage any adverse signs and symptoms they may be experiencing. The following material covers management of the most common signs and symptoms.

Pain

Perhaps the symptom feared most by patients and caregivers alike is pain. It seems that everyone knows someone who had cancer and who died in excruciating pain. Patients are fearful that this will happen to them. Until recently, many patients with advanced stages of cancer did die in pain. However, with few exceptions, that is not the case now.

Assessment of a patient's pain requires answers to some basic questions. The purpose of these questions is not to determine whether a patient's pain is real or for the patient to convince others that he or she is indeed in pain. The purpose is to gather information so that a plan of care can be formulated. Because of the subjective nature of pain, first and foremost is the tenet that pain exists and is experienced whenever the patient says it is.

Once a patient states that he or she is in pain, the next step is to characterize the pain. This includes determining its location, onset (when did it start), pattern (does it radiate anywhere else), intensity (usually graded on a scale of 0 to 10, with 0 being no pain and 10 being the worst pain ever experienced or imagined), duration (how long does it last), and precipitating and alleviating factors. The next step is to determine how the patient perceives the pain, what if anything the pain prevents the patient from doing, and what the patient's expectations are for relief. Does the patient expect the pain to go away completely, or can he or she describe an acceptable level of tolerance? Once these questions have been answered, the health care team can begin formulating a plan of how to deal with the pain.

Because pain has both physical and emotional components, generally a systematic approach is used in attempts to control it. For patients who have not been receiving narcotics, treatment typically begins with mild narcotics such as acetaminophen with codeine (Tylenol 3 or 4) or acetaminophen with hydrocodone (Vicodin). If these drugs are not effective, acetaminophen with oxycodone (Percocet) or aspirin with oxycodone (Percodan) may be tried. If these do not provide relief, plain codeine or oxycodone may be used. Finally, if the pain still persists, hydromorphone (Dilaudid), oral morphine, sustained-release morphine, or fentanyl (Duragesic) patches may be used. Fentanyl patches are a relatively new way of delivering opioids. The medication on the patch is absorbed through the skin and enters the systemic circulation. For patients who cannot swallow or are having profuse diarrhea, the patch is a practical alternative for delivering pain medication.

The threshold for increasing the amount of pain medication or changing to another drug if the original regimen is not working should be low. For patients already tolerant to narcotics, switching from Dilaudid to oral morphine or vice versa may be useful in controlling an increase in pain, because these two agents are not cross-resistant. Additionally, simply increasing the amount of narcotics a patient is taking can control new pain. However, if a patient requires large doses of intravenous morphine, an attempt should be made to acquire the preservative-free preparation. Large doses of the preservative can cause altered mental status and hallucinations. Additionally, pain mediation should be administered around the clock, not "as needed." Around-the-clock administration ensures a steady blood level of medication and provides the best control.

Patients (and the health care providers) should be assured that addiction is not an issue. It is unacceptable for patients to be in uncontrolled pain. The amount of energy a patient expends trying to control pain is tremendous, and this is energy that could be put into spending time with family members, eating, sleeping, or doing other favored activities. With all the technology available today, there is no reason that cancer patients should be in pain. If a patient is in pain, the health care providers are not doing an adequate job.

In addition to opiates, other medications can be used to control pain. The most well known of these are nonsteroidal antiinflammatory drugs (NSAIDS), such as ibuprofen (Motrin) and naproxen sodium (Naprosyn). Nonsteroidal antiinflammatory drugs are particularly helpful when the cause of the pain is bone involvement. If a nerve process may be contributing to the pain, addition of anticonvulsants and antidepressants may be helpful. As noted earlier, palliation of pain can also include use of chemotherapy and radiation therapy. The latter can be especially useful for pain due to hepatic tumors, which can stretch the capsule of the liver, causing severe pain, or to bone metastases. Other methods to be considered for pain relief include nerve blocks, use of transcutaneous electrical nerve stimulation units, and epidural narcotics. These methods usually require referral to the anesthesiology department, physical therapy department, or a pain clinic.

Additional methods of pain control include distraction, massage, relaxation therapy, application of heat or cold to the affected area, and visualization. These techniques can be useful if the pain is mild; however, it is not reasonable to expect them to relieve moderate or severe pain. They should be thought of as adjunctive therapies that can potentiate or amplify the effect of narcotics.

Administration of morphine, orally or parenterally, is not limited to the treatment of pain. Morphine can also be useful when patients experience shortness of breath, difficulty breathing, or air hunger. The exact mechanism of action is unknown, but the drug may increase the diffusion of oxygen across the alveolar membrane. Patients who receive morphine for relief of respiratory signs and symptoms report that it diminishes the feelings of dyspnea and air hunger. Dosages of morphine used for this

purpose are arbitrary. For patients who have not been taking narcotics, 2–5 mg orally may be sufficient. For patients who have been taking large amounts of narcotics to control pain, higher doses are reasonable.

Nausea and Vomiting

Nausea and vomiting, although less feared than pain, can be just as menacing. A key difference, however, is that objective data can be collected. Vomiting can be witnessed, and the material vomited can be measured and characterized. Distinguishing between nausea and vomiting is important. Either of the two can occur alone or be preceded by the other. Nausea and vomiting may be due to therapy the patient has received, the tumor itself, the release of certain cytokines, metabolic disturbances such as hypercalcemia, central nervous system metastasis, or a physical obstruction.

Treatment varies greatly, depending on the situation. Therefore, the cause of the nausea and vomiting must be determined. Some initial questions to ask include ones about current medications or therapies the patient is receiving. Has the patient experienced any new onset of other signs and symptoms? Patients with obstruction or hypercalcemia may have changes in bowel habits and in the characteristics of their stools. Inquiring about the characteristics of the material vomited is also important. Patients should be asked to describe the contents of the vomitus (what exactly are they throwing up). Does the vomitus contain everything that they are eating or only certain foods? Is there any blood in the material vomited? Does the material vomited resemble coffee grounds? Does it have a foul odor? When does the patient experience the nausea or vomiting? Are the problems continual, intermittent, or precipitated by certain events? What is the patient's nutritional and hydration status? Finally, how does nausea or vomiting or both interfere with the patient's life?

Most treatment of nausea and vomiting is not without side effects. Some medications used to treat nausea and vomiting can cause altered mentation. This side effect may be unacceptable to the patient, so it is useful to evaluate the effect of nausea and vomiting on the patient and to have a sense of the patient's preference for treatment. Methods of treating nausea and vomiting include alternative therapies such as biofeedback and visualization; administration of medications, such as anxiolytics, steroids, and drugs that act centrally and peripherally; manipulation of diet; and treatment of the underlying cause of the nausea and vomiting.

Anorexia

Often, eating is the least important task for a patient coming to terms with a progressing disease. Just as often, feeding someone is the one thing a family member or significant other deems important. This dichotomy frequently causes frustration, anger, and anguish within the family. Food is the source of all life. Many emotions are triggered by feeding someone, and many implications are associated with eating. Not eating can be viewed as a way to exert control over one's environment. Probably more realistically, patients who are terminally ill have neither the appetite nor the need to eat, and their neglect of eating is a visible sign to their families that life may be ending. It is not uncommon for a struggle to erupt in this situation. The family wants desperately for the patient to eat, whereas the patient has no need or desire to do so. Anger, frustration, and, ultimately, anguish may be experienced by the family and the patient.

In this situation, reminding the family that the outcome will be the same whether the patient eats or not can add perspective. Family members should be encouraged to spend whatever time is left enjoying the patient's company, instead of feeling hurt or let down when the patient cannot or will not eat. This companionship is much more rewarding than seeing the patient take two bites of a favorite meal. If a patient wants to eat but has no appetite, and nausea and vomiting are not a problem, then appetite stimulants such as dronabinol (Marinol) may be appropriate. Tetrahydrocannabinol, the active ingredient in marijuana and the basis of dronabinol, has been used as an appetite stimulant in many cancer patients. Another appetite stimulant that may be prescribed is megestrol acetate (Megace), a progestin originally used to treat endometrial and breast cancer. The dose required to increase appetite is much higher than the doses used to treat these two cancers. If the patient cannot tolerate all the pills necessary to provide the recom-

mended dose, a more easily tolerated suspension is available.

Constipation and Diarrhea

Other gastrointestinal signs and symptoms terminally ill patients may experience include constipation and diarrhea. Constipation may be a direct result of narcotics used to control pain. Therefore, patients who are receiving narcotics for pain control should be started on a bowel regimen as well. A typical regimen includes use of a stool softener such as docusate sodium (Colace) and a laxative such as senna (Senokot). Patients should continue their usual diet during this time, focusing on foods that tend to regulate the bowel.

Patients who have diarrhea should be examined to ensure that an infectious agent is not the cause. Severe abdominal cramping, bloating, bloody diarrhea, and elevated body temperature may be indications of an infection. If a patient has these signs or symptoms, stool samples should be obtained for tests for the presence of ova and parasites and for drug sensitivity. Diarrhea may also be an indication of fecal impaction; diarrheal stool seeps around the impacted area. Thorough assessment is necessary to differentiate diarrhea due to infection from diarrhea due to impaction.

Treatment of diarrhea includes adequate hydration and administration of antidiarrheals. Some commonly used medications are diphenoxylate and atropine (Lomotil) and loperamide (Imodium). Over-the-counter drugs are generally not useful in controlling diarrhea in dying patients. In severe cases, opioids may be required. Denatured tincture of opium is often used with good results.

HELPING THE FAMILY COPE

Family members of a patient who is dying may require help in coping throughout the patient's illness and for several months after the patient's death. In the beginning, just coming to grips with the diagnosis of cancer and the subsequent treatment may seem overwhelming.

Hope abounds during this time that the patient will become well and even be cured. Once it becomes clear that cure is not possible, and the decision is made to change treatment goals from aggressive to palliative, the family understandably begins grieving the loss of the patient.

The expression of that grief may range from searching endlessly for new, more radical treatments that are "sure cures" to totally giving up and withdrawing from the patient. If the patient is in a hospice program and wishes to die at home, the patient's family members must be involved in every step to ensure the success of this goal. They need to know exactly what they can expect from the hospice team. Some family members feel uncomfortable and awkward and need instruction on what they can do to help. As the family prepares for the death of a loved one at home, they are also preparing for the loss of that person. When they are able to give the patient permission to "let go" and die, they are in fact giving themselves permission to let go of the loved one.

One way to help family members with this process is to explore other losses they have experienced. This includes eliciting feelings and determining previous coping mechanisms. Unresolved issues of previous losses may need to be addressed before the family can grieve the loss of the patient. Unresolved personal issues with the patient may also need to be addressed, so that there are no regrets or guilty feelings after the patient has died. Family members should be encouraged to communicate with the dying person, expressing their thoughts, feelings, and emotions. Looking at an album of photographs or asking family members to recall special events or family history are ways nurses can help facilitate this communication.

Once the patient has died, attention turns to the remaining family members. The structure of bereavement counseling differs among hospice programs. Although such counseling is a required component of all Medicare-certified hospices, the policies pertaining to it are unique to each hospice program. The purpose of bereavement counseling is to help the family adjust to the loss of a family member. Four tasks are necessary for the normal grief process to proceed (Worden, 1982):

1. Accept the reality of the loss.

2. Experience the pain of grief.

3. Adjust to the environment in which the deceased is missing.

4. Withdraw emotional energy and place it in another relationship.

The time it takes for someone to accomplish these tasks varies. Bereavement counseling attempts to ensure that the family is moving in the right direction. The counseling usually includes a bereavement assessment; regularly scheduled visits; and, for those with complicated or abnormal grief reactions, referral to a professional counselor.

Complicated or abnormal grief reactions are usually manifested in one of three ways (Worden, 1982): (1) The reaction may be prolonged. (2) The reaction may be masked in behavioral or physical signs or symptoms (e.g., pain, sexual impotence, "acting out"). (3) The reaction may be an exaggerated or excessive expression of normal grief reactions, such as excessive anger, sadness, or depression. It is important that the members of the hospice team recognize these indicators of abnormal grief. Abnormal grief has been associated with many physical and emotional illnesses, including increased risk of suicide. Again, caregivers should be aware of cultural differences in the grief process and take care not to assume that someone is exhibiting signs of abnormal grief when, in fact, it is his or her custom to behave in such a manner.

BIBLIOGRAPHY

Bedell, S. E., Pelle, D., Maher, P. L., et al. (1986). Do-not-resuscitate orders for critically ill patients in the hospital: How are they used and what is their impact? *Journal of the American Medical Association, 256*(2), 233–237.

Boring, C., Squires, T., Tong, T., & Montgomery, S. (1994). Cancer statistics 1994. *CA—A Cancer Journal for Clinicians, 44*(1), 7–26.

Martinez, J., & Wagner, S. (1993). Hospice care. In S. Groenwald, M. Frogge, M. Goodman, & C. Yarbro (Eds.), *Cancer nursing: Principles and practice* (pp. 1432–1450). Boston: Jones and Bartlett.

Mills, D. (1992). Changes in oncology health care settings. In J. Clark & R. McGee (Eds.), *Core curriculum for oncology nursing* (2nd ed., pp. 205–220). Philadelphia: Saunders.

Vitelli, C. E., Cooper, K., Rogatko, A., et al. (1991). Cardiopulmonary resuscitation and the patient with cancer. *Journal of Clinical Oncology, 9*(1), 111–115.

VonGunten, C. (1991). CPR in the hospitalized patient: When is it futile? *American Family Physician, 4,* 2130–2134.

Wadill, G. (1991). Advanced directives. *Hospice, 2,* 10–11.

Worden, J. (1982). *Grief counseling and grief therapy.* New York: Springer.

STUDY QUESTIONS

Chapter 12

Questions 82–87

82. Which of the following is characteristic of patients with advanced stages of cancer?

    a. They have been cured by their treatment.
    b. Despite treatment, cure is not possible
    c. They had a large tumor at the time of diagnosis.
    d. They all have lymph node involvement.

83. Palliative care includes all of the following *except:*

    a. Treatments that prolong life
    b. Treatment that alleviates suffering
    c. Aggressive management of signs and symptoms
    d. Treatment aimed at promoting a painless death

84. Which of the following statements about advance directives is correct?

    a. Advance directives are federally mandated for hospice programs, clinics, and health care agencies.
    b. If advance directives are not filled out before a patient enters a hospice program, care will be denied.
    c. Advance directives limit patients' rights.
    d. Once signed, an advance directive cannot be revoked.

85. Features frequently offered by hospice programs include:

    a. Aggressive therapy such as treatment of the tumor
    b. Prophylactic intubation when the patient becomes tachypneic
    c. Bereavement counseling
    d. Transfer to the intensive care unit when necessary

86. Which of the following is *not* a sign or symptom often experienced by patients who are terminally ill?

    a. Pain
    b. Nausea and vomiting
    c. Anorexia
    d. Excessive energy

87. The purpose of bereavement counseling for family members of a cancer patient who has died is to do which of the following?

    a. Help the family adjust to the loss of a family member
    b. Provide additional funding for hospice programs
    c. Make sure all the leftover bills get paid
    d. Remove any extra supplies that were left at the patient's house.

CHAPTER 13

CANCER IN CHILDREN

CHAPTER OBJECTIVE

After completing this chapter, the reader will be able to recognize and discuss the key concepts of cancer in children.

LEARNING OBJECTIVES

After studying this chapter, the reader will be able to

1. Recognize the stages of growth and development associated with various age groups in children.

2. Specify the most common solid tumor that occurs in children.

3. Recognize common initial signs and symptoms associated with cancer in children.

4. Specify the age at which most cases of acute lymphocytic leukemia in children occur.

5. Recognize the concepts of death characteristic of children of various ages.

6. Specify the percentage of children with cancer who are cured.

7. Recognize risk factors that increase the chance that a second malignant tumor will develop in survivors of childhood cancer.

INTRODUCTION

Children 60% cured

Malignant tumors in children are rare and account for approximately 1% of the cancers diagnosed in the United States annually. Cancer in children differs from cancer in adults and is generally more responsive to therapy. Approximately 7,800 new cases of cancer in children less than 15 years old and 3,500 new cases in adolescents 15–19 years old are diagnosed each year. Approximately 60% of children are cured of their cancer. Once thought of as an acute disease, cancer in children is now considered a chronic illness. Even those children who die of cancer often live much longer than was once the norm for children with this disease. Cancer remains the second leading cause of death in children, second only to accidents. However, the number of long-term survivors continues to increase because of advances in medical technology, cancer treatments, and supportive care.

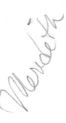

OVERVIEW OF GROWTH AND DEVELOPMENT

Children grow and develop rapidly, especially during the first few years of life. The diagnosis of a potentially life-threatening illness, such as cancer, can have an effect on the child's growth and development. Nurses can help children who have cancer by keeping in mind the children's developmental status (Table 13-1). Being aware of the developmental stage assists in anticipating reactions of a child and in planning age-appropriate strategies. It is important to keep children informed and to provide a forum for discussions of feelings. Interventions may occur indirectly through a parent or directly with the child.

Children who are hospitalized often regress. For example, a toddler who is toilet trained may suddenly revert to needing diapers. This is a normal coping mechanism. It is important for nurses to allow appropriate periods of regression and still remember the importance of promoting normalcy whenever possible. Many children may exhibit signs of magical thinking. They may think that they caused their illness and are being punished for bad thoughts. Until a child understands what does and does not cause cancer, it is easy for him or her to think that anything could have caused it—even words or a fall: for example, "My brother and I were fighting. I wished he were dead. Today we found out that he has cancer."

Throughout the course of cancer, children experience a variety of emotions. Nurses can help by being sensitive to children's needs. It is important to remember to be creative when assessing a child. Assessment provides a better understanding of the child's behavior and makes it possible to help the child and his or her family cope with the diagnosis of cancer and its treatment.

A thorough assessment should include the following:

- The child's developmental status.

- The child's previous experience with illness, cancer, and hospitalization (a child brings the sum total of his or her past experience to each new situation).

- Comfort measures (e.g., the child's favorite toy).

- Previous coping strategies.

- Current coping and adjustment.

- Family structure.

- The child's relationships within the family constellation.

- The boundaries of the family (open or closed).

- Available resources (neighbors, church, school) and how the child interacts with them.

- The child's grade in school (if applicable).

- Activities.

Communication is a potential barrier to obtaining an assessment, especially in young children, because their verbal skills may not be well developed. Use of books, play, and drawings are methods of obtaining information from children in a nonthreatening way. These methods can be useful in both assessment and implementation. They act as springboards for discussion between child and adult. Public libraries are great sources of age-appropriate books.

Because play centers on the self and on stressful situations as perceived by the child, repetition of play enables the child to practice and deal with the stressful situation again and again. Use of dolls or puppets is an example of play activities. Medical play provides children with opportunities to be prepared for what to expect during treatment and to act out medical information they have been given or situations they have observed.

Table 13-1
Concepts of Growth and Development

Age Group	Psychosocial Development (Erikson)	Cognitive Development (Piaget)	Behaviors
Infants (birth to 1 year)	Trust vs. mistrust	Sensorimotor (birth to 2 years)	Response to environment through senses Enjoyment of lights, color, and motion Sucking major source of gratification Separation anxiety
Toddlers (1-3 years)	Autonomy vs. shame and doubt	Sensorimotor and preoperational: preconceptual	Toilet training major task Development of vocabulary (by 24 months, uses about 300 words and speaks in phrases of 2-3 words) Magical thinking Rituals
Preschoolers (3-5 years)	Initiative vs. guilt	Preoperational: intuitive phase	Imaginary friends Expansion of vocabulary Concrete thinking and expression Recognition of sex differences Egocentricity Magical thinking Fear of unknown, dark, being left alone, bodily injury, and mutilation
School agers (6-12 years)	Industry vs. inferiority	Concrete operational (7-11)	Interest in how body works Development of physical abilities Establishment of new relationships Fear of bodily injury and mutilation Beginning of logical thinking
Adolescents (12-19 years)	Identity vs. role confusion	Formal operational	Body image important Control important Peer relationships important Development of sense of own identity Formation of sexual identity Beginning of abstract thinking

Source: Education Committee of the Association of Pediatric Oncology Nurses. (1992). *Pediatric oncology nursing study guide.* Richmond, VA: Phenix Corp., pp. 103-107, and Maul-Mellott, S., & Adams, J. (1987). *Childhood cancer: A nursing overview.* Boston: Jones and Bartlett, pp. 4-10.

Drawings are valuable in eliciting additional information, because they do not depend on a child's willingness to communicate or his or her ability to verbalize. A child can draw pictures about family members, feelings, and perceptions of what is happening and what it is like to visit the hospital. Children should be encouraged to talk about their pictures. The process itself, without interpretation, can be a therapeutic intervention.

Throughout the course of illness, children need the following:

- Parental availability, including clear and frequent messages of what is happening and what to expect.

- Maintenance of routines (e.g., school, bedtimes, nap times, mealtimes). This is especially important in young children.

- Security (e.g., consistent and familiar caretakers).

- Opportunities to express feelings, fears, hopes, and anxieties as they arise. Having the opportunity to discuss feelings plays an important role in adaptation.

- Maintenance of peer relationships.

Nurses are in a unique position to facilitate adaptation to the diagnosis of cancer by providing education, support, and referrals to appropriate resources. The goal should be to assist children and their families in integrating the cancer experience into their lives. When medically possible, treatment and procedures should be scheduled around important life events, such as a birthday, prom, or graduation. Because school is an important developmental task for children, school reintegration is an essential goal. A visit to the child's school to explain the child's diagnosis to classmates and answer questions is helpful to the child's adaptation. Another part of growing up for many children is attending camp during their summer vacations. For children with cancer who are receiving treatment, going to camp could be difficult. However, the development of camps equipped to handle the special needs of children with cancer has made summer camp possible for these children. The goal of nursing care should be to promote normalcy throughout the course of the child's illness.

COMMON CANCERS IN CHILDREN

A variety of tumors develop in children (Figure 13-1). Unlike cancer in adults, neoplasms in children arise primarily from the mesodermal germ layer and the neuroectodermal layer. Leukemias, brain tumors, lymphomas, embryonal tumors, and sarcomas are the most common malignant tumors in children. Dramatic improvements in survival have occurred since the 1970s. The greatest improvements have been in the treatment of Hodgkin's disease, Wilms' tumor, non-Hodgkin's lymphoma, and leukemia. The goals of cancer treatment in children are to eradicate the disease, preserve function, and minimize long-term sequelae.

Leukemias

Leukemias are an abnormal proliferation of immature leukocytes or white blood cells. Leukemias can be classified as acute or chronic. The most common ones in children are the acute leukemias, which account for approximately 85–90% of the leukemias diagnosed.

Acute Lymphocytic Leukemia. Acute lymphocytic leukemia, the most common malignant tumor in children, is the abnormal proliferation and incomplete maturation of lymphoid stem cells. This tumor accounts for 75% of the leukemias diagnosed in children, with approximately 2,000 new cases diagnosed annually. The peak age at onset is 4 years. Acute lymphocytic leukemia is more common in males and in whites than in females and nonwhites.

Signs and symptoms of acute lymphocytic leukemia are related to infiltration of bone marrow and other organs by leukemic cells. The initial signs and symptoms are generally vague and nonspecific. Parents may think the

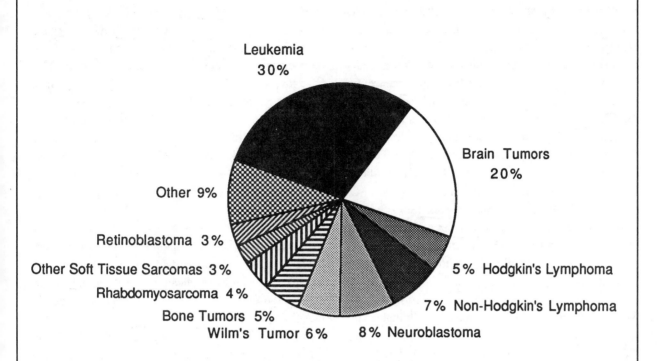

Leukemia
30%

Brain Tumors
20%

Other 9%

Retinoblastoma 3%

Other Soft Tissue Sarcomas 3%

Rhabdomyosarcoma 4%

Bone Tumors 5%

Wilm's Tumor 6%

5% Hodgkin's Lymphoma

7% Non-Hodgkin's Lymphoma

8% Neuroblastoma

Figure 13-1. Distribution of Common Pediatric Malignancies.

child has the flu. Signs and symptoms include fever, recurrent infection, anemia, fatigue, malaise, easy bruising, petechiae, bleeding, pallor, bone pain, and anorexia. Patients with involvement of the central nervous system at the time of diagnosis account for less than 10% of cases. These patients may be asymptomatic or may have signs and symptoms related to increased intracranial pressure, including headache, vomiting, and visual disturbances. Some degree of hepatosplenomegaly is present at the time of diagnosis in most children. The diagnosis is confirmed by results of bone marrow aspiration and biopsy, lumbar puncture, and laboratory tests (complete blood cell count [CBC], blood chemistries, immunophenotyping, cytogenetic assays). Acute lymphocytic leukemia is further characterized by the cell of origin and the stage of differentiation (e.g., T cell, pre-B cell).

A number of prognostic factors have been recognized. Prognosis is good for children 2–9 years old whose white blood cell count is less than 10,000 cells/mm^3. Prognosis is poor for children who are less than 2 years old or more than 10 years old; are black; and have an in-

itial white blood cell count of less than 50,000 cells/mm^3, certain B- and T-cell immunologic subtypes, low hemoglobin levels, low platelet counts, low levels of immunoglobulins, and slow response to therapy (more than 4–6 weeks to achieve remission). On the basis of prognostic factors, children are assigned to low, standard, or high-risk groups for treatment. Tumor lysis syndrome in response to the rapid breakdown of tumor cells is common in patients in the high-risk group.

The primary method of treatment is chemotherapy. Treatment is divided into several phases: induction, consolidation, and maintenance. The goal of induction is to achieve a remission, the goal of consolidation is to eradicate any residual tumor, and the goal of maintenance is to sustain a complete remission. In the maintenance phase, drugs are usually administered over a 2- to 3-year period. The number and dosage of chemotherapeutic agents vary, depending on the prognostic factors and the patient's risk category.

Common chemotherapeutic agents for treatment of acute lymphocytic leukemia include vincristine (Oncovin), prednisone (Deltasone), asparaginase (L-asparaginase, Elspar), and methotrexate (MTX, Amethopterin). Bone marrow is the most common site of relapse. Bone marrow transplantation is a treatment option for patients in second remission after a bone marrow relapse. Two sanctuary sites for acute lymphocytic leukemia, the central nervous system and the testes, affect survival rates. For treatment and prevention of central nervous system disease, children are given drugs prophylactically throughout the course of their therapy. Prophylaxis usually consists of intrathecal medications such as methotrexate, cytosine arabinoside (Ara-C, cytarabine, Cytosar), and hydrocortisone (Solu-Cortef), alone or in combination, or high doses of methotrexate. Patients with central nervous system relapses often receive craniospinal radiation in addition to intrathecal medications.

Ninety-five percent of children with acute lymphocytic leukemia have a remission. Overall prognosis is good; 80% are cured. When the cancer recurs, the prognosis varies, depending on the site of the recurrence (e.g., bone marrow, central nervous system, testes) and whether the relapse occurred when the patient was on or off therapy. Subsequent remissions are generally easy to achieve; however, the duration of remission may be variable.

Acute Myelogenous Leukemia. Acute myelogenous leukemia is an abnormal proliferation and incomplete maturation of the myeloid stem cells. It can occur in any of the myeloid cell lines. It is less common than acute lymphocytic leukemia and accounts for 15–20% of the leukemias diagnosed in children. Unlike the case in acute lymphocytic leukemia, the occurrence of acute myelogenous leukemia has no peak with regard to the patient's age and no sex or racial differences. Subtypes of acute myelogenous leukemia have been recognized.

At the time of diagnosis, children with acute myelogenous leukemia can have a variety of signs and symptoms along a continuum from none to potentially life-threatening complications (e.g., hemorrhage, disseminated intravascular coagulation). Most children are asymptomatic. Clinical features are related to signs and symptoms associated with neutropenia (e.g., fever, sore throat, infection, sepsis), thrombocytopenia (e.g., petechiae, bruising, epistaxis, gingival bleeding), and anemia (e.g., pallor, dyspnea, fatigue, weakness, congestive heart failure). Some patients have disseminated intravascular coagulation, and approximately 10–25% have involvement of the central nervous system, which may be asymptomatic, at the time of diagnosis. Hepatomegaly, splenomegaly, or both are present in approximately 50% of cases. The diagnosis of acute myelogenous leukemia is based on results of bone marrow aspiration and biopsy, lumbar puncture, and laboratory tests (CBC, chemistries, immunophenotyping, cytogenetic assays).

Treatment includes combination chemotherapy. Before therapy begins, interventions are directed at controlling any life-threatening complications present at the time of diagnosis. Common agents used to achieve remission include cytosine arabinoside, daunomycin (daunorubicin) and Adriamycin (doxorubicin). Treatment may also include additional agents such as vincristine, prednisone, 6-thioguanine, cyclophosphamide (Cytoxan), and 5-azacytadine.

Approximately 70–80% of children achieve a remission, which is generally shorter in duration than that in patients with acute lymphocytic leukemia. Once a remission is achieved, patients receive therapy designed to eradicate any residual disease. Although the risk of central nervous system relapse is much lower than in acute lymphocytic leukemia, most regimens include prophylaxis with intrathecal cytosine arabinoside or methotrexate with or without craniospinal radiation. Bone marrow transplantation is often recommended for patients during their first remission. Several studies are currently comparing the advantages of bone marrow transplantation and conventional chemotherapy in producing successful long-term survival. Prognosis is still poorer for acute myelogenous leukemia than for acute lymphocytic leukemia; however the survival rate for the former has increased to approximately 40%. Children who relapse while off therapy have a better prognosis than those who do not achieve a remission or who relapse while receiving therapy.

Central Nervous System Tumors

Brain tumors account for approximately 20% of the cancers diagnosed in children, with 1200–1500 new cases annually. Brain tumors are the most common solid tumor in children and the second most common malignant tumor in this age group. The overall occurrence is not affected by race or sex. Brain tumors can occur in children of any age; however, different types are more prevalent at different ages. Classification of brain tumors in children remains controversial. Approximately 50% of the tumors occur in the posterior fossa and 50% above the tentorium.

The signs and symptoms associated with brain tumors are variable. They are determined by the location and rate of growth of the tumor and the age of the child. Signs and symptoms are usually related to increased intracranial pressure and can include headache (usually in the morning), morning vomiting, visual problems, irritability, behavioral problems, ataxia, and lethargy. Other signs and symptoms related to the location of the tumor may include personality changes, apathy, depression, fatigue, seizures (uncommon), papilledema, and developmental delays or regression of developmental milestones. Initial signs and symptoms in infants are irritability, vomiting, loss of developmental milestones, lethargy, failure to thrive, and enlarging head circumference. School-aged children may have vague complaints of headache, personality change, decreased school performance, altered sensorium, fatigue, and clumsiness. The diagnostic workup includes a physical examination with neurologic assessment and magnetic resonance imaging with or without contrast material. Other studies may include computed tomography and positron emission tomography. Many of the studies used to evaluate brain tumors require the patient to hold still. Sedation may be required to obtain meaningful results.

Treatment of brain tumors depends on the child's age, the histologic features and location of the tumor, and the presence of disseminated disease (rarely outside the central nervous system). Surgery is the primary intervention; the goal is total resection. Although radiation is highly effective in the treatment of brain tumors in children, long-term sequelae often occur, especially in children whose brain is still developing. Consequently, children less than 4 years old often receive only chemotherapy after surgery; the goal is to delay the use of radiation to allow development of brain tissue.

The role of chemotherapy in the treatment of certain tumor types is increasing. The challenge in using chemotherapy is to administer doses that are high enough to cross the blood-brain barrier but are not so high that they cause unacceptable toxic effects to the body. Radiosensitizers, phototherapy, bone marrow transplantation, and biologic response modifiers (e.g., interferon, monoclonal antibodies) are being explored as treatment options. Late sequelae of therapy are common. Children treated for brain tumors generally need rehabilitation, which should begin at the time of diagnosis of the tumor.

Prognosis depends on the type, location, and grade of the primary tumor and the presence or absence of metastatic disease. Long-term survival rates are 55% for medulloblastoma, 94% for juvenile pilocytic cerebellar astrocytoma, 58–88% for low-grade astrocytoma, and 20% for brainstem glioma.

Lymphomas

Hodgkin's Disease. Hodgkin's disease is an indolent tumor that arises from the lymphoid tissues of the lymphatic system. It accounts for about 5% of the cancers diagnosed in childhood. Approximately 350 new cases are diagnosed each year. Hodgkin's disease is rare in children less than 5 years old and appears to peak in children between the ages of 15 and 19 years. Before adolescence, the tumor occurs more often in boys than in girls; however, the ratio of males to females is about the same in adolescence. Four histologic subtypes have been recognized and are used for classification. The nodular sclerosing type is the most common in children.

At the time of diagnosis, 60–90% of patients with Hodgkin's disease have a painless, firm, movable cervical or supraclavicular lymph node. Additionally, 50% of children with this tumor have a mediastinal mass. Approximately 30% of children have systemic signs and symptoms, which indicate a poor prognosis. These include anorexia, unexplained weight loss of more than 10%, malaise, fatigue or lethargy, fevers, and night sweats. Children with systemic signs and symptoms are considered to have "B" disease. Those who are asymptomatic are considered to have "A" disease. Diagnostic workup includes lymph node biopsy to confirm the diagnosis and laboratory studies (CBC, erythrocyte sedimentation rate, level of copper, hepatic and renal tests, levels of alkaline phosphatase). Gallium scans, computed tomography, magnetic resonance imaging, and bone marrow biopsy are done to establish the extent of the disease.

Because lymphadenopathy often develops as a result of adenitis, children frequently are treated with antibiotics before Hodgkin's disease is diagnosed. Once the diagnosis of cancer has been confirmed and the tumor has been staged, treatment of the tumor begins. Treatments include radiation and combination chemotherapy. Patients with stage I disease generally receive radiation only. A variety of combination chemotherapy regimens have been developed and are currently being studied for efficacy. These include MOPP (nitrogen mustard [mechlorethamine], vincristine [Oncovin], procarbazine [Matulane], prednisone), COPP (cyclophosphamide, Oncovin, procarbazine, prednisone), A-COPP (Adriamycin, cyclophosphamide, Oncovin, procarbazine, prednisone), and ABDV (Adriamycin, bleomycin [Blenoxane], dacarbazine, vinblastine [Velban]). MOPP is the traditional regimen for treatment of Hodgkin's disease. Often these regimens are alternated to decrease the development of drug resistance.

The prognosis for Hodgkin's disease is good. The overall survival rates are more than 90% for children with stage I or II A disease and 80% for those with stage III disease. The rate for children with stage IV continues to improve and is approaching 70%. The survival rate for patients who have relapsed is approximately 49%.

Non-Hodgkin's Lymphoma. Non-Hodgkin's lymphoma is an aggressive malignant tumor that arises from the lymphoid tissues of the lymphatic system. Four histologic subtypes are recognized and are used to classify this tumor. Non-Hodgkin's lymphoma accounts for approximately 7% of the cancers diagnosed in childhood. Approximately 550 new cases are diagnosed each year in children from infancy to adolescence. The peak occurrence is between the ages of 7 and 11 years; the

male-to-female ratio is 3:1. Although the exact etiology of non-Hodgkin's lymphoma is unknown, children with certain congenital immunodeficiency syndromes (e.g., Wiskott-Aldrich syndrome) and acquired conditions (e.g., HIV infection) appear to have an increased risk for this tumor.

Clinical features at the time of diagnosis depend on the site and extent of disease; however, manifestation of signs and symptoms is rapid. The most common site of disease at the time of diagnosis is the abdomen. Signs and symptoms include abdominal cramping, change in bowel habits, nausea and vomiting, partial or complete obstruction of the bowel, intussusception, and ascites. Often, patients mistakenly think they have the flu. The second most common site of disease at the time of diagnosis is the mediastinum. Signs and symptoms include cough, fever, dyspnea, respiratory distress, and facial edema. Patients may have tracheal compression.

The diagnostic workup includes history and physical examination, biopsy of tissue, bone marrow aspiration, lumbar puncture, computed tomography of the chest and abdomen, bone scan, gallium scan, and laboratory studies (e.g., CBC, hepatic and renal function tests). Additional studies are ordered depending on the results of the diagnostic studies and the site of disease. Approximately 20% of children have evidence of tumor cells in the bone marrow at the time of diagnosis. The amount of time used for diagnostic workup is generally short, because this tumor grows rapidly and it is important to start therapy as quickly as possible.

Most patients have large tumor burdens at the time of diagnosis, and the disease is usually classified as stage III or stage IV. Because of the large tumor burden and the rapid response to therapy, patients with non-Hodgkin's lymphoma, especially the Burkitt's type, are at risk for tumor lysis syndrome. This syndrome is due to the cellular contents released when the malignant cells are rapidly destroyed by therapy. Before therapy begins, patients should be rigorously hydrated with fluids and begin taking allopurinol.

Treatment of non-Hodgkin's lymphoma consists primarily of combination chemotherapy (e.g., vincristine, prednisone, Adriamycin, and cytosine arabinoside). Prophylaxis to prevent involvement of the central nervous system is used in patients with advanced stages of non-Hodgkin's lymphoma. Treatment regimens are usually less intensive for patients with localized disease. The key for patients with advanced stages of disease appears to be administering the cycles of chemotherapeutic agents as rapidly as possible. Patients going through these intensive regimens require a tremendous amount of support and rehabilitation.

A large tumor burden and the presence of disease in the central nervous system indicate a poor prognosis. Overall survival rates are 90% for patients with localized disease and 60–70% for those with advanced stages of disease. Higher than normal serum concentrations of lactate dehydrogenase may be an indicator that the disease has recurred. Prognosis is poor for patients who relapse. Bone marrow transplantation may be used in patients who have relapsed.

Embryonal Tumors

Neuroblastoma. Neuroblastoma, a malignant embryonic neoplasm arising from neural crest tissue, can develop at any point along the sympathetic nervous system. It accounts for approximately 8% of the cancers diagnosed in children and is the most common neoplasm in infants. Approximately 600 new cases are diagnosed annually. The median age at the time of diagnosis is 2 years; the tumor is diagnosed in 36% of patients before the age of 1 year, in 79% by age 4 years, and in 97% by age 10 years. Neuroblastoma is slightly more common in boys than in girls and is more common in whites than in nonwhites. Cases of familial neuroblastoma have been reported. Since its discovery as an amplification gene in neuroblastoma cells, a number of studies have examined the usefulness of the oncogene N-*myc* for establishing diagnosis and prognosis of this tumor.

Neuroblastoma is a slow-growing encapsulated tumor that often impinges on other organs. The tumor is generally discovered by the patient or the patient's caretaker and is usually quite large at the time of diagnosis. Clinical features vary, depending on the location of the primary tumor and the presence or absence of metastatic disease. Signs and symptoms may arise secondary to compression of vital structures. Common primary sites include the abdomen (65–70%), thorax (15%), and neck (5%). Patients with abdominal tumors may have anorexia, changes in bowel and bladder habits, abdominal pain, anorexia, weight loss, and paralysis due to compression of the spinal cord. Patients with mediastinal tumors may have cough, neck or facial edema, dyspnea, respiratory distress, superior vena cava syndrome, and feeding difficulties (in infants). Patients with neck tumors may have facial paralysis, ptosis, earache, dysphagia, and hoarseness. Other signs and symptoms that may be present at the time of diagnosis include weight loss, irritability, fatigue, low-grade fevers, lymphadenopathy, and generalized aches and pains. Approximately 70% of children with neuroblastoma have metastasis at the time of diagnosis.

Disseminated disease results in site-specific signs and symptoms. For example, bone metastasis may be manifested as bone pain, limping, refusal to walk, or pathologic fracture. Skin metastasis may produce blue or purplish "blueberry muffin" nodules (most common in infants). Involvement of the soft tissues behind the eyes may produce periorbital edema and ecchymosis.

The diagnostic workup includes diagnostic imaging (chest radiography, computed tomography of the primary site, skeletal survey, bone scan, gallium scan, iodine 131-metaiodobenzylguanadine scan), laboratory studies (CBC, liver and renal function tests, serum levels of ferritin, levels of urinary catecholamines, N-*myc* amplification of tumor cells), and bone marrow aspiration and biopsy. Approximately 90% of patients have increased levels of urinary catecholamines.

Treatments include surgery, chemotherapy, and radiation. The goal of surgery is to establish the diagnosis and resect the tumor if possible. Common chemotherapeutic agents include cyclophosphamide, Adriamycin, vincristine, etoposide, teniposide, dacarbazine, and cisplatin. Radiation is used for local control. Neuroblastoma is aggressive and presents challenges. Bone marrow transplantation is being used to treat this disease. The role of immunotherapy is still being studied.

Good prognostic factors include age less than 1 year at the time of diagnosis, stage of disease I, II, or IV-s, and, some clinicians think, location of primary sites in the neck and thorax. Poor prognostic factors include tumors that cannot be completely resected, age more than 1 year at the time of diagnosis, stage IV disease, multiple copies of N-*myc* (more than 10), DNA diploidy, and histologic features characteristic of undifferentiated tissue. In general, children less than 1 year old who have localized disease (stages I and II) have a survival rate of approximately 90%.

Stage IV-s is a stage unique to neuroblastoma. Patients with stage IV-s tumors are infants less than 1 year old with disseminated disease. Unlike children with stage IV neuroblastoma, this group of patients has a better prognosis than what would be expected. Also characteristic of patients with stage IV-s disease is an increased number of spontaneous remissions. As a result, children with stage IV-s neuroblastoma may not receive treatment initially. They are often closely monitored for a spontaneous remission. Approximately 70–80% are cured.

Wilms' Tumor. Wilms' tumor is a rapidly growing and highly malignant embryonal cancer of the kidney that can occur in one or both kidneys. Some cases involve an inherited form. The inherited form is transmitted as an autosomal dominant trait and has been associated with chromosomal abnormalities (e.g., deletion of a suppressor gene located on the short arm of chromosome 11). A variety of congenital anomalies (e.g., aniridia, hemihypertrophy, genitourinary anomalies) have also been associated with an increased risk for Wilms' tumor. The median age at the time of diagnosis is 2–3 years. The disease rarely occurs in children more than 7 years old. Wilms' tumor occurs slightly more often in girls than in boys in the United States, and African-Americans appear to have a slightly increased risk.

Clinical manifestations include an enlarging, usually nontender, abdomen. The mass is generally discovered by the patient or the patient's caretaker and is usually quite large. Additional signs and symptoms include hypertension (30–60% of cases), fever, hematuria, anorexia, and abdominal pain. Diagnostic workup includes an abdominal sonography, computed tomography, and

magnetic resonance imaging to determine the location and extent of the primary tumor. Additional studies include computed tomography of the lungs and chest radiography to detect pulmonary nodules, laboratory studies (e.g., CBC), and urinalysis. Because the wall that encapsulates the tumor is thin and easily torn, palpation of the mass should be avoided to preserve the membrane and to keep the tumor enclosed. Confirmation of the diagnosis and staging are done during surgical resection.

Treatment is primarily surgery (nephrectomy) and adjuvant chemotherapy (e.g., vincristine, actinomycin D, Adriamycin, cyclophosphamide). For patients with unilateral involvement, the affected kidney is removed, and the unaffected kidney is examined to ensure absence of disease. In patients with bilateral involvement, the most involved kidney is removed, and the remaining tumor in the other kidney is resected. Wilms' tumor is highly responsive to chemotherapy and radiation. For patients with a favorable prognosis (disease stages I and II), chemotherapy alone after surgery is effective in achieving long-term survival. Patients with stage III and stage IV disease receive chemotherapy and radiation.

Prognosis depends on the stage of disease at the time of diagnosis, histologic features of the tumor, and involvement of lymph nodes. The national Wilms' tumor study group has developed a five-group staging classification system. Patients who meet the criteria for inclusion in groups I and II have an excellent prognosis, because in their cases, the tumor is completely removed. The overall survival rate is 95%. For patients with pulmonary metastases or unfavorable histologic features, the survival rate is 80%. Even patients with advanced stages of disease, recurrent disease, or disease in both kidneys have greater than a 50% chance of survival.

Retinoblastoma. Retinoblastoma is a rare congenital embryonic malignant tumor that arises from the retina of the eye. This tumor accounts for 5% of childhood blindness. Approximately 40% of the retinoblastomas are due to hereditary factors; in these cases, the tumor usually occurs in both eyes. The other 60% are not due to hereditary factors and usually affect only one eye. Approximately 200 new cases of retinoblastoma are diagnosed annually.

The most common clinical feature at the time of diagnosis is leukokoria, which is also called cat's eye reflex. The next most common indication of retinoblastoma is strabismus. A later indication is a red painful eye. Although often present at birth, retinoblastoma usually is not diagnosed until the patient is about 2 years old. At that time, the parent notices an abnormality of one or both of the eyes and seeks medical attention. Diagnostic workup includes an ophthalmoscopic examination. The child is given a general anesthetic so the eye can be fully examined and the location and size of the retinoblastoma lesions can be mapped. Imaging studies might include sonography, computed tomography, and magnetic resonance imaging.

Treatment is individualized, and planning is critical to determine which therapy will be optimal. Treatment depends on the size and extent of the lesions; however, the primary objective is to preserve vision. Treatments include surgery (enucleation of the eye), radiotherapy, phototherapy, and cryotherapy. A staging classification for retinoblastoma categorizes patients into five different groups according to the extent of disease.

Overall the prognosis for retinoblastoma is good. Children with small lesions confined to the retina have about a 95% chance of long-term survival. Children with metastatic disease usually die within 5–6 months despite treatment. Children with retinoblastoma in both eyes appear to be at an increased risk for the development of second malignant tumors. Genetic counseling is important, especially for children with the inherited form of retinoblastoma. Hereditary retinoblastoma is an autosomal dominant genetic disorder and is associated with a deletion of the short arm of chromosome 12. Offspring of persons with the deletion have a 50% chance of inheriting the gene for retinoblastoma.

Sarcomas

Sarcomas are divided into two categories: bone and soft tissue. They are named according to their tissue and type. Bone tumors account for 5% of cancers in children and soft-tissue sarcomas for 7%.

Osteogenic Sarcoma. Osteogenic sarcoma arises from the mesenchymal cells that produce bone and is the most common bone tumor in children. It occurs primarily in the second decade of life, between the ages of 10 and 20 years. The average age at onset is 15 years. The tumor occurs twice as often in males as in females and is slightly more common in whites than in nonwhites. It occurs primarily in the ends of long bones, such as the distal part of the femur, the proximal part of the tibia, and the proximal part of the humerus.

Most patients have swelling or pain not associated with a traumatic injury. The average duration of signs and symptoms before diagnosis is 3 months, but the signs and symptoms can exist for much longer. Patients seek medical attention because of the development of pain or an injury. Other signs and symptoms include limitation of movement in adjacent joint, pathologic fractures, and erythema. Approximately 10–20% of patients have metastatic disease at the time of diagnosis. The most common site of metastasis is the lungs. Diagnostic workup includes a history and physical examination, biopsy of the mass, radiologic imaging (computed tomography, magnetic resonance imaging, bone scan), laboratory studies (CBC, chemistries, serum levels of alkaline phosphatase and lactic dehydrogenase). The results are used to determine treatment and to establish a prognosis.

Treatment includes surgery and combination chemotherapy. The goal of surgery is local control of disease. This is achieved by either limb salvage procedures or amputation. Chemotherapeutic agents include high doses of methotrexate, Adriamycin, cisplatin, and bleomycin. Chemotherapy may be given before surgery to reduce the size of the tumor. Chemotherapeutic agents have been administered intraarterially with this intent. Adjuvant chemotherapy is begun within 2–3 weeks after surgery. Radiation therapy is not used because osteogenic sarcoma is radioresistant.

Prognostic factors include location of the primary tumor (distal is more favorable), size of the tumor, rate of tumor growth, degree of bone destruction, and presence or absence of metastatic disease. Patients with distant primary lesions and no evidence of metastatic disease have a 65% survival rate. Children who have metastatic disease at the time of diagnosis have a poor outcome. Local control can be achieved despite persistent pulmonary nodules. Patients often have multiple surgeries to resect pulmonary nodules. This provides patients with disease-free time. Unfortunately, the nodules generally reappear, and patients eventually die of the tumor. Currently, treatment is aimed at improving the long-term outcome.

Ewing's Sarcoma. Ewing's sarcoma is the second most common bone tumor in children. It is more common in males after puberty and is rare in blacks. Its peak occurrence is in children 5–15 years old. The most common sites are the pelvis, tibia, and fibula. Patients usually have a soft-tissue mass over the affected bone and pain. Unlike the case in osteogenic sarcoma, patients often have constitutional signs and symptoms such as anorexia, fever, malaise, fatigue, and weight loss. Approximately 10–30% have metastatic disease to the lungs, bone marrow, or other bones at the time of diagnosis. The diagnostic workup includes a physical examination, biopsy of the primary lesion, radiologic imaging (chest radiography, computed tomography, magnetic resonance imaging, bone scan), bone marrow aspiration and biopsy, and laboratory studies (CBC, serum levels of lactic dehydrogenase).

Ewing's sarcoma is highly radiosensitive. Treatment includes surgery or radiation for local control of the primary tumor and adjuvant chemotherapy. Commonly used chemotherapeutic agents are vincristine, cyclophosphamide, Adriamycin, actinomycin D, ifosfamide (Ifex), and etoposide. Treatment regimens often consist of chemotherapy followed by radiation and/or surgery once the tumor has decreased in size. The overall prognosis for patients with primary tumor in a distal site and no metastatic disease is approximately 60%. Prognosis is poor for patients with disseminated disease.

Rhabdomyosarcoma. Rhabdomyosarcoma is the most common soft-tissue sarcoma. The origin of this tumor is the embryonic cells that give rise to striated muscle. Rhabdomyosarcoma accounts for 4% of the cancers in children. Approximately 300 new cases are diagnosed each year. Peak occurrences are in children 2–5 years old and in adolescents 15–19 years old. The tumor is more common in males than in females and in whites than in nonwhites.

Signs and symptoms correlate with the location of the tumor and can include a painless, enlarged mass. The head and neck, including the orbit, are the most common sites (40% of cases). Signs and symptoms of tumors in these sites include otitis, sinusitis, nose bleeds, orbital edema, ptosis, pain, and difficulty breathing. The next most common site is the genitourinary tract (21%). Signs and symptoms for this site include hematuria, urinary obstruction, pain, vaginal bleeding, weight loss, and disturbances with bowel and bladder function. The diagnostic workup includes biopsy or surgical resection of the primary tumor, imaging studies (computed tomography, magnetic resonance imaging, bone scanning, skeletal survey), laboratory studies (CBC, urinalysis, renal and liver function tests), bone marrow aspiration and biopsy, and lumbar puncture (for head and neck primary tumors).

Clinical staging is essential for determining treatment. The current staging criteria place patients into four different groups according to the extent of the disease. Most patients have stage III or stage IV disease at the time of diagnosis, and 18% have metastases. Common sites of metastasis are the lungs, bone, bone marrow, brain, spinal cord, lymph nodes, liver, and heart. Treatment of rhabdomyosarcoma includes surgery (if possible), chemotherapy (vincristine, cyclophosphamide, actinomycin D, Adriamycin, ifosfamide, etoposide), radiation (control of local disease), and combination therapy.

Survival varies greatly; however, children less than 5 years old who have tumors with favorable histologic features, no metastases, and a primary site in the head or neck tend to have a better prognosis. Overall survival is about 50%. Only 10% of patients who have tumors that extend into the central nervous system survive.

THE DYING CHILD AND THE CHILD'S FAMILY

Even with all the advances in treatment and supportive care for children with cancer, some children die of cancer. When no further treatment is practicable, the goals of care shift from cure to palliation. Nurses play an important role in facilitating this transition. The care needs of the patient's family change as the impending death approaches.

Talking About Death

To provide optimum care to children who are dying and to the children's siblings, nurses must be familiar with how children develop concepts related to death (Table 13-2). A child's concept of death is influenced by his or her psychosocial and cognitive development and his or her experiences with death. Because the verbal skills of younger children are not well developed, they tend to communicate through actions and symbols. Books, play, and drawings are three nonthreatening ways of communicating with children.

Strategies for talking with children about death include the following:

- Open discussions with the child. Have the child describe death in his or her own words.

- Encourage expression of emotions of loss and grief; however, do not force the child to express these emotions. Children will share their feelings when they are ready and when the atmosphere is conducive.

- Listen carefully to the child's questions. Ask clarifying questions if you do not understand the child's question or reflect the question back to the child. When you respond, keep your reply simple and to the point. When you have answered the question, stop. Do not give more information than the child is requesting.

- Remember that honesty is the best policy when talking with children. Avoid telling a child an untruth that will need to be corrected later. Telling a lie could influence the trusting relationship the child has with you. Avoid fairy tales and half-truths.

- Take advantage of children's curiosity. One way to discuss death is to associate it with things they can understand (e.g., the life cycle of a flower, death of a pet).

- Avoid associating sleep with death. Children might experience difficulties sleeping.

- Do not tell children that the dead person was taken away. They may fear that someone will take them away.

- Do not tell children that the dead person has gone on a long trip. They may wonder when the dead person will return.

- Carefully explain that sometimes when someone becomes ill, he or she does not get better and may die. It is important for children to understand that not everyone who gets ill will die.

- Try not to talk about the loss of someone. Small children do not understand this concept and may worry that if they "get lost," they will die.

- Spend time in responsive listening to the needs of the child. Pay particular attention to the child's nonverbal communication. Play is one method that can be used to explore a child's thoughts and feelings.

Patients' Needs

The needs of a dying child are physical and psychosocial. The primary goals of interventions are to control signs and symptoms, promote comfort, and facilitate a dignified death. Pain is one of the most challenging problems and is the one symptom that children and their

Table 13-2
Children's Concepts of Death

Age Group	Beliefs	Reactions
Infants	Have no concept of death Begin to experiment with separation (e.g., peek-a-boo)	Experience separation anxiety
Toddlers (1-3 years)	Have no concept of death Fear separation and abandonment	React to loss, experience separation anxiety
Preschoolers (3-5 years)	View death as temporary or reversible View death as a departure or separation View death as punishment for a wrongdoing Are influenced by magical thinking	Often ask when the dead person will return Are ritualistic ? Are curious about death May ask questions about what happens when you are dead (e.g., Are you cold?)
School agers (6-12 years)	Personify death as God, bogeyman, ghost Associate death with old age Begin to understand finality of death (by age 8 or 9)	Act out death and funeral scenes explicitly Fear own death May use rituals to cope
Adolescents (12-19 years)	View death as irreversible Think death will not happen to them	Behave much as adults do Lose control Increase risk-taking behaviors

Source: Education Committee of the Association of Pediatric Oncology Nurses. (1992). *Pediatric oncology nursing study guide*. Richmond, VA: Phenix Corp., p. 108; Fochtman, D., & Mooney, K. (Eds.). (1993). *Nursing care of the child with cancer* (2nd ed.). Philadelphia: Saunders, pp. 450-454; and Maul-Mellott, S., & Adams, J. (1987). *Childhood cancer: A nursing overview*. Boston: Jones and Bartlett, pp. 173-175.

parents have the most concern about managing effectively. Pharmacologic and nonpharmacologic measures can be used to relieve pain. Nurses can assist children and the children's family members by preparing them for the physical changes that occur before death. Dying children may have difficulty sleeping, especially at night. Fears are often enhanced at night when all is quiet and dark.

Dying children need time to grieve the losses they are experiencing and will experience. Some children find that making a will and saying good-byes are helpful. It is important for children to maintain a sense of normalcy and control in their lives for as long as possible. This can be accomplished through maintaining friendships, attending school, and participating in activities important to them. It is sometimes challenging to balance the needs of a child, especially an adolescent, and the needs of the child's parents.

Parents' Needs

The point of no further treatment is the final crisis point for parents. The time from diagnosis to this point can be short or long and often includes several recurrences of cancer. It is important to ascertain parental wishes, support parental decisions, and prepare parents for the eventual deterioration and death of their child. Maintaining open communication, especially active listening, between nurses and parents is essential. Parents generally spend time talking about the child's life. They often express feelings of helplessness and the desire that their child's death be peaceful and comfortable. Nurses can help parents by assisting them in providing comfort and support to the child.

Although expected, the actual moment of death can be a shock. Making funeral arrangements before the child's death often makes the days after the death a little easier. Bereavement is generally long. It is important to families that their child be remembered by nurses and staff members. Sending a card on the anniversary of the child's death or having annual bereavement ceremonies lets the family know their child is not forgotten.

Siblings' Needs

Children often have short attention spans and do not grieve in the same way as adults. As a result, their behaviors may seem inappropriate to adults. For instance, a young child may ask questions about the dying sibling or the dead sibling one moment and the next moment be playing. This does not mean that the child does not have feelings for the sibling. It is important for the family and health care provider to observe the siblings of dying or dead children for behaviors that would indicate that the siblings are having difficulties coping with the situation. Referrals should be made as needed. Siblings can be encouraged to say good-bye to the dying or dead child.

LONG-TERM EFFECTS OF TREATMENT

It is estimated that 1 in 1000 persons in the United States between the ages of 15 and 45 years survived cancer during childhood. The number of survivors continues to grow, and it is estimated that by the year 2000, the number will be 1 in 900 persons. With children surviving longer from the time of diagnosis and more than 60% being cured, the late sequelae of cancer treatment and their impact on the quality of life have received increased attention. Recognition of late sequelae has resulted in the refinement of treatment regimens and interventions to minimize toxic effects. Although not every child treated for cancer will experience late sequelae, children and their families should receive information about long-term effects that may develop as a result of the cancer therapy the children received and the particular circumstances. Many treatment centers have created follow-up or late-effects clinics that specialize in monitoring, determining, and treating long-term effects.

Many clinicians think of late or long-term effects of cancer treatment as being physical (the result of damage caused by treatment). However, the effects can be physical (occurring in any body system), psychosocial, and financial (Table 13-3). The onset can occur from months to years after therapy. The manifestation may be overt, subtle, or subclinical. Signs and symptoms that are subtle or subclinical may initially be overlooked. It is therefore important that children receive a systematic assessment during follow-up appointments. Nurses are involved in screening patients for potential long-term effects, providing education, counseling, and making referrals as appropriate. It is important that any problems that arise be addressed. Because many children are young at the time cancer is diagnosed, they may not realize the importance of health maintenance and long-term follow-up. Nurses play a key role in educating this population of patients.

Table 13-3
Long-Term Effects of Childhood Cancer

Effects	Manifestations
Physical	
Cardiovascular	Cardiomyopathy, congestive heart failure, left ventricular dysfunction, coronary artery disease, arrhythmias, risk of sudden death
Central nervous system	Neuropsychologic skills (e.g., intelligence, academic performance, learning disabilities, visual spatial skills, fine motor skills, memory, attention), structural damage to central nervous system, vision (e.g., cataracts), hearing
Endocrine	Growth (stature and loss of bone growth), gonadal dysfunction (males: azoospermia, decreased testicular function, delayed puberty; females: ovarian failure, amenorrhea, delayed puberty), hypothyroidism
Gastrointestinal	Hepatic fibrosis, cirrhosis, chronic enteritis
Musculoskeletal	Scoliosis, kyphosis, asymmetry, spinal shortening, short stature, dental problems
Pulmonary	Interstitial pneumonitis, pulmonary fibrosis
Renal	Nephritis, chronic cystitis, bladder fibrosis, atypical bladder epithelium, renal tubular necrosis, hemorrhagic cystitis
Psychosocial	Inability to form relationships, inability to plan for the future, difficulties with performance (e.g., school, work), discrimination, fear of late sequelae, changes in body image (e.g., physical disabilities, obesity)
Financial	Difficulty obtaining health insurance, disability insurance, employment; altered occupational achievement capabilities

Source: Education Committee of the Association of Pediatric Oncology Nurses. (1992). *Pediatric oncology nursing study guide.* Richmond, VA: Phenix Corp., pp. 96–101, and Pizzo, P., & Poplack, D. (Eds.). (1993). *Principles and practice of pediatric oncology* (2nd ed.). New York: Lippincott, pp. 1091–1114.

Second Malignant Tumors

Survivors live with the uncertainty that the original cancer may recur or a second malignant tumor develop. Fears are often heightened around the time of annual follow-up appointments. The actual risk that a second malignant tumor will develop is small, 3–12% during the first 20 years after treatment. The patient's primary cancer, age, treatment regimen, and genetic conditions influence the incidence. A variety of risk factors appear to increase the chance of a second malignant tumor. These include treatment with alkylating agents (e.g., in Hodgkin's disease), radiation therapy, genetic predisposition (e.g., retinoblastoma), and some genetic conditions (e.g., neurofibromatosis).

The most common second malignant tumor in patients who received alkylating agents is acute myelogenous leukemia. The peak onset is 5 years after therapy. The risk appears to be related to the amount of drug administered or the total cumulative dose of alkylating agents received. The larger the cumulative dose, the greater is the risk. Patients treated for Hodgkin's disease are at greatest risk for treatment-related acute myelogenous leukemia. The most common second malignant tumor in patients who received radiation therapy is sarcoma (bone and soft tissue). The peak onset is 15–20 years after therapy. Patients who have been treated for retinoblastoma have a 17% risk for treatment-related sarcoma. Osteosarcoma is the most common tumor. Patients with bilateral retinoblastoma, a family history of retinoblastoma, or a chromosomal deletion of 13 or 14 are at greater risk. Although second malignant tumors are uncommon, nurses should be aware of predisposing factors. Clinical manifestation of second malignant tumors is similar to the manifestation of any tumor.

BIBLIOGRAPHY

Education Committee of the Association of Pediatric Oncology Nurses. (1992). *Pediatric oncology nursing study guide*. Richmond, VA: Phoenix Corp.

Foley, G., Fochtman, D., & Mooney, K. (1993). *Nursing care of the child with cancer*. Philadelphia: Saunders.

Hockenberry, M., & Coody, D. (1986). *Pediatric oncology and hematology: Perspectives on care*. St. Louis: Mosby.

Hockenberry, M., Coody, D., & Bennett, B. (1990). Childhood cancers: Incidence, etiology, diagnosis, and treatment. *Pediatric Nursing, 16,* 239–246.

Klopovich, P., & Cohen, D. (1984). An overview of pediatric oncology for adult oncology nurses. *Oncology Nursing Forum, 11,* 50–63.

Maul-Mellott, S., & Adams, J. (1987). *Childhood cancer: A nursing overview*. Boston: Jones and Bartlett.

Miles, R. (1990). Caring for families when a child dies. *Pediatric Nursing, 16,* 346–347.

Moore, I. M., Kramer, R., & Perin, O. (1986). Care of the family with a child with cancer: Diagnosis and early stages of treatment. *Oncology Nursing Forum, 13,* 60–68.

Pizzo, P., & Poplack, D. (1993). *Principles and practice of pediatric oncology*. New York: Lippincott.

Schwab, M., Alitalo, K., Klempnauer, K. H., et al. (1983). Amplified DNA with limited homology to *myc* cellular oncogene is shared by human neuroblastoma cell lines and a neuroblastoma tumor. *Nature, 305,* 245–248.

Spinetta, J., & Deasy-Spinetta, P. (1981). *Living with childhood cancer*. St Louis: Mosby.

Whittham, E. (1993). Terminal care of the dying child. *Cancer, 17,* 3450–3462.

Wingo, P., Tong, T., & Boldem, S. (1995). Cancer statistics 1995. *CA—A Cancer Journal for Clinicians, 45,* 8–31.

STUDY QUESTIONS

Chapter 13

Questions 88–97

Questions 88 and 89: Janie is a 4-year-old who comes to your clinic for her routine checkup. You notice that she has bruises and petechiae on her extremities.

88. Which of the following cancers would be part of the differential diagnosis?

   a. Neuroblastoma
   b. Rhabdomyosarcoma
   c. Leukemia
   d. Wilms' tumor

89. What is Janie's psychosocial developmental state?

   a. Initiative versus guilt
   b. Trust versus mistrust
   c. Autonomy versus shame and doubt
   d. Industry versus inferiority

90. Most cases of acute lymphocytic leukemia in children occur in children of what age?

   a. Less than 2 years
   b. 4 years
   c. 8 years
   d. 15 years

91. What is the most common solid tumor in children?

   a. Osteosarcoma
   b. Neuroblastoma   –?brain
   c. Central nervous system tumors
   d. Rhabdomyosarcoma

92. Johnny is a 16-year-old white male who comes to the emergency department because of increasing leg pain and difficulty walking that are not associated with an injury. He has had intermittent swelling and pain above his right knee for 4 months. Which of the following cancers would be part of Johnny's differential diagnosis?

   a. Wilms' tumor
   b. Osteogenic sarcoma
   c. Neuroblastoma
   d. Retinoblastoma

93. What is the most common site of metastasis of osteogenic sarcoma?

   a. Lungs
   b. Brain
   c. Liver
   d. Skin

94. What is the most common clinical indication of retinoblastoma?

   a. Visual disturbance
   b. Dilated pupils
   c. Eye erythema
   d. Leukokoria

95. Which of the following statements about pre-schoolers' concept of death is correct?

    a. They have no concept of death. *Toddler*

    b. They think death is a punishment for a wrongdoing.

    c. They associate death with old age. *School age*

    d. They view death as irreversible. *Adolescent*

96. What percentage of children treated for cancer are cured?

    a. 40

    b. 50

    c. 60

    d. 70

97. Which of the following risk factors increases the likelihood that a survivor of childhood cancer will have a second malignant tumor?

    a. Treatment with alkylating agents

    b. Biotherapy

    c. Rhabdomyosarcoma primary

    d. Lower socioeconomic status

CHAPTER 14

PROFESSIONAL ISSUES FOR NURSES IN CANCER CARE

CHAPTER OBJECTIVE

After completing this chapter, the reader will have a basic understanding of the professional issues of oncology nursing, including ethical challenges, occupational stress and burnout, and grieving by caregivers.

LEARNING OBJECTIVES

After studying this chapter, the reader will be able to

1. Specify ethical issues associated with the care of cancer patients.

2. Recognize the definition of burnout.

3. Specify the physical effects of stress.

ETHICAL ISSUES

When caring for patients who have cancer, nurses often are confronted with ethical issues. These issues may be related to advances in technology, values on death or dying, decision making, or allocation of health care resources. Value orientations usually provide the ethical foundations for determining what is good or right in nursing practice (Baird, McCorkle, & Grant, 1991). Nursing values should be analyzed by nurses as a professional group as well as by nurses as individuals, so that each nurse can best assist and advocate for patients without confusion between his or her own values and the values of others.

Ethics is a philosophical study of moral conduct. It examines not what we do, but what we ought to do. It is hoped that some congruency exists between what we actually do and what we ought to do (Ashwanden, Belcher, Mattson, Moskowitz, & Riese, 1990). Ethics and moral questioning are not new phenomena in nursing. As long as there have been nurses, there has been reflective thinking about implications of care (Ashwanden et al., 1990).

In recent years, nurses have seen more of a professional focus on ethical issues. This change may have occurred because more than ever before, nurses feel less sure about what ought to be done. Several factors may contribute to this degree of uncertainty:

- New technologies make a wider range of possibilities available for care and treatment of patients.

- Values on death and dying may differ among a patient, the patient's family members, and the health care team.

- Values on who should make decisions about care and treatment may also vary among a patient, the patient's family members, and the health care team.

- Allocation of health care resources may be incongruent with the values of the persons involved.

Rapid technologic advances have occurred in the diagnosis and treatment of cancer. These advances bring with them new capabilities to maintain and sustain life. Nurses are faced with new challenges and questions related to these changes. How are life and death defined? When is no further treatment appropriate? When should the shift be made from treatment to palliative care? Continuous advances in technology make these questions more difficult to answer (Ashwanden et al., 1990).

Decision making is an integral part of the cancer experience. Decisions are made by patients, their family members, and the health care team. Each of these persons holds a set of values. Each decision requires a combination of facts and a set of values that helps determine what ought to be done (Baird et al., 1991). Determining these values is essential in ethical decision making.

A key role in the nurse-patient relationship in cancer care is the role of advocate. Advocacy is often defined as active support of an important cause, or asserting a patient's choices or desires (Baird et al., 1991). This requires a clear understanding of the patient's values.

Each nurse must also be aware of his or her own set of values. This determination of values will help the nurse clarify true advocacy for the patient's choices versus the nurse's personal wishes. Occasionally, the nurse may find those values in conflict. Clear determination of values can help avoid confusion in decision making and clarify the ethical issue.

Ethical issues in oncology take many forms. Three common areas of ethical decision making are informed consent, clinical trials, and no-code decisions (Clark & McGee, 1992).

Informed consent refers to having full knowledge and understanding of risks, benefits, and available options about various treatment alternatives in order to make a decision. In the past, the ethical focus of informed consent was on disclosure of information. Was the patient provided the information? Now, the focus has changed to patient's understanding of the information and how to enable patients to make an autonomous decision (Groenwald, Frogge, Goodman, & Yarbro, 1990).

Clinical trials in oncology are studies or experiments in humans to evaluate the efficacy of research or investigational methods that may have therapeutic implications for patients. Several ethical principles in nursing practice can be applied to decision making related to clinical trials in oncology: justice, autonomy, beneficence, and nonmaleficence. In clinical trials, justice refers to the investigators treating the patient or client fairly. Autonomy focuses on the right of the patient to make independent decisions about his or her well-being and personal affairs. Beneficence is the obligation of the health care providers to do good for the patient. Closely related to the principle of beneficence, the principle of nonmaleficence is the obligation of the health care providers to do no harm to the patient.

On the basis of these ethical principles, the role of nurses in clinical trials may involve the following (Clark & McGee, 1992):

- Ensuring that informed consent is obtained and documented.

- Assessing the response to treatment.

- Managing signs and symptoms related to treatment.

- Providing physical and psychosocial care.

- Collaborating with the investigational or research team.

- Documenting the response to treatment.

- Maintaining current knowledge of drugs, procedures, and treatments used.

- Encouraging patient's autonomy throughout the research period through reiteration of patient's rights.

A third common ethical issue in oncology is no-code decisions. A no-code status refers to a decision made by a patient or the patient's legal representative that cardiopulmonary resuscitation will not be attempted in the event that the patient's heartbeat and respirations cease. Many variations of no-code decisions exist. Some may include other aspects or details of treatments or care measures that can be used. The purpose of a no-code status or other advance directive is to validate agreement between the patient, the patient's family members, and the health care team about the right to die without resuscitation or under certain situations (Clark & McGee, 1992).

In these situations, nurses often are involved in providing an environment for clear, open communication between patient's, the patient's family members, physicians, and other health team members. A determination of patient's cultural values of death and dying, as well as their personal values, is important. Nurses also play a key role in ensuring clear documentation of patients wishes so that other health care team members will know what the wishes are.

Future trends in nursing ethics will include a wide variety of issues. One primary issue is allocation of health care resources. Nurses and other health care providers are grappling with questions of fair allocation of limited health resources, such as "Who should receive what

kind of care?" These questions are not easily answered, because they often create potential conflict among a person's own values.

Every health care decision has a value component (Groenwald et al., 1990). Understanding the nature of values and ethical principles is fundamental to oncology nursing. With increasing responsibility and expanding areas of professional decision making, oncology nurses are more aware than ever of the importance of being prepared to participate in ethical issues and decision making.

AVOIDING BURNOUT

Providing nursing care to cancer patients is both stressful and satisfying. When asked about the parts of oncology nursing that are rewarding, nurses often say that the sources of rewards are also the sources of difficulty and stress (Carroll-Johnson, 1994). This special nature of cancer nursing makes occupational stress and burnout great concerns for health professionals.

Any health professional who has worked with cancer patients for more than 6 months knows that the energy, compassion, and wisdom needed in this profession are cyclical. Some weeks nurses may be filled with a kind of missionary zeal and other weeks find themselves asking what possessed them to ever consider this kind of work (Hill, 1989). This kind of perspective is not that different from the perspective of a cancer patient's experience with disease. Nurses thoughts and feelings related to caring for cancer patients' often echo those of patient's (Table 14-1).

Oncology nurses become close to patients and patient's families. The nature of the disease provides nurses the opportunity and challenges of helping through some rough times (Meyer, 1992). Nurses share triumphs and failures with patients and patient's families. This sharing can be a great source of reward as well as a source of stress.

Table 14-1
Similarities in the Feelings of Cancer Patients and Their Caregivers

Patients' Comments	Caregivers' Comments
Loneliness has been the hardest part . . . I'm still searching for other survivors to talk to.	Sometimes I feel that my professional life has isolated me from the rest of the world . . . No one wants to hear about my work, and I need to talk about it.
Having had cancer means that you are never the same. Life is so different now . . . I look at people and events and problems, at just about everything, in a changed way. It's important to me to make my life count.	Working in oncology changes people. Regular life problems seem less important. You become impatient with things that seem to be a waste of time. You recognize that your hold on life is tenuous and that you have to make the most of each day.
It was only after it was over . . . after the daily trips for radiation, after the chemotherapy, and the seemingly endless nausea and fatigue, after practically living at the hospital for months . . . that I realized what had happened to me. After it was over, I cried and cried and cried.	I worked in oncology for a long time. I think that I did a pretty good job and coped well. But after . . . I left oncology, I walked around for weeks with the tears streaming down my face. After I left oncology, I cried and cried and cried.

Source: Hill, H. L. (1991). *Journal of Psychosocial Oncology, 9*(2), 97-112.

Stress is necessary for life. It demands physical, emotional, and intellectual adaptation. Stress becomes a problem when the level of stress exceeds a person's ability to respond effectively or is perceived to be taxing beyond the normal ability of the person to cope (Baird et al., 1991; Clark & McGee, 1992). Burnout is described as an extreme outcome of unrelieved stress. It is exhaustion related to excess demands on energy, strength, and resources (Carroll-Johnson, 1994; Clark & McGee, 1992).

Burnout is a familiar problem to health care professionals in oncology. The nature of the work exposes them to ongoing emotional, intellectual, and physical demands. Professional stress requires adaptation in the performance of a person's professional role (Clark & McGee, 1992). Vachon (1987) found that stress affects caregivers of all ages. Physical effects linked with chronic stress and burnout include fatigue, headaches, gastrointestinal disturbances, weight loss, insomnia, depression, low morale, job turnover, and impaired job performance (Carroll-Johnson, 1994). The impact of stress can be intensified by the following (Clark & McGee, 1992):

- Suddenness of onset.

- Chronicity of stressor(s).

- Degree of intensity.

- Significance of the stressor to the individual.

- Vulnerability of the individual.

- Occurrence of multiple stressors.

Coping effectively with stress is important not only for maintaining the health of individual caregivers but also for providing better nursing care for patients (Carroll-Johnson, 1994).

CARING FOR THE CAREGIVER

Because cancer is an experience that demands a great deal from both patients and caregivers, stress is inevitable. Finding ways to cope and deal with stress as a caregiver can contribute greatly to the length and satisfaction of a career in oncology nursing.

Coping can involve recognizing job stressors. A variety of stress management strategies can be used once stressors are recognized. An understanding of these strategies is essential for both health care professionals and health care organizations. Vachon (1987) suggested both individual and organizational strategies for managing stress.

Individual strategies include the following:

- Having a sense of competence, control, or pleasure in work.

- Having control over aspects of practice.

- Managing one's lifestyle in a healthy way.

- Developing a personal philosophy of illness, death, and professional role.

- Leaving the work situation.

- Distancing oneself from patients and their families.

- Increasing education.

- Having an outside support system.

- Having a sense of humor.

Another important finding in this study was recognizing the need for every normal person to have both love and work. Erikson (1963) also recognizes this need. He states that work and productiveness should not preoccupy persons to the extent that they lose the right or capacity to be loving beings.

Organizational strategies for managing stress include the following:

- Team philosophy and support building.

- Staffing policies.

- Administrative policies.

- Collegial relationships.

- Formalized ways of handling decisions.

- Good orientation and educational programs.

- Job flexibility.

- Support groups.

As with individual coping strategies, the key for organizational strategies is the determination of stressors. Recognizing the stressful nature of oncology can only help caregivers in preparing for and dealing with the inevitable stressors.

GRIEVING BY THE CAREGIVER

Several myths have been dispelled about oncology nursing through research. It has been discovered that even in the shadow of cancer, great rewards can be inherent in oncology nursing (Carroll-Johnson, 1994). Cancer nurses often feel privileged to be with patients and families during some difficult times. One nurse stated, "I've received far more than I've ever given" (Meyer, 1992).

Those who provide care to patients with cancer also need support (Zwingler, 1994). Because of their experiences, oncology nurses can easily feel different and separate from the rest of the world (Hill, 1991). This feeling of separation is especially common among office-based oncology nurses and home health care nurses. These groups provide a great deal of psychosocial support for patients and families yet are isolated from support themselves (Zwingler, 1994).

Nurses working with cancer patients need to allow or create time for grieving and support for themselves. Regardless of a patient's prognosis or outcome, nurses should be aware of the impact being a caregiver can have on their lives. Nurses who have an outlet for stress will be happier and less prone to burnout and, in turn, will be better able to support patients (Zwingler, 1994).

Supportive outlets for nurses to grieve or reflect on the caregiving experience can take many forms. Some support can come from family and friends. However, rarely can this support network completely understand the experience of those who care for cancer patients. Oncology nursing organizations or groups can be another excellent source of support. These groups can provide a network for nurses with similar professional experiences to reflect, grieve, support, and grow with one another.

Oncology nurses have shared life-and-death experiences with patients. The emotions and stressors related to these events must not be ignored or displaced. They will only be manifested as burnout and despair (Hill, 1991). Nurses must seek out the support needed to maintain a healthy, long professional career in caring for cancer patients.

BIBLIOGRAPHY

Ashwanden, P., Belcher, A. E., Mattson, E. A., Moskowitz, R., & Riese, N. (1990). *Oncology nursing: Advances, treatments and trends into the 21st century.* Rockville, MD: Aspen.

Baird, S. B., McCorkle, R., & Grant, M. (1991). *Cancer nursing: A comprehensive textbook* (pp. 313-337, 1065-1075). Philadelphia: Saunders.

Carroll-Johnson, R. M. (1994). The meaning of oncology nursing: Results of the Life Cycle Research Project. *Oncology Nursing Forum, 6*(8 Suppl.), 5-47.

Clark, J. C., & McGee, R. F. (1992). *Oncology Nursing Society: Core curriculum for oncology nursing* (2nd ed., pp. 221-250). Philadelphia: Saunders.

Erikson, E. (1963). *Childhood and society* (2nd ed.). New York: Norton.

Groenwald, S. L., Frogge, M. H., Goodman, M., & Yarbro, C. (Eds.). (1990). *Cancer nursing: Principles and practice* (2nd ed., pp. 1201-1215). Boston: Jones and Bartlett.

Hill, H. L. (1989). To fill a heart: Oncology over the long haul. *Journal of Psychosocial Oncology, 7*(3), 145-152.

Hill, H. L. (1991). Point and counterpoint: Relationships in oncology care. *Journal of Psychosocial Oncology, 9*(2), 97-112.

Meyer, C. (1992). The richness of oncology nursing. *American Journal of Nursing, 92,* 71-74, 76, 78.

Nash, E. S. (1989). Occupational stress and the oncology nurse. *Nursing RSA, 4*(8), 37-38.

Vachon, M. L. S. (1987). *Occupational stress in the care of the critically ill, the dying, and the bereaved.* New York: Hemisphere.

Zwingler, R. (1994). Cancer update 94. *Nursing 94, 24*(4), 59-61.

STUDY QUESTIONS

Chapter 14

Questions 98–100

98. Which of the following refers to having full knowledge and understanding of risks, benefits, and available options about various treatment alternatives in order to make a decision?

    a. Competence
    b. Informed consent
    c. Articulateness
    d. Ethics

99. Ethical principles associated with clinical trials include all of the following *except:*

    a. Justice
    b. Autonomy
    c. Unlimited resources
    d. Nonmaleficence

100. Which of the following is described as an extreme outcome of unrelieved stress related to excess demands on energy, strength, and resources?

    a. Stress
    b. Moral conduct
    c. Grieving
    d. Burnout

BIBLIOGRAPHY

For Chapter 1-3, 5, 7 and 9

Ahmann, F. R. (1984). A reassessment of the clinical implications of the superior vena cava syndrome. *Journal of Clinical Oncology, 2,* 961–969.

Arbeit, J. (1990). Molecules, cancer, and the surgeon. *Annals of Surgery, 212,* 3–13.

Baird, S. B., McCorkle, R., & Grant, M. (Eds.). (1991). *Cancer nursing: A comprehensive textbook.* Philadelphia: Saunders.

Bajorunas, D. R. (1990). Clinical manifestations of cancer-related hypercalcemia. *Seminars in Oncology, 17,* 16–25.

Balch, C. (1990). The surgeon's expanded role in cancer care. *Cancer, 65,* 604–609.

Barstow, J. (1985). Safe handling of cytotoxic agents in the home. *Home Healthcare Nursing, 3,* 46–47.

Besarb, A., & Caro, J. F. (1978). Mechanisms of hypercalcemia in malignancy. *Cancer, 41,* 2276–2285.

Bick, R. L. (1988). Disseminated intravascular coagulation and related syndromes: A clinical review. *Seminars in Thrombosis and Hemostasis, 14,* 299–338.

Brager, B. L., & Yasko, J. M. (1984). *Care of the client receiving chemotherapy.* Reston, VA: Reston Publishing.

Burnet, F. M. (1970). The concept of immunological surveillance. *Progress in Experimental Tumor Research, 13,* 1–27.

Callahan, R., & Salomon, D. S. (1993). Oncogenes, tumour suppressor genes and growth factors in breast cancer: Novel targets for diagnosis, prognosis and therapy. *Cancer Surveys, 18,* 35–56.

Cassileth, B., & Brown, H. (1988). Unorthodox cancer medicine. *CA—A Cancer Journal for Clinicians, 38,* 176–186.

Chernecky, C. C., & Ramsey, P. W. (1984). *Critical nursing care of the client with cancer.* Norwalk, CT: Appleton-Century-Crofts.

Clark, J. C., & McGee, R. F. (Eds.). (1992). *Oncology Nursing Society: Core curriculum for oncology nursing* (2nd ed.). Philadelphia: Saunders.

DeVita, V. J., Hellman, S., & Rosenberg, S. A. (Eds.). (1991). *Biologic therapy of cancer.* Philadelphia: Lippincott.

DeVita, V. T., Jr., Hellman, S., & Rosenberg, S. A. (Eds.). (1989). *Cancer: Principles and practice of oncology* (3rd ed.). Philadelphia: Lippincott.

Elias, G. (1989). *Handbook of surgical oncology.* Boca Raton, FL: CRC Press.

Fidler, I. J., & Balch, C. M. (1987). The biology of cancer metastasis and implications for therapy. *Current Problems in Surgery, 24,* 129–209.

Fidler, I. J., & Nicolson, G. L. (1987). The process of cancer invasion and metastasis. *Cancer Bulletin, 39,* 126–131.

Fischer, D. S., & Tish-Knobf, M. K. (1989). *The cancer chemotherapy handbook* (3rd ed.). Chicago: Year Book Medical.

Fiscus, J. A., Hayes, N. A., Rostad, M. A., & Whedon, M. A. (1989). *Safe handling of cytotoxic drugs.* Pittsburgh: Oncology Nursing Society.

Fojo, A. T., Ueda, K., Slamon, D. J., et al. (1987). Expression of a multidrug-resistance gene in human tumors and tissues. *Proceedings of the National Academy of Sciences of the United States of America, 84,* 265–269.

Foon, K. A. (1989). Biologic response modifiers: The new immunotherapy. *Cancer Research, 49,* 1621–1639.

Glover, D. J., & Glick, J. H. (1987). Oncologic emergencies. *CA—A Cancer Journal for Clinicians, 37,* 302.

Goldie, J. H., & Coldman, A. J. (1979). A mathematic model for relating the drug sensitivity of tumors to their spontaneous mutation rate. *Cancer Treatment Reports, 63,* 1727–1733.

Goldie, J. H., & Coldman, A. J. (1984). The genetic origin of drug resistance in neoplasms: Implications for systemic therapy. *Cancer Research, 44,* 3643–3653.

Groenwald, S. L., Frogge, M. H., Goodman, M., & Yarbro, C. (Eds.). (1990). *Cancer nursing: Principles and practice* (2nd ed.). Boston: Jones and Bartlett.

Gullo, S. M. (1988). Safe handling of antineoplastic drugs: Translating the recommendations into practice. *Oncology Nursing Forum, 15,* 595–601.

Hiller, G. (1987). Cardiac tamponade in the oncology patient. *Focus on Critical Care, 14,* 19–23.

Holleb, A. I., Fink, D. J., & Murphy, G. P. (Eds.). (1991). *American Cancer Society textbook of clinical oncology.* Atlanta: American Cancer Society.

Howard-Ruben, J., & Miller, N. (1984). Unproven methods of cancer management: II. Current trends and implications for patient care. *Oncology Nursing Forum, 11,* 67–74.

Howland, W. S., & Graziano, C. C. (Eds.). (1985). *Critical care of the cancer patient.* Chicago: Year Book Medical.

Meriney, D. K. (1990). Diagnosis and management of acute promyelocytic leukemia with disseminated intravascular coagulopathy: A case study. *Oncology Nursing Forum, 17,* 379–383.

Miller, N., & Howard-Ruben, J. (1984). Unproven methods of cancer management: I. Current trends and implications for patient care. *Oncology Nursing Forum, 10,* 46–54.

National Cancer Institute. (1987). *Closing in on cancer.* Bethesda, MD: Author.

Occupational Safety and Health Administration. (1986). *Work practice guidelines for personnel dealing with cytotoxic (antineoplastic) drugs.* Washington, DC: Author.

Rodriguez, M., & Dinapoli, R. P. (1980). Spinal cord compression with special reference to metastatic epidural tumors. *Mayo Clinic Proceedings, 55,* 442–448.

Rosenberg, S. A., Lotze, M. T., Muul, L. M., et al. (1985). Observations on the systemic administration of autologous lymphokine activated killer cells and recombinant interleukin-2 to patients with metastatic cancer. *New England Journal of Medicine, 313,* 1485–1489.

Schimke, R. T. (1984). Gene amplification, drug resistance, and cancer. *Cancer Research, 44,* 1735–1742.

Schnipper, L. E. (1986). Clinical implications of tumor-cell heterogeneity. *New England Journal of Medicine, 314,* 1423–1431.

Shimm, D. S., Logue, G. L., & Rigsby, L. C. (1981). Evaluating the superior vena cava syndrome. *Journal of the American Medical Association, 245,* 951–953.

Sirica, A. E. (Ed.). (1989). *The pathobiology of neoplasia.* New York: Plenum.

Tenenbaum, L. (1989). *Cancer chemotherapy: A reference guide*. Philadelphia: Saunders.

Vogt, P. K. (1993). Cancer genes. *Western Journal of Medicine, 158,* 273–278.

Wittes, R. E. (1989). *Manual of oncologic therapeutics 1989/1990*. Philadelphia: Lippincott.

Woodruff, M. (1990). *Cellular variation and adaptation in cancer: Biological basis and therapeutic consequences*. New York: Oxford University Press.

Yarbro, J. W. (1992). Oncogenes and cancer suppressor genes. *Seminars in Oncology Nursing, 8,* 30–39.

GLOSSARY

Acral erythema: Redness of the skin occurring over the extremities.

Adenoma: Benign epithelial neoplasm of glands.

Adenocarcinoma: One type of malignant epithelial cell tumors of the glands.

Adjuvant treatment: Treatment given in addition to another treatment or therapy.

Advocacy: Active support of an important cause; asserting a patients choices or desires.

AJCC staging: American Joint Committee on Cancer system of staging cancer that groups disease into four stages (I–IV).

Alopecia: A thinning or complete loss of hair. It can occur anywhere on the body.

Anaplasia: Lack of differentiation.

Anemia: A reduction below normal in the number of red blood cells in the blood, in the amount of hemoglobin, or in the hematocrit; occurs when equilibrium between blood loss and blood production is disturbed.

Apheresis: Any procedure in which blood from a donor is separated into individual components (e.g., platelets, leukocytes), part is retained, and the remainder is retransfused into the donor.

Aspiration biopsy: A procedure in which the biopsy specimen to be examined is removed via a needle and syringe; also called fine-needle aspiration. Generally, the cells removed are examined by using cytologic techniques.

Atypia: Condition of being irregular or not conforming to type. In cancer, cells that are abnormal and may characterize certain precancerous lesions.

Benign: Not malignant or recurrent; favorable for recovery.

Biopsy: Removal and examination of tissue, cells, or fluid from the living body; done to establish a precise diagnosis.

Bone marrow: The soft organic material that fills the cavities of the bones; the site where blood cells are produced and mature.

Bone marrow aspiration and biopsy: Procedure in which a sample of the bone marrow is removed and examined.

Bone marrow transplantation: Procedure in which high doses of chemotherapy are given and bone marrow cells, either from a compatible donor (allogeneic) or from the patient's own bone marrow (autologous), are transplanted to enable the hematopoietic system to recover and make new blood cells.

Burnout: An extreme outcome of unrelieved stress; exhaustion related to excess demands on energy, strength, and resources.

Cancer: Common term for all malignant tumors.

Carcinogenesis: Production of cancer.

Carcinoma: Malignant neoplasm or tumor made up of epithelial cells.

Carcinoma in situ: Malignant neoplasm composed of epithelial cells that has not invaded the basement membrane of the tissue; the cancer cells are still within their site of origin.

Cell cycle time: Time between successive episodes of mitosis.

Cellular kinetics: Dynamics, or rate of change, of cells; refers to growth and division of cells.

Chemotherapy: Therapy in which drugs or chemical agents are used to treat disease.

Chromosomes: The threadlike structures in the nucleus of an animal cell that function in the transmission of genetic information.

Chronic myelogenous leukemia: A form of leukemia characterized by increased numbers of granulocytes and megakaryocytes.

Clinical trials: Studies or experiments in humans to evaluate the efficacy of research or investigational methods that may have therapeutic implications for patients.

Contralateral: On the opposite side.

Cryotherapy: The freezing of tissue to treat disease.

Cytopathology: The study of cells in disease.

Dedifferentiation: Process whereby cells lose characteristics of normal cells; anaplasia.

Deletion: In genetics, an aberration in which a part of a chromosome or any DNA segment (e.g., a gene) is lost.

Differentiation: In cancer, an increase in morphologic or chemical heterogeneity; extent to which parenchymal cells differ from comparable normal cells both morphologically and functionally.

DNA (deoxyribonucleic acid): Genetic material contained in the nucleus of each cell.

Doubling time: Time required for a population of cells to multiply by two.

Dysplasia: Recognizable morphologic alteration in a tissue that includes loss of normal orientation and mutation, proliferation, and cytologic changes; may be precursor of cancer and may be reversible.

Endocrine factors: Hormonelike factors capable of affecting many cells systemically.

Epithelium: Covering of the internal and external organs of the body; consists of cells bound together by connective tissue.

Excisional biopsy: Removal of an entire lesion, including a margin of contiguous normal-appearing tissue.

Frozen section: In surgical pathology, rapid freezing and examination of a sample of tissue; may be used to determine a preliminary diagnosis while the patient is still in the operating room.

Gland: An aggregation of specialized cells that secrete or excrete materials not related to their ordinary metabolism.

Grade of tumor: Degree of differentiation and classification of the severity of a tumor.

Granulocytopenia: A decrease in the number of granulocytes in the blood; characterized by an increase in the risk for infection; also called agranulocytosis.

Growth factors: Hormones that regulate growth of selected tissues or types of cells.

Hematopoiesis: Formation and development of blood cells.

Herpes simplex virus (HSV): A group of DNA viruses that can cause infection, often involving the skin or nervous system.

Histology: A branch of anatomy that deals with the structure of tissues as discerned with a microscope.

Hodgkin's disease: A type of lymphoma, or malignant tumor, of the lymphoid tissue.

Hormonal therapy: Use of hormonal agents to treat or prevent disease.

Hyperplasia: The abnormal multiplication or increase in the number of normal cells in normal arrangement in a tissue.

Hypertrophy: Abnormal increase in cell size.

Immune surveillance: A hypothesized monitoring function by which the immune system recognizes and destroys tumor cells on an ongoing basis.

Incidence: The number of new cases of a specific disease occurring during a specified period.

Informed consent: Having full knowledge and understanding of risks, benefits, and available options about various treatment alternatives in order to make a decision.

Initiation: The first step in carcinogenesis; irreversible, but not directly resulting in cancer; mutagenic kind of activity.

Intraperitoneal delivery: The delivery of fluids, drugs, or other agents directly into the peritoneal cavity; also called "belly bath."

Intravesical delivery: The delivery of fluids, drugs, or other agents directly into an organ with a cavity or into a cavity-containing lesion.

Invasion: Process by which cells of one type penetrate into the interior of a tissue containing cells of a different type; infiltration and destruction of surrounding tissue.

Ipsilateral: Occurring on the same side.

Leukokoria: A condition characterized by the appearance of a whitish reflex or mass in the pupillary area behind the lens; also called cat's eye reflex. In cases of retinoblastoma, observed when white light is shined into the pupil and the light source, the tumor, and the pupil are aligned.

Leukopenia: A decrease in the number of white blood cells or leukocytes in the blood.

Limb salvage: A surgical procedure in which bone is removed and replaced with a prosthesis.

Localized disease: In staging tumors, disease confined to the organ of origin.

Long-term effect or late effect: A toxic effect of cancer treatment that occurs months to years after completion of therapy. A long-term effect can be physical, nonreversible, or psychosocial.

Long-term survivor: A patient who has remained disease-free for 5 years and whose cancer treatments have been completed for at least 2 years.

Lumpectomy: Surgical removal of only the palpable lesion and adjacent tissue in breast cancer, with removal of axillary lymph nodes through a second incision; also called segmental or partial mastectomy.

Lymphatic spread: Spread of tumor cells through the lymphatic system.

Lymphedema: Swelling of the extremities due to the accumulation of lymph in soft tissues.

Lymph node dissection: Removal of regional lymph nodes.

Lymph node sampling: Removal of regional lymph nodes at various levels.

Mastectomy: Surgical removal of the breast.

Metaplasia: Change in a tissue in which one type of adult cells is replaced by another type of adult cells not normal for that tissue; predisposing factors for metaplasia may also induce malignant transformation.

Metastasis: Spread of neoplasm to distant parts of the body, with the development of similar cancer in the new location.

Mitosis: Process by which cells grow and divide.

Modified radical mastectomy: Surgical procedure in which the entire breast and axillary lymph nodes are removed, with preservation of the pectoral muscles.

Moist desquamation: A skin reaction associated with radiation therapy that resembles a second-degree burn.

Mucositis: A generalized inflammation of the mucous membranes that can progress to ulceration. Examples include stomatitis, esophagitis, pharyngitis, and vaginitis.

Nadir: The lowest point. In myelosuppression, the maximum point of bone marrow depression.

Neoplasm: Any new and abnormal growth; abnormal mass of tissue that grows independently from that of normal tissues, not subject to the usual rules of tissue organization.

Neutropenia: A decrease in the number of neutrophils and bands in the blood; characterized by an increase in the risk for infection; also called granulocytopenia.

No-code status: A decision made by a patient or the patient's legal representative that cardiopulmonary resuscitation will not be attempted in the event that the patient's heartbeat and respirations cease.

Node negative: In tumor staging, no involvement of regional lymph nodes.

Non-Hodgkin's lymphoma: Any of several malignant lymphomas or cancers of the lymphoid tissue that lack the giant Reed-Sternberg cells characteristic of Hodgkin's disease.

Non–small-cell lung cancer: Any of several pulmonary tumors composed of cells larger than and different from the cells characteristic of small-cell lung cancer.

Nucleus: The central controlling body within a living cell that contains the genetic codes for life, growth, and reproduction of the cell.

Oncogenes: Genes that regulate proliferative processes.

Pluripotent stem cells: The most primitive cells of the bone marrow. These cells are capable of giving rise to any blood cell lineage.

Postsurgical/pathologic staging: Staging that includes pathologic examination of resected tissue for evidence of disease.

Prevalence: The number of cases of existing disease at a designated point in time, regardless of when the disease began or was diagnosed.

Primary tumor: The original tumor, especially in cases of metastasis; refers to the organ where the tumor originated.

Prognosis: The prospect for recovery from a disease.

Prognostic indicators: Any factors that affect prognosis.

Proliferating cells: Cells that are multiplying.

Promoter: Nontumorigenic agent that will induce tumors in initiated cells; causes reversible changes.

Protecting factors: Substances or agents that may protect the host from carcinogens.

Radical mastectomy: Surgical removal of the breast, pectoral muscles, and axillary lymph nodes.

Regional disease: In staging, disease that extends beyond the organ of origin to surrounding tissues or lymph nodes.

Reversing factors: Agents that inhibit the effects of promoting factors.

Sarcoma: Malignant neoplasm of mesenchymal origin.

Screening: Assessment of asymptomatic individuals or populations for risk factors or presence of disease.

Seeding: Spread of tumor cells in a natural body cavity.

Staging: Classification of the extent of cancer.

Stomatitis: An inflammation of the mucous membranes lining the oral cavity.

Strabismus: Deviation of the eye that is not controlled by the patient. For example, when the patient is looking forward, one eye may drift inward.

Stress: Stimuli requiring adaptation.

Surgical evaluative staging: Staging of the extent of disease done after surgical exploration or biopsy.

Thrombocytopenia: Abnormal decrease in the number of platelets in the blood.

TNM classification: System of staging tumors in which *T* refers to the tumor, *N* to involvement of lymph nodes, and *M* to metastases.

Transformation: Multistep process by which normal cells change into neoplastic cells.

Tumor: A swelling or growth that arises from preexisting tissue and is unrelated to the normal rate of growth for that particular tissue. **Benign** tumors are noncancerous, that is, noninvasive and nonmetastatic. **Malignant** tumors are cancerous, able to invade and destroy adjacent normal tissue.

Tumor lysis syndrome: A process that occurs when a large number of tumor cells rupture and release their contents. This can occur when cells in a large tumor die either by natural cell death or as the result of response to cancer treatment. The syndrome is characterized by electrolyte imbalances and potential renal failure.

Tumor markers: Antigens, enzymes, or other substances used to assess the progress of certain cancers.

Xerostomia: Dryness in the mouth caused by injury to the salivary glands; can be a side effect of radiation therapy to the head and neck.

X-ray: Electromagnetic radiation of wavelength 10 nm or less.

INDEX

A

ABCD (for melanoma), 159-160
Absolute granulocyte count (AGC), 92
Acute lymphocytic leukemia, 184-186
Acute myelogenous leukemia, 186
Acute nausea/vomiting, 83
Adenocarcinoma, 132-133
"A" disease, 188
Administration,
    basic concepts of chemotherapy, 55
    methods of chemotherapy, 53-54
    safe handling during, 56-58
Advanced cancer,
    advance directives and, 172-173
    hospice care during, 173-175
    overview of, 171-172
    palliative care for, 172
Advance directives, 172-173
Advocacy, 202
AIDS, 161
Alcohol, 136, 138
Alkylating agents, 48-49
Allogeneic bone marrow transplantation, 66, 68
Alopecia (hair loss),
    as cancer side effect, 99-100
    due to chemotherapy, 52-53
    due to radiation therapy, 39
Amputations, 21
Anemia, 51, 96-97
Ann Arbor staging system, 156
Anorexia, 87, 177
Anthracycline drugs, 52
Anticipatory nausea/vomiting, 83-84
Anticonvulsants, 103
Antimetabolites, 48-49, 80
Antitumor antibiotics, 48, 80
Anxiety, 121
Appetite suppression, 87
Autologous bone marrow transplantation, 65, 67-68

B

"B" disease, 188
Bereavement counseling, 178
Bethesda staging system, 148
Bilateral orchiectomy, 152
Bilateral salpingo-oophorectomy, 22
Biological response modifiers (BRMs), 61-62
Biopsy,
    for brain/CNS cancers, 154
    for breast cancer diagnosis, 136
    for colorectal cancer, 142
    for head/neck cancer diagnosis, 139
    for melanoma, 160
    needle, 16
    prior to radiation therapy, 111
    for prostatic cancer, 150
Biotherapy, 10-11, 61-64, 78, 80
Bladder cancer, 143-144
"Body bath" administration, 53-54
Bone marrow transplantation,
    collection/infusion for, 67-69
    complications of, 68-69
    future trends in, 69-70
    for leukemia, 158
    overview/goals of, 64, 67
    process for allogeneic, 66
    process for autologous, 65
    types of, 67-68
Bone metastasis, 151
Bone sarcomas, 163-165
Brachytherapy, 33-36
Brain tumors, 152-154, 187
Breast cancer,
    classification of, 136
    epidemiology/etiology of, 135-136
    implant therapy for, 34
    nursing care for, 137-138
    prognosis for, 137
    surgery for, 18-19, 137

PRETEST ANSWER KEY

1.	a	Chapter 1
2.	c	Chapter 1
3.	c	Chapter 2
4.	c	Chapter 2
5.	d	Chapter 3
6.	b	Chapter 3
7.	a	Chapter 4
8.	c	Chapter 4
9.	a	Chapter 5
10.	c	Chapter 5
11.	c	Chapter 6
12.	d	Chapter 6
13.	c	Chapter r 7
14.	c	Chapter 7
15.	a	Chapter 8
16.	c	Chapter 8
17.	a	Chapter 9
18.	c	Chapter 9
19.	a	Chapter 11
20.	a	Chapter 12
21.	a	Chapter 12
22.	d	Chapter 13
23.	c	Chapter 13
24.	c	Chapter 14
25.	d	Chapter 14